Primary Care

KF trainins

www. outreach.psu.edu/
Sport Camps /
7/18 — 7/23

PRIMARY CARE

Balancing Health Needs,
Services, and Technology

Barbara Starfield

New York   Oxford
OXFORD UNIVERSITY PRESS
1998

Oxford University Press

Oxford   New York
Athens   Auckland   Bangkok   Bogotá   Buenos Aires   Calcutta
Cape Town   Chennai   Dar es Salaam   Delhi   Florence   Hong Kong   Istanbul
Karachi   Kuala Lumpur   Madrid   Melbourne   Mexico City   Mumbai
Nairobi   Paris   São Paulo   Singapore   Taipei   Tokyo   Toronto   Warsaw

and associated companies in
Berlin   Ibadan

This book is a revision of Barbara Starfield's *Primary Care: Concept, Evaluation, and Policy*
published by Oxford University Press 1992.

Library of Congress Cataloging-in-Publication Data
Starfield, Barbara.
[Primary care]
Primary care : balancing health needs,
services, and technology/Barbara Starfield.
p.   cm. Rev. ed. of: Primary care.
New York : Oxford University Press, 1992.
Includes bibliographical references and index.
ISBN 0-19-512542-8 (cloth. — ISBN 0-19-512543-6 (paper)
1. Primary care (Medicine)   2. Primary care (Medicine)—United States.
3. Medical care.   I. Title.
R729.5.G4S72   1998
362.1—DC21   98-10794

1 3 5 7 9 8 6 4 2

Printed in the United States of America
on acid-free paper

PREFACE

In the six years since the book *Primary Care: Concept, Evaluation, and Policy* was published, the world of health services has undergone myriad changes. Health care reform characterizes almost every country, even those with health systems that had been stable for decades. A large part of the impetus for reform stems from ever-increasing costs of care consequent to aging of the population, better survival of the chronically ill resulting from improved medical treatments, and the increasing role of expensive technology in the diagnosis and management of illness. Few countries can afford to absorb the increased costs without serious consideration of alternatives. Because of the commonality of concerns across countries and the centrality of primary care within them, there is a convergence of interest in the nature of primary care and its role within health systems. Thus, this book draws heavily on knowledge and experiences from a wide variety of countries.

The book is intended to help readers understand the role of primary care as an organizing focus of health systems, to provide the available scientific evidence on its utility, and to help further its development and growth. However, growing threats to quality of care and increasing social inequities that threaten to worsen even further the disparities between socially advantaged and socially disadvantaged populations bring a new urgency to the topic of effectiveness and equity of health services and the role of primary care in enhancing them.

In its most highly developed form, primary care is the point of entry into the health services system and the locus of responsibility for the care of patients and populations over time. There is still a prevalent belief that the substance of primary care is essentially simple. Nothing could be further from the truth, and this book is testimony to its challenges.

The book has five main sections: Primary Care and Health; Primary Care Practice; Accountability in Primary Care; Patients and Populations for Primary Care; and Health Policies and Primary Care.

- Primary Care and Health. Three chapters address the relationship between primary care and health, trace the history of the development of primary care as a concept, and lay the groundwork for thinking about the how the contributions of primary care have been and might be assessed.
- Primary Care Practice. Three chapters describe the characteristics of primary care

practice and types of practitioners and examine primary care as a component of health service systems.

- Accountability in Primary Care. Five chapters address measurement and evaluation of the essential components of primary care. Four describe the importance of each of the major features of primary care, approaches to assessing their attainment, and their important policy implications; another explores the importance of patient–practitioner interactions in primary care.
- Patients and Populations for Primary Care. Three chapters explore the interrelatedness of patient-focused and population-focused approaches to achieving high-quality, effective, and equitable primary care.
- Health Policies and Primary Care. The last four chapters explore various systems of primary care in western industrialized nations, the importance of information systems in primary care, research needs that might be adopted as a national strategy and be undertaken by research organizations or individual researchers, and a policy agenda to achieve greater effectiveness and equity.

The book is for those challenged by critical thinking about what primary care is, what it should be, and what it can contribute to improving health. This includes many clinicians who practice it, educators who teach it, researchers who study and evaluate it, patients who use it and want to understand it, and policy makers interested in improving it. The book attempts to serve five audiences: practitioners of primary care who want to understand what they do and why; educators of primary care practitioners who want a basis for thinking about their approaches to learning; researchers who might find frameworks, concepts, and clues to guide their work; policy-makers who would benefit from a better appreciation of the difficulties and challenges of primary care and its importance; and consumers of health services who may find it helpful in understanding and interpreting their own experiences.

The earlier book was written on the eve of impending health care reform in the United States in the hope of bringing greater attention to primary care in those efforts. Therefore, the examples were largely from this country. The situation has now changed; almost all countries are struggling with their own reforms, and the principles apply everywhere. The results of studies in other countries, largely written in the English language, are now incorporated in this book to a much greater extent. Because the literature dealing with primary care is still sparse, many of the chapters in this book incorporate findings cited in the earlier book along with evidence that has been added during the 1990s. Thus the book serves as a source of accumulated information concerning the development and assessment of primary care in the twentieth century.

The book is oriented largely toward care provided by physicians. This is not to suggest that other personnel, especially nurses, have little responsibility in primary care. Rather, the thesis is based on the assumption, generally considered as accurate for industrialized nations, that it is the physician who bears the responsibility for seeing to the totality of primary care. Other personnel may assume responsibility for certain of its aspects, even for some highly central ones, but it is the physician who must oversee all of its aspects. Recognition of the importance of other types of professionals comes in the form of the use of the word *practitioner* throughout the book. Practitioner, instead of physician, is used wherever the particular function under consideration is sometimes or might be assumed by a non-physician professional. Although the special expertise of primary care physicians makes them "specialists" in their area of practice, the book adopts the more conventional designation of non-primary care practitioners as "specialists" or "subspecialists." Readers should understand that this is merely "shorthand," since primary care physicians are indeed specialists in primary care.

Primary care is complex. Its challenges will require concerted efforts at research and systematic translation of knowledge into policy. Although primary care has become increasingly recognized as a critical feature of health systems, it still suffers from a lack of appreciation of its characteristics and contributions, and its functions are at constant threat of being trivialized in the zeal to economize on health services. Strong primary care is essential to a strong health system. If this book conveys this to readers, it will have achieved its goals.

ACKNOWLEDGMENTS

Many people have contributed in many ways to this analysis of the importance of primary care within health service systems. By far the best contributions have been from my colleagues and friends who have thought deeply about the subject of primary care in the context of health systems. I am especially indebted to Juan Gérvas and Mercedes Perez Fernandez, whose sustaining friendship and colleagueship have exposed me to new ways of thinking and inquiry. Their stewardship of the BBC (Bibliografico CESCA), an invaluable monthly annotated international bibliography, is responsible for my awareness and appreciation of a larger body of information than otherwise would have been the case.

My early exposure to the writings of Kerr L. White and then the opportunity to work as a faculty member in his department were certainly seminal in my thinking about primary care, a term that would not exist but for its introduction by Kerr in the early 1960s. His writings were the first to make real sense to me, as a young clinician struggling to understand what I was doing. Kerr's challenge to the health care system to convert data to information to intelligence to wisdom are as pertinent today as they were 40 years ago.

I thank also my special colleagues at Johns Hopkins, who continue to make research collaboration truly exciting. Jonathan Weiner, Don Steinwachs, Chris Forrest, and Anne Riley come especially to mind because of our joint work on subjects related to primary care, case–mix measures, and child and adolescent health status assessment.

I am also grateful to Margorie Bowman, who helped me considerably with the clinical vignettes, and to Karen Rappaport.

Not enough can be said about the enormous willingness of my international colleagues to share information and ideas—their special contributions are noted, with gratitude, in Chapter 15.

As always, my family deserves special mention. My wonderful mother, Eva Starfield, took on the role of reactor and unofficial editor of my book after the death of my wonderful father. My husband, Neil Holtzman, served as official sounding board, despite the discomforts of having to live through the irritability that accompanies any intense endeavor such as book writing. I give my special thanks to Rob and April, Jon and Beth, and Susan and Steven for providing me with emotional as well as intellectual diversion in the form of five exceptional grandchildren and to Deborah, for just being herself.

Finally, I give extreme gratitude to my assistant Ruth Hurd, who didn't blink an eyelash at the interminable changes, who stayed perfectly calm through what must have seemed like hundreds of drafts, and whose help was simply invaluable.

CONTENTS

— I —
Primary Care and Health

— 1 —

Primary Care and Its Relationship to Health

> ... the failure to recognize that the results of specialized observation are at best only partial truths, which require to be corrected with facts obtained by wider study.
> ... No more dangerous members of our profession exist than those born into it, so to speak, as specialists.   Osler, 1892

There are two main goals for any health services system. The first is to optimize the health of the population by employing the most advanced state of knowledge about the causation of disease, illness management, and health maximization. The second and equally important goal is to minimize the disparities across population subgroups so that certain groups are not at a systematic disadvantage with regard to their access to health services and achievement of optimal health.

In recognition of the rising social and health inequities in almost all countries, the World Health Organization adopted a set of principles with which to build the primary care base of health services. Known as the Ljubljana Charter, it proposes that health care systems should be

- Driven by values of human dignity, equity, solidarity, and professional ethics
- Targeted on protecting and promoting health
- Centered on people, allowing citizens to influence health services and to take responsibility for their own health
- Focused on quality, including cost effectiveness
- Based on sustainable finances, to allow universal coverage and equitable access
- Oriented toward primary care

The European Community adopted these principles in 1996; they build on a long tradition of a striving toward equity and "solidarity" in most European nations (BMJ, 1996). Unfortunately, not all nations subscribe to these principles.

As knowledge accumulates, professionals increasingly tend to sub-specialize in order to cope with and manage the volume of new information. Therefore, in almost every country, we see the health professions becoming more fragmented, with increasing narrowing of interests and competence and a focus on specific diseases or types of diseases rather than on the overall health of people and communities. In some countries, there are more subspecialists than primary care specialists. Specialty care often commands more resources than does basic care because emphasis is placed on the development and deployment of expensive technology to keep ill people alive rather than on programs to prevent illnesses or reduce discomfort from more common, non-life-threatening ailments. While it may be that the tendency toward specialization based on the most current knowledge provides highly efficacious care of individual diseases, it is unlikely to produce highly effective basic care. Why is this so? Specialization oriented toward the treatment of disease cannot maximize health because prevention of illness and promotion of optimal functioning transcend specific diseases and require a broader perspective than can be achieved by the disease specialist. Effective medical care is not limited to the treatment of disease itself; it must consider the context in which the illness occurs and in which the patient lives. Moreover, diseases rarely exist in isolation, especially when experienced over time. Thus, disease specialists may provide the most appropriate care for the specific illnesses within their area of special competence, but a primary care practitioner is required to integrate the care for the variety of health problems that individuals experience over time.

A health system oriented toward subspecialization has another problem: It threatens the goals of equity. No society has unlimited resources to provide for health services. Subspecialty care is more expensive than primary care and is therefore less accessible to individuals with fewer resources to pay for it. Moreover, the resources needed for highly technical disease-oriented care compete with those required to provide basic services, especially for people unable to pay for them.

In contrast, primary care involves managing patients who often have multiple diagnoses and puzzling complaints that cannot be fit into known diagnoses and providing treatment that improves overall quality of life and functioning. The European region of the World Health Organization proposed that *health* be defined as "the extent to which an individual or group is able, on one hand, to realize aspirations and satisfy needs and, on the other hand, to cope with the environment. Health is therefore seen as a resource for everyday life, not the objective of living; it is a positive concept embracing social and personal resources as well as physical capacities."

"Health" has many types of determinants (Fig. 1.1) Highly influential is a gene structure that has been evolving for millions of years and that determines the limits on what health services can achieve in improving health. The gene structure continues to evolve, and tomorrow's situation, in terms of the potential for health, is likely to be different from that of today. This is becoming increasingly the case because scientists are learning how to tamper with genes in order to alter states of health. In addition, modern technology makes it increasingly possible to interfere with the expression of genes by such means as modifying the environment, altering behavior, and using certain types of medical care. The other determinants of health—social and physical environment, individual behaviors, and health services (medical practice)—as superimposed on the gene structure (genotype) are shown in Figure 1.1. As indicated in this figure, the health of an individual or a population is determined by its gene pool, but heavily modified by the social and physical

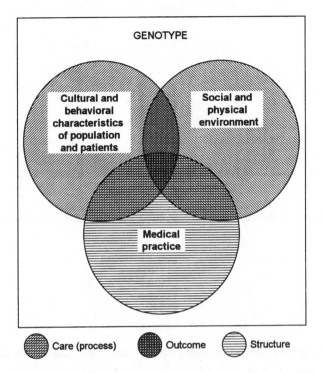

Figure 1.1. Determinants of health status. Source: Starfield (1973).

environment, by behaviors that are culturally or socially determined, and by the nature of the health care provided.

Figure 1.2 provides the likely pathway for these major determinants according to current knowledge. The chain of causation is complex. It involves antecedent factors, such as the environmental context, social conditions and social relationships, and genetic risk factors. Some of these operate directly (such as contaminated water or safety hazards in homes), and some operate indirectly through mediating factors involving behaviors, social stresses, social isolation, and access to medical care. All risks interact in various ways (many of them unknown) in their effect on health.

This view of the determinants of health pertains both to the individual and to populations of individuals. That is, the state of health of a population is determined by the same factors acting at the ecological (population) level rather than the individual level. Thus the state of health of a community is determined by the environmental characteristics of that community, the behavioral characteristics of its population, and the sense of coherence and degrees of social cohesion in the community. The same is the case for social conditions such as levels of income and wealth in the population, the general level of education in the community, and the characteristics of work opportunities available to its members.

In most industrialized nations there are systematic differences in ill health

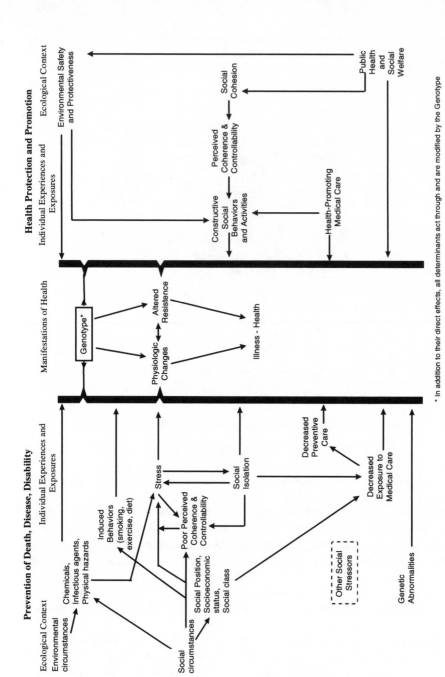

Figure 1.2. Determinants of health and illness. Adapted from Starfield (1990).

* In addition to their direct effects, all determinants act through and are modified by the Genotype

across communities, with higher concentrations among the socially disadvantaged, regardless of the measure of morbidity (mortality, objectively ascertained morbidity, self-assessed health, the presence of limitations from chronic illness, or simply the presence of chronic illness). Many studies have shown that morbidity concentrates more among the socially disadvantaged, and this is the case in every country where it has been studied. However, the disparities vary from country to country, being much worse in some (such as the United States) than in others (such as the Netherlands) (Wagstatf and Van Doorslaer, 1993). Using mortality of men aged 35–64 as the indicator of health, Kunst (1997) found persistent and even increasing socioeconomic disparities in health between the 1970s and the 1980s in several industrialized nations, but the absence of consistency across different causes of mortality led him to conclude that life-style factors, such as smoking and alcohol intake, are also likely to play a role in explaining the differences across countries. In his report, he explicitly recognized that these life-style factors may be heavily influenced by antecedent social and economic differences among individuals and communities, as predicted by models of the determinants of health represented in Figure 1.2.

Greater national wealth does not guarantee the social and economic conditions that produce a high level of health. The United States, for example, is among the wealthiest countries, but its population does not reap the benefit of this in terms of better health. The lack of consistent relationship between various aspects of health status and a country's overall wealth is well documented. For example, there are substantial differences in survival of children among countries with similar levels of overall wealth and similar survival in some countries with very different levels of health. Within the group of nations with a Gross Domestic Product (GDP) of more than 20,000 U.S. dollars per capita, the variation in survival rates for children under 5 years of age ranges from about 990 per 1,000 in the United States to 995 per 1,000 in Finland, Sweden, and Iceland. Among nations with a GDP between 1,000 and 2,000 U.S. dollars per capita, the range is from under 900 per 1,000 in Swaziland and Papua New Guinea to 990 per 1,000 in Cuba, which has the same child survival rate as the United States with a GDP one-twentieth as great.

Countries also differ widely in the gaps in income between poor and affluent individuals within each country. The Luxembourg Income Studies demonstrate the disparity in family after-tax income between children whose families are poorer than 90% of the households in the country and those in the most affluent 10% of the population within each of 18 western industrialized nations. The family income of the most affluent 10% of children is more than six times as great as the poorest 10% in the United States—by far the most socially inequitable among the countries. The gap is about four times in Italy, Canada, and Australia. It is three to four times in the United Kingdom, France, Germany, and Switzerland, but less than three times as great in Finland, the Netherlands, Sweden, and Austria. The same is the case when all people, not only children, are considered; the United States is by far the most inequitable, and Finland, Sweden, and the Netherlands the least inequitable. However, the inequities are worse for all individuals than for just children in the case of France, Austria, Norway, Denmark, Sweden, and Finland, suggesting that these countries make special efforts to provide social supports for disadvantaged children, but less so for adults. In contrast, inequities are worse for children than for all individuals in the United States, Italy, Canada, and Germany (Rainwater and Smeeding, 1995; Smeeding, 1996).

As noted above, health is directly associated with social advantage in absolute terms. The more the social resources of individuals and communities, the greater the likelihood of better health. Moreover, relative rather than absolute social deprivation is also associated with poorer health. That is, the greater the disparities in wealth within any population, the greater the disparities in health. This has been demonstrated by a variety of approaches to assessment. Wagstaff and Van Doorslaer (1993) used data from population surveys in which people were asked to report on their health. The greater the income inequality within countries, the greater the health inequality. Differences in extent of disparities in income, as measured by the percent of after-tax and benefit income for the least well-off 70% of the population, are related to differences in life expectancy. The less the income disparity, that is, the more equitable the distribution of income in the population, the longer the average life expectancy, even when the *average* levels of income in the country are similar (Wilkinson, 1992, 1996, 1997).

The same relationship has been shown to exist within countries and for other indicators of health. For example, data from the 50 U.S. states show a very notable relationship between indices of income inequality in the state and age-adjusted mortality; infant mortality; heart disease mortality; mortality from cancers; deaths from all infectious diseases combined and from tuberculosis, and pneumonia and bronchitis separately; and homicides. The findings persisted even when differences in rates of smoking were taken into account (Kennedy et al., 1996). In another study using a different measure of income inequality, the findings were the same. In addition, greater income inequality was also found to be associated with a higher percentage of liveborn infants weighing less than 2,500 grams and higher rates of disability among the population (Kaplan et al., 1996). That is, the more the income inequality, the greater the rates of health-related problems regardless of the particular measure of income inequality.

Health services, as one of the direct determinants, can play a role in improving health, even in the face of marked inequities in the distribution of wealth. Because the overall level of spending on health services is not uniformly associated with better levels of health, any effect of health services on health must be a consequence of specific characteristics of those health services. On theoretical grounds alone, it is likely that the achievement of effectiveness and equity requires the health system to have a strong primary care orientation.

For primary care to optimize health, it must focus on people's health in the constellation of the other determinants of health, that is, on the social and physical milieu in which people live and work rather than only on their individual diseases. Primary care facilities achieve equity by providing care at the most appropriate level; it thus releases resources that can be used to narrow disparities in health between more deprived and less deprived segments of the population.

Primary care is that level of a health service system that provides entry into the system for all new needs and problems, provides person-focused (not disease-oriented) care over time, provides care for all but very uncommon or unusual conditions, and coordinates or integrates care provided elsewhere or by others. It thus is defined as a set of functions that, in combination, are unique to primary care. Primary care also shares characteristics with other levels of health systems: accountability for access, quality, and costs; attention to prevention as well as therapy and rehabilitation; and teamwork. Primary care is *not* a set of unique clinical tasks or activities; virtually all types of clinical activities (such as diagnosis, prevention, screening, and various strategies for clinical management) are characteristic of all levels of care. Rather, primary care is an approach that forms the basis for and determines the work of all other levels of health systems. Primary care addresses the most common problems in the community by providing preventive, curative, and rehabilitative services to maximize health and well being. It integrates care when there is more than one health problem and deals with the context in which illness exists and influences the responses of people to their health problems. It is care that organizes and rationalizes the deployment of all resources, basic as well as specialized, directed at promoting, maintaining, and improving health.

Vuori (1985) suggested four ways of viewing primary care: as a set of activities, as a level of care, as a strategy for organizing health care, and as a philosophy that permeates health care. Because there are few activities that are unique to primary care, the first approach is inappropriate. Levels of care, strategies for organizing health care, and a "philosophy" are inter-related, and the definition of primary care used in this book captures their inter-relationships.

Primary care is distinguished from short-term consultative care (secondary care) and long-term disease management (tertiary care) by several characteristics. Primary care deals with more common and less well-defined problems, generally in community settings such as offices, health centers, schools, and homes. Patients have direct access to an appropriate source of care, which continues over time for a variety of problems and includes needs for preventive services.

Compared with subspecialty medicine, primary care is less intensive of both capital and labor and is less hierarchical in organization. Therefore, it is inherently more adaptable and capable of responding to changing societal health needs. In specialty care, patients have typically been referred by another physician who has already explored the nature of the patient's problem and has initiated preliminary diagnostic work. The diagnostic process results in a precise definition of pathophysiology; interventions are directed primarily at that pathophysiological process. In primary care, in contrast, the patient is usually known to the physician, and entry into the system is usually patient initiated, often with poorly specified and vague complaints. The major task is elucidation of the patient's problem and elicitation of information that leads to a diagnosis and choice of the most appropriate management. Primary care physicians, compared with other specialists, deal with a broader range of problems, both with individual patients as well as across their practice population. Because they are located closer to the patient's milieu than are specialists, they are in a better position to appreciate the role played by the multiple and interacting determinants of illness and health.

The Historical Context of Primary Care

In 1920, 8 years after the institution of national health insurance in Great Britain, a "white paper" was released (Lord Dawson of Penn, 1920) dealing with the organization of the health services system. It distinguished three major levels of health service: primary health centers, secondary health centers, and teaching hospitals. Formal linkages among the three levels were proposed, and the functions of each were described. This formulation was the basis for the concept of regionalization: a system of organization of services designed to respond to the various levels of need for medical services in the population. This theoretical arrangement subsequently provided the basis for the reorganization of health services in many countries, which now have clearly defined levels of care each with an identifiable and functioning primary medical care sector.

In 1977, at its thirtieth annual meeting, the World Health Assembly decided unanimously that the main social target of member governments should be "the attainment by all citizens of the world by the year 2000 of a level of health that will permit them to lead a socially and economically productive life." Now known as "Health for All by the Year 2000," this declaration set in motion a series of activities that have had a major impact on thinking about primary care. The principles were enunciated at a conference that was held in Alma-Ata and dealt with the topic of "primary health care." The consensus reached there was confirmed by the World Health Assembly at its subsequent meeting in May 1979. *Primary health care* was defined as

> Essential health care based on practical, scientifically sound, and socially acceptable methods and technology made universally accessible to individuals and families in the community by means acceptable to them and at a cost that the community and the country can afford to maintain at every stage of their development in a spirit of self-reliance and self-determination. It forms an integral part of both the country's health system of which it is the central function and the main focus of the overall social and economic development of the community. It is the first level of contact of individuals, the family and the community with the national health system, bringing health care as close as possible to where people live and work and constitutes the first element of a continuing health care process.
>
> World Health Organization, 1978

Primary health care was recognized as an "integral, permanent, and pervasive part of the formal health care system in all countries, and not as an *add-on*"(Basch, 1990). The Alma-Ata conference further specified that the core components of PHC were health education; environmental sanitation, especially of food and water; maternal and child health programs, including immunization and family planning; prevention of local endemic diseases; appropriate treatment of common diseases and injuries; provision of essential drugs; promotion of sound nutrition; and traditional medicine.

Although these concepts of primary health care were intended to apply to all countries, there is disagreement about the extent to which they are applicable in industrialized nations as well as about the impediments to applying them (Kaprio,

1979). The concept of primary health care, which, in its emphasis on "nearness to the people," seems alien in countries with health systems based on technology, specialization, the primacy of the hospital, and medical school curricula that are under the control of hospital-based specialists. Furthermore, the principle that health care should be "needs-related" is not easily understood in countries with well-established health systems but with no information system to systematically document health needs or to evaluate the impact of health services on them. Community orientation has little historical basis in the health systems of most industrialized nations.

However, some countries have reorganized their health services to consolidate the medical and health aspects of primary care. For example, the new "family doctors" in Cuba live where they work. They are therefore members of the community they serve, and it is to their advantage to act as agents of change when there are environmental or social circumstances that need improvement (Gilpin, 1991). This integration of conventional medical services with social and environmental services fits the model envisaged at Alma-Ata.

Many of the specific goals defined at Alma-Ata are already achieved in industrialized countries (Vuori, 1984). Most such countries can point with pride to long-standing programs for most of the activities: food and safety of water supply, maternal and child health, immunization, prevention and control of endemic diseases, basic treatment of health problems, and provision of essential drugs. When primary health care is viewed as "accessible" services, many of these countries can justly claim to have achieved the goals because of availability of medical care services. It is only when nations view primary health care as a strategy to integrate all aspects of health services that it becomes equally applicable as a goal in industrialized nations. This view requires that a health care system be organized to stress social justice and equality, self-responsibility, international solidarity, and acceptance of a broad concept of health (Vuori,201984).

The changes required to convert conventional primary medical care in industrialized nations to broader primary health care as defined at Alma-Ata are described in table 1.1. All the directions of change are part of the goals of primary care as conceived in this book, which uses the term *primary care* to connote conventional primary medical care striving to achieve the goals of primary health care. The intent is to suggest that increasing the orientation of primary care services toward meeting the needs of communities as well as those of individuals who appear for care will bring conventional primary medical care closer to primary health care as envisaged at Alma-Ata and toward greater equity.

Primary Care as a Focus of Policy Interest

In many parts of the world, the benefits of primary care have long been assumed on faith. As noted above, the Dawson Report in 1920 laid out an organizational structure based on different levels of care in which the most basic was the primary health care center, buttressed by a secondary level consisting of specialists who provided consultative care that, in turn, was supported by a tertiary level based in

Table 1.1. From Primary Medical to Primary
Health Care

Conventional	New
Focus	
Illness	Health
Cure	Prevention, care, and cure
Content	
Treatment	Health Promotion
Episodic care	Continuous care
Specific problems	Comprehensive care
Organization	
Specialists	General practitioners
Physicians	Other personnel groups
Single-handed practice	Team
Responsibility	
Health sector alone	Intersectoral collaboration
Professional dominance	Community participation
Passive reception	Self-responsibility

Adapted from Vuori (1985).

teaching hospitals for care of more uncommon and complicated illnesses. The
Alma-Ata Declaration 1978 codified the "sanctity" of primary health care as a
principle for all health systems of the world.

It is only recently, however, that empirical evidence of the benefits of primary
care has been sought and found.

International comparisons

Not all countries have organized their health systems around a strong base of
primary care. The technological imperative of the twentieth century has been responsible for a tendency toward specialism, to the disadvantage of generalism, and
this imperative has been stronger in some countries than in others. To what extent
are these differences in primary care orientation associated with better health, lower
costs, and satisfaction of people with their health system? A comparison among 12
different western industrialized nations indicates that countries with a stronger orientation to primary care indeed are more likely to have better health levels and
lower costs (Starfield, 1994).

A score for strength of primary care orientation was developed using five health
system characteristics thought to be associated with strong primary care and six
characteristics of practice that reflect strong primary care. The five system characteristics were the extent to which health professionals and facilities were regulated so that they were distributed geographically approximately according to degree of need; the type of physician designated as the primary care physician; the

professional earnings of primary care physicians relative to other specialists; the number of primary care physicians relative to other specialists; and the extent of insurance coverage for health services.

The six practice characteristics were the extent to which people first sought care from their primary care physician before going elsewhere; the strength of relationships between people and their primary care physician; the extent to which primary care practice dealt with common needs regardless of their type; the degree of coordination between primary care and other health services; family orientation of primary care; and community orientation of primary care.

Each country was assigned a score of 0, 1, or 2 depending on the presence and strength of the characteristic. Countries were then ranked on their average scores for the 11 characteristics. The measures of health and costs consisted of the following:

1. Rank of the rates for 14 health indicators obtained by comparable methods and from a single data source. The indicators included neonatal mortality; postneonatal mortality; infant mortality (neonatal and postneonatal combined); life expectancy at age 1 year (to eliminate the contribution of infant mortality) and at ages 20, 65, and 80 years, each for males and females separately); age-adjusted death rates; and years of potential life lost before age 65 as a result of preventable conditions. They also included a measure of morbidity: low-birthweight percentage.
2. Rank for total health systems expenditures per capita, as expressed in purchasing power parities. As is the case with the other rankings, the "best" rank is 1.
3. Ranks for each population's satisfaction with its health system, as obtained by a telephone survey in which people rated their country's health system according to the extent to which it needed improvement. The ranking was based on the difference between the percentage of the population sample reporting that major changes were needed and the percentage who said their system needed only minor changes to make it better.
4. Ranks for expenditures per person for prescribed medications in purchasing power parities, with 1 given to the country with the lowest costs of prescribed medication.

Figure 1.3 shows that the stronger the country's primary care system, the better the rank for the combined impacts. Figure 1.4 shows the rankings for primary care strength on one axis and the rank for total health care costs per capita on the other axis, with 1 given to the country with the lowest total costs. The graphs make it clear that the countries with stronger primary care do better on both outcomes and costs.

Three other important facets of this comparison are important. First, the scores for the system characteristics and for the practice characteristics were highly related, that is, countries in which health policies were conducive to primary care were those countries in which the practice characteristics also reflected strong primary care (Fig. 1.5) Second, the advantages accruing from strong primary care were much greater for young age groups, that is, during in infancy and childhood than in adulthood (Starfield, 1993). Third, the group of countries with health sys-

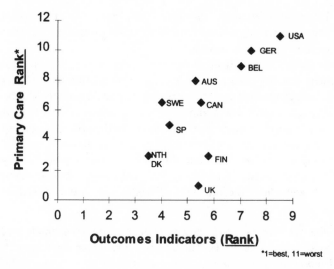

Figure 1.3. Relationship between strength of primary care and combined outcomes.

tems that attempt to distribute resources according to need rather than demand (the "market") achieve better health levels than other countries (Starfield, 1993).

Other evaluations of the impact of primary care

The earliest of these evaluations measured the impact of primary care by examining a variety of outcome measures in areas more and less well endowed with primary care physicians and specialists.

Using data from all counties within the contiguous United States for 1978–1982, Farmer and colleagues (1991) were the first to demonstrate consistently lower age-specific mortality rates in counties with higher ratios of primary care physicians to populations. Although rates of poverty (but not rural areas, percentage female-

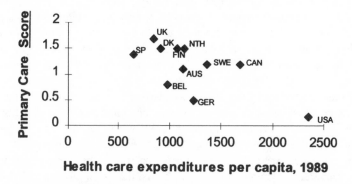

Figure 1.4. Relationship between strength of primary care and total health care expenditures.

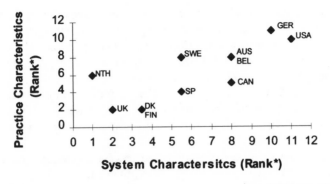

*1=best, 11=worst

Figure 1.5. Relationship between health system policies and practice characteristics related to primary care.

headed households, percentage of population with fewer than 12 years of education, or percentage minority) were also consistently related to mortality rates, the primary care physician to population ratio had an independent effect.

Shi (1994) extended this approach by examining the effect on "life chances" (total mortality rates, heart disease mortality rates, cancer mortality rates, average life expectancy at birth, neonatal mortality, and low birth weight) of primary care physicians to population ratios, specialists to population ratios, state ranking on socioeconomic indicators (unemployment rate, educational level, pollution index, per capita income), and state rankings on life-style indicators (seatbelt non-use, obesity, and smoking rates). Table 1.2 summarizes the findings, which show that the more primary care physicians per population and the fewer the number of other specialists per population, the better the life chances, independent of the effect of other influential factors such as per capita income.

Table 1.2. Major Determinants of *Outcomes* (overall mortality, mortality from heart disease, mortality from cancer, neonatal mortality, life span, low birth weight) in 50 U.S. States

Specialty physicians	More: All outcomes worse
Primary care physicians	Fewer: All outcomes worse
Hospital beds	More: Higher total, heart disease, and neonatal mortality
Education	No relationship
Income	Lower: Higher heart and cancer mortality
Unemployment	Higher: Higher total mortality, lower life span, more low birthweight
Urban	Lower mortality (all), longer life span
Pollution	Higher total mortality
Life-style	Worse: Higher total and cancer mortality, lower life span
Minority	Higher total mortality, neonatal mortality, low birth weight, lower life span

Note: All variables are ecologic, not individual.

Source: Shi (1994).

Shea and colleagues (1992) used a case-control approach to examine the impact of having a primary care physician. Men appearing at an emergency room in a large metropolitan area were characterized as having complications of hypertension or as having another condition while incidentally also having hypertension that was uncomplicated. Those men whose hypertension was the cause of their visit were much less likely to have a regular source of primary care than men whose hypertension was an incidental finding. The presence of a source of primary care was the most notable difference between the two groups—even more important than insurance coverage.

Welch and colleagues (1993) examined claims for services provided to individuals over age 65 years in the entire United States to explore the reasons for geographic variation in expenditures for physicians' services. Although expenditures were not related to the total number of physicians per population, they were lower in areas with a higher proportion of primary care physicians, even after controlling for the additional effects of rates of admission to hospitals and high payment rates. The findings of this study were further refined by demonstrating that a greater supply of family physicians and general internists was significantly associated with lower expenditures for physician services, even after controlling for the effect of a number of sociodemographic and health system supply variables. In contrast, the greater the supply of non-primary care specialists, the higher the expenditures.

More recent assessments of the benefits of primary care have addressed more directly the characteristics of primary care itself rather than the type of practitioner who presumably provides them. Because they require an understanding of the specific characteristics of primary care and methods to assess them, they are discussed later on in Chapter 13.

References

Basch P. Textbook of International Health. New York: Oxford University Press, 1990.

BMJ. The Ljubljana charter on reforming health care. BMJ 1996; 312(7047):1664–5.

Farmer F, Stokes S, Fiser R, Papini D. Poverty, primary care, and age-specific mortality. J Rural Health 1991; 7:153–69

Gilpin M. Update—Cuba: On the road to a family medicine nation. J Public Health Policy 1991; 12(1):83–203.

Kaplan GA, Pamuk ER, Lynch JW, Cohen RD, Balfour JL. Inequality in income and mortality in the United States: Analysis of mortality and potential pathways. BMJ 1996; 312:999–1003.

Kaprio L. Primary Health Care in Europe. Copenhagen: Regional Office for Europe, World Health Organization, 1979.

Kennedy BP, Kawachi I, Prothrow-Stith D. Income distribution and mortality: Cross sectional ecological study of the Robin Hood index in the United States. BMJ 1996; 312: 1004–7.

Kunst A. Cross-National Comparisons of Socio-Economic Differences in Mortality. Rotterdam: Erasmus University, 1997.

Lord Dawson of Penn. Interim Report on the Future Provisions of Medical and Allied

Services. United Kingdom Ministry of Health. Consultative Council on Medical Allied Services. London: Her Majesty's Stationery Offices, 1920.

Osler, Sir William. Remarks on specialism. Boston Med Surg J 1892; 126:457–9.

Rainwater L, Smeeding T. U.S. doing poorly—compared to others. National Center for Children in Poverty. News and Issues, Fall/Winter 1995.

Shea S, Misra D, Ehrlich M, Field L, Frances C. Predisposing factors for severe, uncontrolled hypertension in an inner-city minority population. N Engl J Med 1992; 327: 776–81.

Shi L. Primary care, specialty care, and life chances. Int J Health Serv 1994; 24:431–58

Smeeding T. America's income inequality: Where do we stand? Challenge, Sept/Oct 1996.

Starfield B. Health services research: A working model. N Engl J Med 1973; 289:132–6.

Starfield B. Social factors in child health. In Green M, Haggerty R (eds): Ambulatory Pediatrics IV, Philadelphia: WB Saunders, pp 30–36. 1990.

Starfield B. Primary care. J Ambulatory Care Manage 1993; 16(4):27–37.

Starfield B. Primary care: Is it essential? Lancet 1994; 344:1129–33.

Vuori H. Primary health care in Europe—Problems and solutions. Community Med 1984; 6:221–31.

Vuori H. The role of schools of public health in the development of primary health care. Health Policy 1985; 4:221–30.

Wagstaff A, Van Doorslaer E. Equity in the finance and delivery of health care: Concepts and defintions. In Van Doorslaer E, Wagstaff A, Rutten F (eds): Equity in the Finance and Delivery of Health Care: An International Perspective. Oxford: Oxford University Press, 1993, pp 7–19.

Welch WP, Miller M, Welch G, Fisher E, Wennberg J. Geographic variation in expenditures for physicians' services in the United States. N Engl J Med 1993; 328:621–7.

Wilkinson RG. Income distribution and life expectancy. BMJ 1992; 304:165–8.

Wilkinson RG. Unhealthy Societies: The Afflictions of Inequality. London: Routledge, 1996.

Wilkinson RG. Socioeconomic determinants of health. Health inequalities: Relative or absolute material standards? BMJ 1997; 314(7080):591–5.

World Health Organization. Primary Health Care. Geneva: World Health Organization, 1978.

World Health Organization. Health promotion: A discussion document on the concept and principles. Copenhagen: WHO Regional Office for Europe: 1984.

— 2 —

A Framework
for Measuring Primary Care

Primary care, as defined in Chapter 1, provides the philosophical underpinnings for the organization of a health services system. But the general definitions provide no help when the task is to determine whether a given system merits the description *primary care*. More specificity is required.

Historically, primary care has been defined by the type of physician providing it; even now it is common for it to be characterized as that which is provided by general practitioners (or family physicians). The problem with this characterization is that the norm for primary care becomes that which describes the practices of family medicine. Since this may vary from place to place and country to country, a better alternative to specifying its functions is needed.

Primary care might be distinguishable from other types of care by clinical characteristics of patients and their problems. These characteristics include the variety of diagnoses or problems seen, an identifiable component devoted to prevention of illness, and a high proportion of patients who are already known to the practice.

Primary care practitioners are ordinarily believed to be distinguished from their secondary and tertiary counterparts by the variety of the problems encountered. Over the totality of problems, subspecialists might have a greater variety of diagnoses, because most very rare conditions might be encountered in specialty care and not in primary care. Primary care practitioners would be expected to have a greater variety of the more common diagnoses (e.g., those that comprise 50% of visits, because subspecialists would be expected to see mainly patients with a subset of these common diagnoses who have complications that cannot be dealt with by primary care physicians. In addition, subspecialists by definition limit themselves to only certain types of diagnoses and therefore would care for a narrower range of diagnoses. Thus, primary care practitioners should see a greater variety of types of diagnoses, at least among their most frequent diagnoses, than do subspecialists.

Another way to assess the variety of diagnoses or the variety of presenting problems is to examine the percentage of all diagnoses contributed by the 50 most common diagnoses; this percentage should be lower in primary care practice than in subspecialty practice because primary care practices would be expected to have a greater variety.

Because primary care is the point of first contact into the health care system, its practitioners should encounter a much wider array of presenting problems than is the case in subspecialty care. When these presenting problems are catalogued, a much greater number of problems should comprise any given percentage of all problems in primary care than in specialty care.

Primary care practices might also be assumed to have a larger percentage of visits classified as related to prevention.

Primary care practices should involve a greater proportion of patients who are continuing in care than those coming into care for the first time, and descriptions of primary care and subspecialty practices should demonstrate this difference. A related characteristic that should distinguish primary care is a greater familiarity of primary care practitioners with both the patient and the patient's problems. Both primary care physicians and subspecialists would be expected to see new patients and to see "old" patients with old problems. Primary care practitioners should see more "old" patients with new problems because they have the responsibility for the patient's care over time regardless of what the particular problem is.

This descriptive ("empirical") approach to characterizing medical care was best summarized by White (1973), who distinguished primary, secondary, and tertiary care by the nature of health problems, site of care, referral pattern, duration of responsibility, sources of information, use of technology, orientation of interest, and training need. Table 2.1 presents his framework. As the table indicates, distinctions between the levels of care are made according to the degree of differences for each of the 23 characteristics.

Such approaches, while generally useful for the purpose of illustrating the uniqueness of primary care, do not provide an adequate basis for setting goals for attainment of a high level of performance of primary care services. Newer approaches to evaluating the attainment of better primary care move from a content and task-orientation approach to an approach that considers what primary care should be providing in the context of the characteristics of health service systems. This section shows that the most important functions of primary care can be measured in a way that provides a basis for setting goals and continuous improvement in their achievement.

All evaluations require standards against which performance can be measured either according to a pre-set goal or by comparison of one system (or facility) against another (Parker et al., 1976). This chapter provides a theoretical framework for setting these standards. Subsequent chapters show how this framework can be used to assess each of the major features of primary care.

Attempts to define primary care by its functions date back to the early 1970s. Primary care is now widely accepted as being the delivery of first-contact medicine; the assumption of longitudinal responsibility for the patient regardless of the presence or absence of disease; and the integration of physical, psychological, and social aspects of health to the limits of the capability of the health personnel. Such a description was proposed in the Millis Report (1966) and is consistent with the

Table 2.1. Relative Content of Primary Care and Other Care

	Primary Care	Consultation (Secondary) Care	Tertiary Care
Health Problem			
Rare and complicated	+	+	++++
Infrequent and specific	++	++++	++
Common and nonspecific	++++	++	+
Site of Care			
Community setting	++++	++	+
Inpatient: General care	++	++++	++
Inpatient: Intensive care	O	++	++++
Referral Pattern			
Direct access	++++	+++	O
Referral practice	+	+++	++++
Extent of Responsibility			
Continuing care	++++	+	+++
Intermittent care	+	++++	+
Episode care	+	++	+++
Information Service			
Patient and family	++++	++	+
Epidemiological database	++++	+++	+
Biomedical database	+	++	++++
Use of Technology			
Complex equipment and staff	+	++	++++
Regular laboratory	++++	++++	++
Orientation			
Prevention/health maintenance	++++	++	+
Early diagnosis/disability containment	+++	+++	++
Palliation/rehabilitation	++	++	++++
Training Need			
Broad and general	++++	++	+
Concentrated	++	+++	++
Narrow and highly specialized	O	++	++++

O = not characteristic

+ to ++++ = increasingly characteristic

Adapted from White (1973).

major features of primary care: first contact, longitudinality, comprehensiveness, and coordination (or integration) (Alpert and Charney, 1974; Parker, 1974).

One approach to assessing primary care was suggested by a committee at the Institute of Medicine (1978) that listed the attributes of primary care as accessibility, comprehensiveness, coordination, continuity, and accountability. Of these five attributes, only comprehensiveness was actually defined ("ability of the primary care team to handle problems arising in the population it serves"). Accountability was recognized as a feature not unique to primary care, although essential to it. The committee acknowledged that primary care could not be assessed by descriptive features such as the location of care or by the provider's field of training or by the provision of a particular set of services. But it stated that "professionals who train men and women for primary care should accustom their students to a practice environment that meets or exceeds" the standards of primary care, specified in the form of positive responses to a set of 21 questions that concerned its five attributes. Seven questions were devoted to accessibility, six to comprehensiveness, four to coordination, three to continuity, and one to accountability.

The results of the efforts of this committee were an important milestone in the attempt to devise a normative method for measuring attainment of primary care. However, there are limitations to the checklist of questions. First, most of the indicators in the checklist might be attributes of secondary or tertiary care as well as of primary care; these include the opportunity for patients to schedule appointments; appreciation of patients' culture, background, socioeconomic status, and living circumstances; willingness to admit patients to hospitals, nursing homes, or convalescent homes; provision of simple, understandable information about fees; acceptance of patients without regard to race, religion, or ethnicity; easily retrievable and accessible medical records; provision of a summary of patients' records to other physicians when needed; and assumption of responsibility for alerting proper authorities if a patient's problem reveals a health hazard that may affect others.

Second, many of the indicators require a very high level of performance and allow for no variability and therefore may be difficult to achieve. One example is the requirement that "90% of appropriate requests for routine appointments such as preventive examinations be met within one week."

Third, many of the indicators represent the potential ability to provide a service rather than its actual accomplishment. Some examples are provision of personnel who can deal with patients with special language barriers (rather than actual provision of such services to those who need them), willingness of practitioners to admit patients to other facilities (rather than the degree to which they do so when it is necessary), and willingness of the practice unit to handle the great majority of patients' problems (rather than demonstrating that the unit actually accomplishes this).

An alternative to the method of assessing primary care suggested by the Institute of Medicine assesses the actual *degree* of attainment rather than the *potential* for achievement of first contact, longitudinality, comprehensiveness, and coordination. The standards for assessing adequacy would be based on the degree of improvement from one time to another or by comparing one system against another rather than against an arbitrary absolute standard. As with the Institute of Medicine checklist, the approach facilitates self-evaluation of clinics or practice units, as well as evaluation by an outside agency, to determine the degree to which a facility or health services system provides primary care that meets accepted standards or at least achieves a higher level of performance than others.

To do this, the criteria of the Institute of Medicine were adapted by Smith and Buesching (1986) to ascertain the degree of achievement of primary care. They asked a random sample of people about selected characteristics of their care and derived a primary care score from the responses.

Access was ascertained from responses to statements such as "I could call my principal physician today with chest pain and get a prompt response" and "If I contacted my principal physician with a medical problem that was not an emergency, he or she would see me within a reasonable period of time."

Continuity was reflected in answers such as "My principal physician sees me for regular checkups even if I do not have a specific illness" and "My principal physician provides me with reliable follow-up treatments for illness."

Comprehensiveness was judged by such answers as "My principal physician takes care of most of my medical problems" and "My principal physician has an excellent knowledge of all my current medications."

Coordination responses included "If I have a laboratory test or x-rays, my principal physician explains the results to me" and "If several physicians are involved with my care, my principal physician organizes it."

An additional feature, personalized care, was assessed by means of responses such as "My principal physician has an excellent knowledge of the kind of work I do" and "I can discuss a personal, family, or emotional problem with my principal physician." Satisfaction with care was highly associated with the score derived by combining the responses for these attributes; high primary care scores were also associated with patients who were ill fewer days and who stayed home fewer days due to illness after confounding factors such as perceived health status and reported health problems were taken into account. Specialty of the principal physician was not associated with the primary care score, however, and about 25% of the community sample named a subspecialist as their principal physician.

A more recent Institute of Medicine report on primary care defined it as "the provision of integrated, accessible health care services by clinicians who are accountable for addressing a large majority of personal health care needs, developing a sustained partnership with patients, and practicing in the context of family and community" (Donaldson et al., 1996). Recognizing that the terms in this definition might be open to different interpretations, the report further specified each of the components of the definition, as follows:

Integrated: Comprehensive (addressing any health problem at any given stage of a patient's life cycle); coordinated (ensuring the provision of a combination of health services and information that meets a patient's needs and also involving the connection between these services); continuous (care over time by a single individual or team of individuals and effective and timely communication)

Accessible: Ease of approach and elimination of geographic, administrative, financial, cultural, and language barriers

Health Care Services: Services provided by health care professionals directly or under their direction for the purpose of promoting, maintaining, or restoring health

Clinician: An individual who uses scientific knowledge and has authority to direct the delivery of personal health services to patients

Accountable: Responsible for addressing a large majority of personal health needs

Majority of personal health needs: Clinicians receive all the problems brought by
patients (unrestricted by problem or organ system), and have the training to
diagnose and manage a large majority of those problems when appropriate
Personal health care needs: Physical, mental, emotional, and social concerns that
involve the functioning of an individual
Sustained partnership: Relationship established over time between patient and clinician with the mutual expectation of continuation over time
Patient: An individual who interacts with a clinician because of an illness or for
health promotion and disease prevention
Context of family and community: Understanding of the patient's living conditions,
family dynamics, and cultural background with reference to the community in
which the patient lives

This definition of primary care did not explicitly include "first-contact" care,
although the report, as part of a section on comprehensiveness, recognizes that
"primary care is the usual and preferred route into the health care system" (Donaldson et al., 1996, p. 38). Moreover, it is similar to the earlier Institute of Medicine
definition in including some characteristics that also pertain to other levels of health
systems. For example, accountability applies not only to primary care but also to
the system of which primary care is a part. Sustained partnerships are expected
from specialists who accept responsibility for ongoing management of patients with
rare or unusually complex conditions. Furthermore, many of the concepts mentioned in the definition are open to a variety of interpretations. Just within a year
after the report appeared, two separate groups of researchers (Flocke, 1997; Franks
et al., 1997) made reference to the definition in justifying their approaches to measurement of primary care; these approaches were widely disparate. Furthermore,
"the majority of personal health care needs" is ambiguous and open to the interpretation that it refers to the majority of conditions that are listed in compendia
such as the International Classification of Diseases (see Chapter 16). That is, "majority" (in the report's sense) pertains only to specific individuals rather than to
needs of populations. For populations, it is the concept of meeting all of the common needs that is most relevant.

This most recent Institute of Medicine definition is also especially notable in
its focus on individual patients rather than on organization of health services to
meet population needs. The next section of this chapter emphasizes the importance
of focusing on primary care within a health system context that explicitly addresses
the dual functions to meet the needs of communities as well as of those individuals
who present themselves for care ("patients").

Primary Care from a Health Care System Vantage

The Canadian Medical Association explicitly considers primary care as the entry
point to the health care system and inter-related to the other components of the
system. It defines primary care as consisting of "first contact assessment of a
patient and the provision of continuing care for a wide range of health concerns,

and including the management of health problems, prevention and health promotion; and ongoing support, with family and community intervention where needed.'' It thus differs from the Institute of Medicine report in distinguishing first-contact care as a critical function and in including community interventions in the definition of functions (Canadian Medical Association, 1994).

The Charter for General Practice/Family Medicine in Europe, developed by a working group of the European region of the World Health Organization (1994), explicitly recognizes the role of primary care as a system of care that provides accessible and acceptable care for patients; ensures the equitable distribution of health resources; integrates and coordinates curative, palliative, preventive, and health promotion services; rationally controls secondary care technology and drugs; and increases cost-effectiveness of services through 12 characteristics:

1. General: Not restricted to age groups or types of problems or conditions
2. Accessible: In time, place, financing, and culture
3. Integrated: Curative, rehabilitative, health promotion and disease prevention
4. Continuous: Longitudinality over substantial periods of life
5. Team: Doctor is part of a multidisciplinary group
6. Holistic: Physical, psychological, and social perspectives of individuals, families, and communities
7. Personal: Person- rather than disease-focused care
8. Family oriented: Problems understood in the context of the family and social network
9. Community oriented: Context of life in the local community; awareness of health needs in the community; collaboration with other sectors to initiate positive health change
10. Coordinated: Coordination of all advice and support that the person receives
11. Confidential
12. Advocacy: Patient's advocate on health matters at all times and in relationship to all other health care providers.

It further recognizes that certain structural conditions, organizational improvements, and professional development issues have to be considered in providing high-quality primary care. The structural conditions included the clear definition of a practice population with the right of the members of the population to choose and to change the choice of primary care practitioner, the ability to locate a practice in the community in which the practice population resides, first-contact care in which access to specialists is through the primary care practitioner, and a system of remuneration that is balanced to provide the full range of services needed by the population.

The population- as well as person-focused views of primary care provide a basis for a normative system of measurement of the functions of primary care within a health services system. Furthermore, it introduces the need for considering the structure of health systems as well as the behaviors that reflect the function, both from the population as well as from the individual vantage point.

Figure 2.1 specifies the important components of the health system according to their type: structure, process, and outcome (Donabedian, 1966). The individual

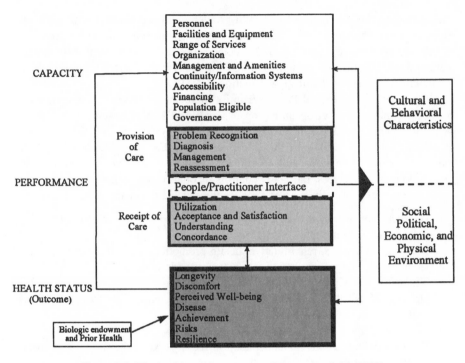

Figure 2.1. The health services system. Source: Starfield (1992).

characteristics within each component differ from place to place and from time to time, but each health services system has a structure (or "capacity") consisting of the characteristics that enable it to provide services, the processes (or "performance") that involve actions by the practitioners in the system as well as the actions of the populations and patients, and the outcome as reflected in various aspects of health status. These components interact with, and are determined by, individual behavior and the social, political, economic, and physical environment in which the health services system exists.

The following pages describe an approach to measuring primary care that is based on certain structures and processes or, as more commonly designated, "capacity" and "performance" within the health services system. This approach to measuring primary care assumes that structural attributes must be in place for important activities to occur. It also assumes the importance of assessing the performance of those activities. Thus, measuring the key features involves measurement of a behavioral characteristic and the structural characteristic on which it depends.

Let us examine, in turn, the capacity and the performance of the health services system to set the stage for choosing those features that are most important in primary care. The next chapter will consider "outcomes," in the context of a discussion of measurement of health status.

Capacity of a Health Services System

The capacity of the health services system is what enables health services to be delivered. The enablers consist of the resources that are needed to provide services. As shown in Figure 2.1, there are at least ten main structural components:

Personnel: This includes all who are involved in providing the services and their education and their training.

Facilities and equipment: These include the buildings (e.g., hospitals, clinics or health centers, and offices) and the physical components of the facilities including such elements as laboratory instruments and technology for diagnosis or therapy.

Management and amenities: These include characteristics of services other than those directly related to clinical care. For example, are laboratory results reported in a timely fashion? Are patients treated with courtesy and respect?

Range of services provided by facilities: This range of services may vary from country to country and from community to community, but every facility has made decisions about the kinds of services that will be available and those that will not be available. The range of services provided is an important consideration for the nature of primary care and is discussed in greater detail in Chapter 10.

Organization of services: Do the personnel work in groups or alone? What are the mechanisms for ensuring accountability, and who is responsible for providing the different aspects of care?

Mechanisms for providing continuity of care: These mechanisms are especially important in primary care because without them there would be no way to deal with problems that require more than one visit or require the transfer of information. Continuity is usually provided in the form of practitioners or teams of practitioners who serve as the primary contact for the patient, but sometimes the only mechanism for continuity is some form of medical record. Continuity is considered in greater detail in Chapter 11.

Mechanisms for providing access to care: There is no point to having personnel, facilities, and equipment if they cannot be reached by persons who need them. There are several types of accessibility: accessibility in time (that is, the hours of availability), geographic accessibility (adequacy of transportation and distance to be covered), and psychosocial accessibility (are there language or cultural barriers to communication between personnel in the facilities and the patients?). Accessibility and its special importance in primary care are considered in greater detail in Chapter 7.

Arrangements for financing: What is the method of payment for services, and how are the personnel remunerated for their work? Of all of the structural features, this one is most likely to differ across countries and therefore a feature of great interest cross-nationally for comparative studies.

Delineation of the population eligible to receive services: Each unit of the health services system should be able to define the community it serves and should

know its important sociodemographic and health characteristics. Members of
the population should be able to identify their source of care and be aware of
its responsibility for providing required services. This structural feature is another critical element for primary care, especially for the feature known as
longitudinality. It is further discussed in Chapter 8.

Governance of the health system: Health systems differ in their accountability to
those they serve. Often they do not involve the population at all in decisions
about the way services are organized or delivered. Sometimes, community
councils serve in an advisory capacity. Rarely is responsibility for decision-
making shared or assumed by community boards.

Approaches to governance are on a continuum from least empowered (the ability to be heard) to most empowered (the ability to control the organization). The
continuum consists of three main types: control, choice, and moral/legal suasion
(Saltman, 1994). Political control, in which people have authority over budgets and
resource allocation, is the most direct form of governance; it also is consistent with
collective, democratic decision-making. Choice, as an alternative form of governance, is a much more indirect method that is based on the principle that allowing
people to choose where and from whom they receive their services will encourage
competition and thus, by default, reach accountability. Carrying the principle of
choice to its logical conclusion, financing of services would allow for people to
seek care from alternative health providers and receive reimbursement as they
would for care received from conventional medical practitioners. (This is the case
in the Netherlands, where the insurance system will reimburse for acupuncture and
other alternative regimens, and in Germany, where therapy in spas is reimbursable.)
The third mechanism of governance is more indirect and is represented by systems
of legal and social redress for inappropriate or harmful services. Satisfaction surveys to determine how people feel about their services operate by moral suasion,
the most indirect measure of control because people have no ability to change
aspects of services that are deemed inadequate.

Performance of a Health Services System

The processes of a health services system are the actions that constitute the delivery
and receipt of services. Thus, there are two components: those that represent activities of the providers of care and those that represent activities of the population.
The providers first must recognize the needs existing both in the community and
in individual patients. This feature is known as *problem* (or *needs*) *recognition* and
is a particularly important consideration for primary care. The problem may be a
symptom, a sign, an abnormal laboratory test, a previous but relevant item in the
history of the patient or of the community, or a need for an indicated preventive
procedure. Problem recognition implies being aware of the existence of situations
requiring attention in a health context. After recognizing the problem, the health
professional generally formulates a *diagnosis* or an understanding of the problem
when no diagnosis is possible. This is necessary to move to the next step in the
process of care, which concerns the instituting of an appropriate strategy for *treat-*

ment or management. Subsequently, an arrangement must be made for *reassessment* of the problem to determine if the original recognition of the problem, the diagnosis, and the therapy were adequate. At this point, the process of care is started on a new cycle of monitoring and surveillance, with recognition of the problems as they now exist.

The processes of care that reflect how people interact with the health system are also important. First, people decide whether and when to use the health care system. If they do use it, they come to an understanding of what providers offer to them and then make decisions about how satisfied they are with their care and whether they will accept the recommendations or instructions of the providers. Subsequently, they decide on the extent to which they participate in the process. They can decide to carry through with the recommendations or to modify them in ways in which they see fit or to disregard them partly or completely. Certain processes of care contributed by patients are an important key consideration in the assessment of primary care, as noted in Chapters 7 and 8.

Measuring the Attainment of Primary Care: The Capacity–Performance Approach

Both the potential for and the achievement of the critical features of primary care can be measured by the capacity–performance approach. Four structural elements of the health services system define the potential, and two process features translate the potential into the important activity.

The four structural elements relevant to primary care are accessibility, range of services, eligible population and continuity. They are defined as follow:

Accessibility involves the location of the facility near the population it serves, the hours and days it is open for care, the degree to which it can tolerate visits made without appointments, and the extent to which these aspects of accessibility are perceived as convenient by the population.

Range of services is the package of services available to the population, as well as those services that the population believes are available.

Definition of the eligible population includes the degree to which a health care service can identify the population for which it assumes responsibility and the degree to which the individuals in the served population know that they are considered to be part of it.

Continuity consists of the arrangements by which care is provided as an uninterrupted succession of events. Continuity may be achieved by a variety of mechanisms: one practitioner who cares for the patient, or a medical record that reflects the care given, or a computer record, or even a client-held record. The extent to which the facility provides such arrangements and the perception of their attainment by the individuals in the population indicate the extent of continuity of care.

Translating the potential into the appropriate activity requires two performance elements of the health services system: utilization of services by the population and recognition of problems by health services practitioners.

Utilization refers to the extent and kind of use of health services. The primary reason for a visit may be to investigate the occurrence of a new problem or to follow up an old one or to receive preventive services. Utilization may be initiated by the patient or be at the request or direction of a health professional, or it may occur as the result of some administrative requirement.

Problem (or *needs*) *recognition* is the step that precedes the diagnostic process. If problems or health needs are not recognized, there will be either no diagnostic process or an inappropriate one. Patients may not complain of problems because they are not aware of them, or they may complain of one thing that masks another. Accurate determination of the patient's or population's health needs is the role of the practitioner.

As previously stated, one of the four elements of structure (accessibility, range of services, eligible population, continuity) and one of the two process elements (utilization, problem recognition) are required to measure the potential for and attainment of each of the attributes of primary care: first-contact care, longitudinality, comprehensiveness, and coordination. Each of the four attributes is of sufficient importance to warrant a separate chapter. The following section briefly describes the elements of structure and process required to measure each one.

First-contact care implies accessibility to and use of services for each new problem or new episode of a problem for which people seek health care. Regardless of what a facility states or perceives its accessibility to be, it does not provide first-contact care unless its potential users perceive it to be accessible and reflect this in their use. Therefore, measurement of first-contact care involves evaluating accessibility (the structural element) and utilization (the process element).

Several important questions concern first-contact care. To what extent does the system provide for easy access, both geographically and by having longer hours of availability? Does the population perceive access to be convenient? To what extent is easier access associated with utilization of the facility by its defined population for new problems? First-contact care is discussed more fully in Chapter 7.

Longitudinality presupposes the existence of a regular source of care and its use over time. Thus, the primary care unit must be able to identify its eligible population and the individuals in that population—who should obtain care from the unit except when outside consultation and referral are required. Moreover, the linkage of the population with its source of care should be reflected in strong interpersonal ties that reflect the mutual affiliation of people and their practitioner.

Several important questions concern longitudinality. Do individuals who are clearly identified as enrollees identify the facility as their regular source of care and use it as such over a period of time? Do all visits, except those initiated by providers, take place at the facility? Does the nature of the interaction between the practitioner and patients reflect their mutual affiliation? Longitudinality is the subject of Chapter 8.

Comprehensiveness implies that primary care facilities must arrange for the patient to receive all types of health care services, even though some may not be provided efficiently within the primary care facility. This includes referrals to secondary services for consultation, to tertiary services for definitive management of specific conditions, and to essential supporting services such as home care and other community services. Although each primary care facility may define its own range of services differently, each should make its responsibility explicit to both its patient population and staff and must recognize situations in which services are available. The staff should provide for, and recognize the need for, preventive services and for services to deal with symptoms, signs, and diagnoses of manifest illness. It should also adequately recognize problems of all types, be they functional, organic, or social. The latter is particularly important because all health problems occur within a social setting that often predisposes to or causes disease.

Several important questions concern comprehensiveness. How inclusive is the benefit package offered? Is it explicit, and is it understood by the population? In providing services, do the practitioners recognize a broad spectrum of needs within the population? Do they refer to other specialists when appropriate? Comprehensiveness is the subject of Chapter 10.

Coordination (integration) of care requires some form of continuity, either by practitioners or by medical records or by both, as well as problem recognition (a process element). For example, the status of problems noted in previous visits or problems for which referrals to other practitioners were made should be ascertained at subsequent visits. This recognition of problems will be facilitated if the same practitioner sees the patient on follow up or if there is a medical record that highlights these problems. Thus, both continuity and problem recognition are necessary in assessing coordination of care.

Several important questions concern coordination. To what extent is scheduling arranged to allow patients to see the same provider for all visits? Do the medical records contain information pertinent to the care of patients? Is there an increased recognition of problems associated with improved continuity? Is this increased recognition a function of better records or of regular practitioner continuity or of both? Coordination is the subject of Chapter 11.

Assessing the Effectiveness of Primary Care Attributes

Primary care functions and primary care tasks

Sometimes, primary care functions are confused with tasks that are needed to carry out the functions. Thus, primary care is often characterized by what services it provides in the interests of attaining comprehensiveness. Typical examples of such services are health promotion, disease prevention (including primary prevention as well as secondary prevention, i.e., early detection through screening), diagnosis and management of a wide variety of medical conditions, maternal and child health care, emergency care, rehabilitative care, palliative care, referrals when appropriate, maintenance of the medical record, patient advocacy, health education, and participation in community health programs and health advocacy (Alberta Medical Association, 1996). Defining and measuring primary care by achievement of its cardinal functions will, by the effect of these functions, result in a similar or identical task list. It is the functions that are critical because many of the tasks that are part of primary care (e.g., prevention, emergency care, patient advocacy, health education, rehabilitative care) are tasks that are also part of other levels of care and may even be assumed by other levels of care (e.g., public health activities) instead of being provided in primary care settings.

Essential differences between primary care and care by other specialists

Although primary care and other levels of care often share attributes, there are notable differences in the way the functions are carried out. The following discusses some of the main differences.

1. Accessibility. All services should be appropriately accessible. Access to sub-specialists' services should be ensured for those who need them, and the time constraints should be appropriate to patients' needs and the urgency of their situation. In primary care, however, access should be universal and is not necessarily related to the degree of need because individuals cannot be expected to know the gravity or urgency of many of their conditions before they have sought care.
2. Medical records. All health professionals should maintain complete and accurate records and be responsible for the content they generate. Primary care is special only in that it bears responsibility for knowing about the essential elements of records generated in other levels of care.
3. Utilization of services by populations. Although individuals in populations use all levels of services from time to time, use of primary care is initiated primarily by individuals, whereas in secondary and tertiary care, use is most often generated by the health care professional.
4. Problem recognition. Both primary care and non-primary care must recognize problems that are brought to them. In primary care, these problems and needs are often poorly defined and poorly differentiated, whereas at other levels of care they are better defined because they have already been through a defining "filter."
5. Range of services. Both primary care and other levels of care must specify the range of services that will be provided according to the training, experience, and competence of the practitioner. In primary care, however, the range must be broader because it must encompass all health problems that are common in the population instead of a subset of them.
6. The diagnostic process in primary care differs from that in other levels of care. Because the likelihood of serious illness is lower in primary care, the frequencies of diagnostic testing and prescription of definitive therapy are less. The value of time ("watchful waiting") becomes greater both to better define the presenting problems and to judge the likelihood of success of alternative regimens. Whereas the threats to effectiveness and efficiency of primary care lie in the greater likelihood of overlooking disease when it is there and possible delay in making diagnoses of less common diseases, the threat to effectiveness and efficiency of subspecialty care lies in the greater likelihood of attributing complaints to diseases that are *not* present and the consequent harm as a result of

excessive testing, inappropriate diagnoses and therapy (even temporarily), and unnecessary anxiety on the part of patients. Primary care is more often subject to errors of omissions, whereas specialty care is more prone to errors of commission.

In theory, the structural element of each characteristic should be closely related to the process element. That is, better access should lead to better utilization for each new health problem; better identification with a regular source of care should be associated with more consistent use of that regular source of care over time and better practitioner–patient interactions; a broader range of available services should be associated with better recognition of the need for those services; and better continuity of care should lead to better coordination of care as measured by greater recognition of information about patients. In practice, there is little research that specifically tests the theory.

Furthermore, the unique features of primary care are not always clearly separable. If there is a relationship between a practitioner and patient that transcends the presence of particular problems or types of problems (longitudinality), it is more likely that the practitioner will be the one from whom care is initially sought for a new problem (first-contact care). Similarly, longitudinality should also be related to comprehensiveness, as a practitioner or facility that provides care over time regardless of the type of problem should also be providing a greater breadth of services. Similarly, the greater the range of services that are provided, the greater the burden of coordination, especially if some of these services have to be provided elsewhere rather than in the primary care site itself. Despite these interrelationships, the four unique characteristics of primary care are conceptually distinct; it is only when they are put into operation in practice that the potential for overlap becomes evident. The extent of overlap is, in fact, of high priority for research.

The ability to measure the important features of primary care makes it possible to set goals for their achievement and to measure their attainment. It also makes it possible to ascertain whether particular facilities or professionals qualify for the designation as primary care providers. Services qualifying as primary care can be compared with other forms of care with regard to the impact of the services. Knowledge about the relative importance of each feature in contributing to desired outcomes can result from research using this approach to measurement. Is the attainment of a satisfactory level of first-contact care associated with increased satisfaction among patients as well as with better problem resolution? Is longitudinality associated with better problem recognition, better understanding, and participation of patients, and does it result in fewer days of disability and discomfort? Is comprehensiveness associated with different utilization patterns, fewer episodes of new illness, or more rapid resolution of problems? Is coordination associated with less overall utilization, better understanding and increased patient participation in their care, and more rapid problem resolution with fewer new problems? Does primary care return patients more quickly to optimum levels of activity, comfort, and satisfaction with their health, and does it do a better job helping people achieve their full potential and maximal resilience against threats to their health? Are each of the four characteristics equally important, or are some more important than others?

No primary care system can attain perfect performance in all of its four essential components: first contact, longitudinality, comprehensiveness, and coordination. If standards are too high, patients will be disappointed and professionals will be frustrated. But justification for primary care need not depend on the attainment of optimum standards; it is sufficient only to demonstrate that the goals of primary care are better served by practitioners trained and organized to provide primary care than by practitioners trained to focus on particular illnesses, organ systems, or pathogenetic mechanisms and that the attainment of the goals progressively improve over time.

References

Alberta Medical Association. Primary Medical Care. Edmonton, Canada: Alberta Medical Association, June 1996.

Alpert J, Charney E. The Education of Physicians for Primary Care. Pub. No. (HRA) 74-3113. Rockville, MD: U.S. Department of Health, Education, and Welfare, Public Health Service, Health Resources Administration, 1974.

Canadian Medical Association. Strengthening the Foundation: The Role of the Physician in Primary Health Care in Canada. Ottawa: Ontario Canadian Medical Association, 1994.

Donabedian A. Evaluating the quality of medical care. Milbank Q 1966; 44(pt 2):166–206.

Donaldson M, Yordy K, Lohr K, Vanselow N (eds). Primary Care: America's Health in a New Era. Institute of Medicine. Washington, DC: National Academy Press, 1996.

Franks P, Clancy C, Nutting P. Defining primary care: Empirical analysis of the national ambulatory medical care survey. Med Care 1997; 35:655–68.

Flocke S. Measuring attributes of primary care: Development of a new instrument. J Fam Pract 1997; 45:64–74.

Institute of Medicine. A Manpower Policy for Primary Health Care: Report of a Study. IOM Pub. No. 78–02. Washington, DC: National Academy of Sciences, 1978.

Millis JS (Chairman). The Graduate Education of Physicians. Report of the Citizens Commission on Graduate Medical Education. Chicago: American Medical Association, 1966, p 37.

Parker A. The Dimensions of Primary Care: Blueprints for Change. In Andreopoulos S (ed): Primary Care: Where Medicine Fails. New York: Johns Wiley and Sons, 1974, pp 15–80.

Parker A, Walsh J, Coon M. A normative approach to the definition of primary health care. Milbank Q 1976; 54:415–38.

Saltman RB. Patient choice and patient empowerment in Northern European health systems: A conceptual framework. Int J Health Serv 1994; 24(2):201–29.

Smith W, Buesching D. Measures of primary medical care and patient characteristics. J Ambulatory Care Manage 1986; 9:49–57.

Starfield B. Primary Care: Concept, Evaluation, and Policy. New York: Oxford University Press, 1992.

White KL. Life and death and medicine. Sci Am 1973; 229:23–33.

World Health Organization. A Charter for General Practice/Family Medicine in Europe. Regional Office for Europe. Geneva: World Health Organization, working draft, 1994.

— 3 —

Morbidity
in Primary Care

Most approaches to characterizing health status in clinical practice are based on the frequency of individual diagnoses or on individual diagnoses grouped by organ system. This may not be the best approach for primary care practice. Many individuals have more than one diagnosis, and some diseases predispose to others. Thus, disease-by-disease approaches fail to capture morbidity experiences of individual patients or of populations of patients. Since primary care is focused on patients and on patient populations rather than on their diseases, approaches that characterize morbidity according to the different manifestations of health and illness would be more useful in primary care. This chapter discusses the challenges to characterizing morbidity patterns in these different ways.

Characterizing Health and Illness

Assessment of health and illness (health status) serves four purposes: to facilitate the delivery of clinical care, to document differences across populations and subpopulations to inform public health activities and health policy, to deploy and manage resources according to extent of need, and to measure the impact (outcomes) of health services.

Facilitating the delivery of clinical care

Clinical care is generally more predictable and more effective when interventions are targeted toward interrupting the pathogenetic pathway, that is, by attacking a link in the chain of events between a determinant of the illness and the illness itself. The "diagnosis," or name given to the illness, serves an important function in medical care because it usually implies a likely etiology and course of the illness and thus suggests a strategy for treatment. Diagnoses are the conventional way of specifying morbidity in clinical care, although not necessarily the most appropriate in primary care.

35

Assessing and documenting the health of populations and subpopulations

By extension from clinical care, the health of a population or subpopulation could be described by the frequency of individual diagnoses in the population, and different populations could be compared with regard to the incidence (frequency of new occurrences) or prevalence (frequency at any given point in time) of each specific diagnosis. For example, atlases of mortality in different countries, or in different political subdivisions of any given country, portray the frequency of occurrence of deaths due to specific diagnoses (Holland, 1991, 1993).

Knowledge about the incidence or prevalence of specific diseases derives largely from data on patient visits to physicians. However, most new health problems that arise never come to the attention of practitioners (White, 1961). Furthermore, many problems cannot be resolved in one visit; sometimes many visits are required to provide the information necessary to diagnose and resolve a problem. A major conceptual advance in moving beyond visit-based approaches is the episode-of-care–based approach. Physicians indicate which visit in a series of visits is the initial one for a problem, characterize the problem, maintain an accounting of which subsequent visits are for the problem, and indicate the visit in which the problem is considered resolved. (If the problem is an ongoing one, a period of time such as 1 year serves to delineate the episode.) The approach is most useful when it starts with a presenting problem (whether or not it is related to an ongoing disease) and follows it through to its resolution; the problem is designated using a coding system such as the International Classification of Primary Care (see Chapter 16), and the episode is designated by a diagnosis *if and only if* a diagnosis is reached. Lamberts and Hofmans-Okkes (1996) described the nature of primary care practice in the Netherlands by showing that, in a patient population of 15,158 women aged 25–44 years, 11,570 (76%) visited their primary care doctor at least once in a year. The 20 most common new episodes constituted one-third of all new episodes. The 15,158 women had an average of 2.9 new episodes per year, of which 2.4 were new and only 0.5 were old. (For the 11,570 visiting patients, the average number of episodes was 3.8, of which 3.1 were new.) The time to resolution, its correlation with different types of resources used, and the amount of resources for the diagnosis and management of different conditions can be ascertained by applying this episode approach.

However, morbidity, as expressed by an individual's diagnoses, or even the particular symptoms or disabilities, is increasingly recognized as an incomplete and inadequate measure of illness burden. It provides no information on more positive aspects of health as expressed in the most common approaches to defining health (see chapter 1). Moreover, patterns of diagnoses of individual diseases vary from place to place and from time to time. Although there are standard criteria for a few diagnoses, these are not universally used; what is called one disease in one place may not be recognized as the same disease in other places. Thus, although the International Classification of Diseases is used throughout the world to designate causes of death as well as causes of hospitalization and outpatient visits, there is no assurance that the same diagnosis means the same thing in all places because no definitions have been included in past editions. There have been attempts to reduce the variability in style of diagnosis by developing clusters of diagnoses that essentially reflect similar illnesses (Schneeweiss et al., 1983), but these do not include all diseases, nor are they often used for comparisons between practices in different places.

Undoubtedly the main reason for the search for measures other than clinical diagnoses for describing and comparing the health of populations results from the recognition that counting individual diagnoses does not adequately represent health. Many countries conduct household surveys of representative samples of their population. These surveys often elicit information about peoples' perceived health (excellent, very good, good, fair, poor), about their symptoms, and about various illnesses for which they may or may not have sought care. These types of data are becoming important sources of information about the health of different groups within populations and even across populations of different countries. Thus, Wagstaff and Van Doorslaer (1993) used data on reported days of disability from chronic conditions, limitations of activity associated with them, and self-perceived health to show that countries with more equitable health systems had better health. The major drawback of these types of data is possible differences in tendency to report problems in different populations.

Planning and allocating resources

Efficient deployment of resources depends on good information about the existence of problems that are amenable to alteration by health services. The existence of differences in morbidity in different practices provides the basis for allocating resources differentially according to the needs of the population served.

There are three alternatives to dealing with this challenge to resource allocation: the historical, the sociodemographic, and the categorization by diagnoses.

1. The historical approach to characterizing the extent of morbidity in practice: Various factors make the historical approach the most predictive of the present and future situation. Most practices do not change much from year to year, and most practice populations remain relatively constant. The health of their populations also remains relatively constant, except for the gradual increase in diseases of aging as people remain within primary care practices. Because the determinants of health and illness are biological, social, and environmental, the general morbidity mix of individual practices tends to remain constant. Thus, the resources expended in caring for a practice population and the utilization experiences of that population remain relatively constant over time, at least from year to year, in the absence of externally imposed incentives or disincentives to change them. Describing these patterns of use of services in one time period is therefore highly predictive of the patterns of use of resources in the ensuing time period as long as there are no extraneous factors to alter the likelihood of resource use. However, external factors do often arise in the form of newly available technologies for intervention and financial incentives to employ them. Because not all practices will be exposed to or respond similarly to these incentives, resource allocations based on prior use of resources often have to do

with differences in patterns of practice rather than with differences in the needs of the populations served.

2. The sociodemographic approach: Because illness patterns are so highly sensitive to the social and environmental context, the morbidity pattern in any particular practice or groups of practices will be heavily dependent on the sociodemographic characteristics of the practice population. Characteristics of special importance are income and wealth (including housing and nutrition as well as material resources to deal with illnesses that may occur), occupation (with its different health hazards), social structure of the area of residence, and a variety of environmental influences in the area. These types of factors are sufficiently predictive of the level of practice morbidity that resources can be directed differentially according to the nature of the community served. For example, in Sweden and in the United Kingdom, indices of social deprivation are used, sometimes with additional information on health characteristics, to provide different levels of financial support to practices depending on the sociodemographic characteristics of their populations (Diderichsen et al., 1997), as well as for epidemiological studies in practice.

3. The "case-mix" approach: Whereas most aspects of health services delivery (such as numbers of visits, counts of personnel, or money spent) lend themselves to direct quantification, morbidity does not. There is no way to sum the burden of diseases, either for individuals or within a population of individuals, and, even if there were, the sum would be meaningless because the severity of each individual disease component is likely to vary among different individuals and populations (Iezzoni, 1997). Case-mix measures are ways of measuring the total burden of morbidity in a population of patients by combining diagnoses in different ways; they are an important tool for evaluating both quality and costs of care. Many aspects of evaluating quality require comparisons of different practitioners and practices; where outcomes of care are different, it may be because the underlying challenges are greater in one than in the other rather than a result of differences in the quality of care provided. Thus, all comparisons of quality of care require standardization of initial morbidity before evaluating differences in the results that are found. Similarly, differences in the need for and expenditure of resources between health systems, practices, or practitioners may result from differences in the extent of morbidity in their populations. The existence of many thousands of individual diseases, each with greatly varying levels of severity and need for resources, precludes the possibility of simple additions of diagnoses to achieve a description of the level of burden of morbidity.

Summarizing information from clinical practice to provide profiles of the burden of morbidity existing in practices is a difficult challenge. Most practices are composed of patients with hundreds if not thousands of diagnoses; a summary measure that takes them all into account is a daunting challenge.

When populations are reasonably homogenous, particularly with respect to age and social characteristics, morbidity patterns may be sufficiently uniform that frequencies of individual diagnoses can be used to characterize case mix. For example, in a practice population composed mainly of elderly people, the variability in disease distribution will be less than in a mixed-age population because some diseases are much more common in the elderly and the variability in susceptibility to other diseases (such as those for which genetic variability will have resulted in death before old age) will be less so that a more homogeneous pattern of illness results. Case-mix approaches based on the presence of particular diagnoses may therefore be relatively successful in older populations (Ellis et al., 1996). In more heterogeneous populations, the resource needs for individual diagnoses are highly variable. In different areas and in different practices, the variability in severity of individual diagnoses precludes practice profiling and resource allocation based solely on the presence or absence of individual diagnoses encountered in the practice, especially when the practice population is diverse in age and other sociodemographic characteristics.

An approach that combines diagnoses into a manageable number of different categories based on the similarity of their need for resources is more useful under such circumstances. The main source of information to profile practices in this way derives from diagnoses recorded on claims or encounter forms, which also contain information to determine the resources devoted to dealing with them over periods of time. Practices can be compared with regard to the burdens of morbidity in their patients as well as the costs of providing care for them. Case-mix systems also can be used to set capitation rates; if one practitioner has a heavier burden of morbidity, a higher capitation payment may be justified. If certain health care facilities are paid more for caring for population groups that are sicker, the distribution of resources will be fairer and there will be no tendency for a facility or practitioner to try to avoid caring for especially sick individuals. As capitation payments become more widespread, there is likely to be increasing need for such case-mix systems.

Although many case-mix methods exist, most are limited to inpatient care. Those that deal with ambulatory care are based primarily on visits rather than on people.

However, the ACG (Adjusted Clinical Groups, formerly Ambulatory Care Groups) system is a case mix system that characterizes people according to the illnesses they experience in a period of time (usually a year). It does this by combining diagnoses in patient populations into groups that are relatively homogeneous in their resource use over that period of time. This system for categorizing the burden of morbidity as represented by the mix of diagnoses was originally developed to explain patterns of utilization. Prior research had shown that individuals (both children and adults) who were high users of services tended to remain high users over long periods of time (Densen et al., 1959; Starfield et al., 1985). Conversely, those who were low users tended to remain low users over the same long time period. To determine whether these patterns were a result of a predisposition to use health services on the part of families, a result of the presence of particular kinds of illnesses (such as chronic medical problems or mental health problems), or some factor related to morbidity patterns, a method to characterize morbidity was developed. This method conceptualized illness as fitting into one of several types: minor illnesses that are generally self-limited if treated appropriately; illnesses that are more major but also are limited in time if treated appropriately;

medical illnesses that are generally chronic in nature and not curable by medical therapy; illnesses resulting from anatomical problems (such as hearing, vision, and orthopedic problems) that are generally not curable even with adequate intervention; and conditions that are considered psychosocial in nature. Exploration of the relationships between these factors (familial use of services, presence of particular types of illnesses, and the "morbidity burden" measure) indicated that the most salient factor was the latter: burden of morbidity. That is, individuals who had diagnoses fitting into more of the five different types were much more likely to be persistently high users of services, and, conversely, those with lower burdens of morbidity as manifested by having fewer types were more likely to be persistently low users of services.

These studies suggested that an amplification of this approach to "morbidity burden" could be useful for a variety of purposes in primary care in specific, ambulatory care in general, and perhaps even total care of individuals and populations. Tests of this potential indicated that this was, indeed, the case. The approach involved assigning each of the diagnoses in the International Classification of Diseases—Clinical Modification (ICD-CM) into 1 of 32 categories, as listed in Table 3.1. (There were originally 34, but two have been deleted because they had few diagnoses and are now reassigned to other ADGs.) The assigning of the diagnoses to these categories was done by physicians knowledgeable of the clinical presentation and epidemiology of illnesses, using the following criteria, in the order presented:

Likelihood that the condition would persist and the patient would have return visits for it

Likelihood of a specialty consultation or referral, currently and in the future

Expected need and cost of diagnostic and therapeutic procedures associated with the condition

Likelihood of an associated hospitalization

Likelihood of an associated disability

Likelihood of associated decreased life expectancy

The 32 groupings are collapsed into 12 relatively similar groups (CADGs), which are then aggregated according to their most commonly encountered combinations in clinical practice. Each individual in an enrolled population is characterized by the diagnoses that the individual receives in the period of time and placed in that final grouping (the Adjusted Clinical Group [ACG]) that represents the constellation of diagnoses for that patient. The case mix of a health facility, or of any practitioner, can be described according to the pattern of ACG. Practitioners or facilities with greater frequencies of those ACGs that represent sicker patients can be considered to need more resources to care for those patients in their practices.

The important features of the ACG system are that a single ACG is assigned to an individual based on the pattern of morbidity experienced by that individual over a period of time, generally a year. This assignment of morbidity is not dependent on visit rates per se or on the extent of use or cost of diagnostic and

Table 3.1. The Adjusted Diagnostic Groups (ADGs)

 1. Time Limited: Minor
 2. Time Limited: Minor—Primary Infections
 3. Time Limited: Major
 4. Time Limited: Major—Primary Infections
 5. Allergies
 6. Asthma
 7. Likely to Recur: Discrete
 8. Likely to Recur: Discrete—Primary Infections
 9. Likely to Recur: Progressive
10. Chronic Medical: Stable
11. Chronic Medical: Unstable
12. Chronic Specialty: Stable—Orthopedic
13. Chronic Specialty: Stable—Ear, Nose, Throat
14. Chronic Specialty: Stable—Eye
15. Deleted
16. Chronic Specialty: Unstable—Orthopedic
17. Chronic Specialty: Unstable—Ear, Nose, Throat
18. Chronic Specialty: Unstable—Eye
19. Deleted
20. Dermatological
21. Injuries/Adverse Effects: Minor
22. Injuries/Adverse Effects: Major
23. Psychosocial: Time Limited, Minor
24. Psychosocial: Recurrent or Persistent, Stable
25. Psychosocial: Recurrent or Persistent, Unstable
26. Signs/Symptoms: Minor
27. Signs/Symptoms: Uncertain
28. Signs/Symptoms: Major
29. Discretionary
30. See and Reassure
31. Prevention/Administrative
32. Malignancy
33. Pregnancy
34. Dental

therapeutic procedures because only diagnoses are used for the assignment. An individual may have multiple illnesses of one type, yet be assigned to only one category of illness for the year. Thus, the method is not dependent on number of illnesses but on their type as characterized by the criteria for assignment. Each of the 32 basic categories is relatively homogeneous in its likelihood of visits and use of other resources. The resulting ACG categorizations are highly predictive of number of ambulatory care visits and use of ambulatory care resources during the period of time from which the diagnoses were assigned; they are also predictive of use for the next year (Weiner et al., 1991).

The ACGs also have clinical validity in that the patterns of morbidity are relatively stable over time. Individuals in one category are much more likely to stay in that category in the next year than would be expected by chance distributions of illness, and the utilization experiences in the subsequent year are similar within categories (Starfield et al., 1991).

Thus, the ACG system has potential utility for describing differences in the patterns of illnesses in different clinical populations, in serving as a method for stratifying populations into clinically meaningful groups for the purpose of profiling the practices of different practitioners or groups of practitioners, and as a method for studying resource use and planning for resource needs of different populations. It also has applicability in research that seeks to explain the predictiveness of various health system factors on resource use, in that differences in morbidity in different populations can be controlled for when examining the impact of practitioner and system factors on use of services and resources.

The ACG case-mix system is being used widely as a profiling technique in clinical settings to describe and understand differences in practice patterns of clinicians, in providing a means to develop a capitation rate for practices, and in research studies that require a mechanism to control for the effect of morbidity while examining the impact of other factors on resource use. While originally developed and applied only in ambulatory settings, diagnostic codes found for hospitalized patients and resources consumed in hospital care have been added.

Tables 3.2 summarizes major research using ACGs. Each study is described according to its purpose and source of information; the types of characteristics examined; whether the ACG system was used in its ACG form (one pattern of morbidity for each individual in the population), in its ADG form (each type of morbidity for each individual considered individually), or, in some cases, in its CADG form (each of the collapsed groupings for each individual considered individually); and the use of the ACG system in interpreting the major findings of the research.

ACGs in the European context

The ACG system in the U.S. context increasingly has been expanded to encompass all health services use rather than just primary care use because budgeting for health services of individuals and groups takes into account projected use not only for primary care services but also for specialty services and inpatient care. That is, insurance premiums, whether they are part of private insurance or government-provided insurance for the elderly or poor, generally cover a full range of services, albeit often incompletely. In contrast, in Europe, planning and budgeting for services generally is done separately for primary care services and for specialty services (whether they are provided in outpatient clinics of hospitals or as inpatient services). In Europe, interest in the ACG system has been largely in its applicability for describing and understanding primary care.

Developmental work in Spain has shown the applicability of the system to primary care within the context of a national health system. Juncosa and colleagues (1998) used the ACGs to profile 2,467 patients of 13 primary care teams in 9 health centers in the province of Barcelona, Spain. Instead of using all diagnoses made in the 13,269 visits made by these patients, diagnoses (or, if not diagnosis,

Table 3.2. ACGs: Profiling, Capitation Decisions, Research, and Methodological Studies

	Subject	Site	Data Source	Variables	Use of ACGs/ADGs	Findings
	Use of ACGs for Profiling					
Salem-Schatz et al. (1994)	Referral, 38,000 people	Staff model practices	Encounter data	Age, sex, physician, and practice characteristics	ACGs as morbidity control	Case-mix control reduced variability
Weiner et al. (1996b)	Total charges	Various	Medicaid claims data	Physicians and practice characteristics, geographic areas, patient characteristics	As morbidity control	Case-mix control reduced variability
Tucker et al. (1996)	Total charges	21 independent practice associations	Claims data	Age, sex (providers)	Charges generated within ACG groups	Consistency of physician characterization across ACGs; consistency across 2 consecutive years
Green et al. (1996)	Procedure charges	130 nonacademic practices in four states	Claims data	Physician and practice characteristics	As control for morbidity	Creation of database for profiling studies
	Use of ACGs for Capitation Decisions					
Weiner et al. (1996a)	Total charges for groups differentiated by age/gender, disease, and cost group	Physician practices	Medicare data tapes	Age, sex, illness groups, cost groups	Predictor variables (ADGs)	Increased ability to predict subsequent year costs even without consideration of any prior year utilization

(continued)

Table 3.2. ACGs: Profiling, Capitation Decisions, Research, and Methodological Studies—Continued

	Subject	Site	Data Source	Variables	Use of ACGs/ADGs	Findings
Fowler et al. (1996)	Total covered charges	Maryland Medicaid and group-model HMO	Claims data and encounter data	Age, sex, welfare status, different case-mix measures (all except ACGs/ ADGs involve prior use variables)	Predictor variables	Predictive ratios for AGS and ADGs approximately as good as methods based on prior use. Predictive ratios for children and people with chronic conditions poor, but best for ACGs and ADGs in Medicaid population
Use of ACGs for Research						
Starfield et al. (1994)	Quality of care	135 practices of different types	Medical records	Type of site, quality of care criteria, total charges generated	As control for morbidity differences	No consistent relationship between quality and costs; average cost Community Health Centers had generally best quality
Powe et al. (1996)	Quality of care	Practices of different types	Medicaid claims for patients with one or three chronic illness	Patient characteristics, costs, type of practice	To derive iso-cost categories	No relationship between cost and quality
Harlow (1998)	Longitudinal care in medical practice	Practices of different types	Medicaid claims data	Age, type of practice	CADGs as morbidity control	Different types of sites differ in extent of longitudinal care provided

Study	Topic	Setting	Data	Variables	Use of ACGs/ADGs	Findings
Hughes et al. (in preparation)	Resource use in medical practice	Community health centers versus other types of practices	Medicaid claims data	Patient characteristics	As morbidity control	Pending
Blumenthal et al. Unpublished Manuscript	Trends in characteristics of primary care practice	Office-based practice in United States	National Ambulatory Medical Care survey	Practice patterns, physician characteristics, patient characteristics	CADGs used to characterize morbidity in visits	Various publications on trends in primary care practice
Reid (1998)	Referral practices and characteristics	Office-based practices in Alberta, Canada	Claims data for patients with diabetes	Patient and practitioner characteristics	As morbidity control	Characteristics of referrals vary by patient and practitioner characteristics
Briggs et al. (1995)	Resource availability and costs	Health services areas in Iowa	Claims data	Types of insurance coverage, urban/rural, number of physicians, number of hospitals	11 ACGs used to stratify for types of morbidity	Little and inconsistent impact of resource availability on costs once morbidity is controlled
Methodologic Studies of ACGs						
Fowles et al. (1996)	Comparisons of case-mix measures for costs prediction	Network model plan in one geographic area	Claims and encounter data, patient questionnaire	Adults only, age, sex, sociodemographic variables, self-reported health status	As possible explanatory variables	ADGs best predictor at individual patient level; ACGs best predictor at group level

the problem) associated with an episode of care (see above) were used. At the end of a course of treatment, practitioners decided when the episode had begun and assigned only one problem or diagnosis for all of the visits associated with that diagnosis. If there was an intercurrent illness arising during the period between the first visit for the problem and the last, it formed the basis for a different episode, as did all problems arising anew after the episode had finished. Thus, the patients had 7,559 different episodes in the year (December 1993–June 1994), each of which had an associated diagnosis that was assigned to an ADG. The resulting distribution of ADGs was very similar to the distribution found by the original developers of the system, using ambulatory care data from a group-model health maintenance organization in the United States.

Since primary care practices in many countries of Europe use the International Classification of Primary Care (ICPC) rather than the ICD-CM to code problems or diagnoses, the researchers developed a method to assign problems and diagnoses to ADGs using the ICPC instead of the ICD. Although the ICPC is compatible with the ICD, it has fewer codes so that there is not a one-to-one correspondence for individual problems or diagnoses. In some cases, one ICPC code corresponds to more than one ICD-CM code, each of which may be assigned to different ADGs. By means of an iterative process considering the frequencies of the different diagnoses within these codes, the researchers assigned each ICPC code to its most likely ADG. The resulting distribution of ADGs, using the ICPC rather than the ICD, was very similar to that using the ICDs, thus indicating that they can be used interchangeably.

Primary care researchers in the Basque region of Spain (Orueta et al., 1998) have also found a close correspondence between the predictiveness of morbidity groups, whether accomplished using the individual ADGs or ACGs, to those in US studies. That is, the proportion of variance in resource use (considering the costs of visits themselves as well as diagnostic tests associated with them) that is explainable by differences in morbidity ranges between 40% and 50% when diagnoses are assigned by episode (as in the study in Barcelona).

Other researchers in Spain are testing the applicability of the ACG system in a collaborative study involving over 50 practices in different regions of the country. A preliminary report with 22 doctors, including four pediatricians, confirmed the similarity of distributions of ADGs and ACGs and the predictive ability of the system to reflect the number of visits (Carmona et al., 1997).

Thus, a case-mix system that describes the experiences of people with their mix of morbidity appears highly useful in meeting the variety of needs that arise in primary care, wherever it is practiced.

To measure the impact (outcomes) of health services on health

The fourth purpose of health status assessment is to measure the impact of health services. When the effect of medical care is to prevent the occurrence of specific illnesses, the impact of practitioners and facilities can be assessed by measuring the frequency of occurrence of the specific preventable diseases in the patient population. However, most diseases cannot be prevented, and the aim of care is to reduce the duration of the illness or the discomfort and disability associated with it. Thus, the most appropriate health status measures to assess the impact of interventions are those that directly determine the effect of health services in the context of the daily lives and aspirations of people.

Advances in both molecular biology and the social sciences are prompting a change in the way that ill health is viewed and measured. A focus on disease is being replaced by a focus on morbidity, or "dis-ease," which is a much broader representation of ill health.

A century ago and until relatively recently, the genetic basis for disease was thought to be through the action of single genes that, by mutation or inheritance, would "cause" certain conditions in individuals whose cells carry the affected gene. The more that is learned about the mode of action of genetic material, the more it is recognized that this is the case for only a tiny proportion of the afflictions suffered by individuals (Holtzman, 1989). Genetically determined disease is not only more commonly associated with the effects of multiple genes, but is very sensitive to the simultaneous presence or absence of associated factors in the environment (Holtzman, 1989). In a like manner, advances in methods for identifying and measuring the effects of social and environmental factors have made it apparent that risk of disease or its complications depends not on one or a few such factors but, rather, on a complex pattern of their occurrence in time and space. Social class is a well-known and well-documented determinant of illness, yet many individuals in the lowest social class are in good health.

As noted above, educational levels, housing and nutrition, environmental hazards (both physical and social), family dynamics and psychological resources, and exposure to the mitigating effects of medical care interventions are among the myriad "causes" of disease. As a result of this multiplicity of determinants, it is unlikely that the manifestations of disease will be the same in everyone with the disease. Thus, variability in severity and manifestation of any given disease is much more common than is an "average" manifestation of the disease. Most "causes" may not be associated with disease or may be associated with different manifestations of illness (including multiple illness in the same individual), and "causes" do not necessarily "cause" manifest or even occult illness. Figure 3.1 expresses these phenomena, which are known as *penetrance, pleotropism,* and *etiological heterogeneity* (Holtzman, 1989); superimposed on these is the phenomenon of susceptibility, in which both "causes" and diseases may be interrelated and potentiating.

Despite the widespread lack of appreciation (and hence documentation) of the heterogeneity of manifestations and prognosis of most specific diseases, of the clustering of apparently unrelated diseases in individuals already identified as having a specific diagnosis, and of the consequent lack of focus on the subject in the research literature, there is ample evidence that morbidity is not distributed randomly in the population but, rather, that it tends to cluster in certain individuals. Roos et al. (1997) showed that, in an entire population of adult patients with hypertension, only one-third (34%) of visits made by these patients in a year were for that diagnosis; the next most common reason for a visit was diabetes (which accounted for 3% of visits). Thus, a substantial majority of visits (63%) were for

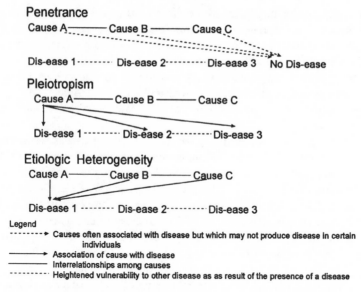

Figure 3.1. The basis for variability in disease causation and manifestations.

a large number of different conditions, no one of them accounting for more than 1% of all visits. Clouse and Osterhaus (1994) demonstrated that adults (aged 18–64 years) with a diagnosis of migraine have 33% greater costs for conditions *unrelated* to migraine than other patients matched for age, gender, length of enrolment, and subscriber or dependent status. In children with chronic illnesses, the observed co-prevalence for the most common pairs of childhood chronic conditions is 140%–380% greater than statistically predicted levels (Newacheck and Stoddard, 1994). Severity of illness generally is *not* related to the biological severity as measured by the likelihood of premature death or level of biomedical indicators of disease. With only a few exceptions for very uncommon diseases, there is as much variability in manifestations and impact of specific diseases as there is between different diseases (Stein and Jessop, 1982).

Thus, health status measured merely by the existence or likelihood of occurrence of a specific disease or even combinations of diseases is an incomplete approach to characterizing the health either of individuals or of populations. Because assessment of health status is necessary for adequate planning and delivery of care, advances in its conceptualization and measurement are important for both health policy and for clinical care.

The World Health Organization's original definition of health (1948) has been criticized on the grounds that it is not only unattainable but also that it provides the wrong thrust in its focus on complete physical, mental, and social well being. If civilization advances as a result of continuous challenge to wrest control from the natural environment, ''complete well being'' is a deterrent to progress. The subsequent proposal from the European Office is more to the point: ''the extent to which an individual or group is able, on the one hand, to realize aspirations and satisfy needs and, on the other hand, to cope with the environment. Health is therefore seen as a resource for everyday life, not the objective of living; it is a positive concept embracing social and personal resources, as well as physical capacities'' (World Health Organization, 1984).

Thus, health is not the absence of disease or predisposition to disease; rather, it is the continual re-definition of potential for maximum functioning to meet the challenges of life in the most positive and productive way. In the future, approaches to profiling morbidity burdens in practice will have to move toward approaches that are not based only on diagnosed disease or diseases.

There are many ways to consider health status and outcomes of care when viewed from this broader perspective (McDowell and Newell, 1996). Most divide health into the components mentioned in the original World Health Organization definition of health: mental, physical, social. Figure 3.2 presents another type of approach. In this conceptualization, health status has seven components, ranging from longevity to resilience:

Longevity: The most common measure of health status especially at the population level is longevity or life expectancy and its converse, mortality. An important characteristic of the health of individuals is their life expectancy; the average life expectancy in a population is an important descriptor of a the health status of a nation. Health care systems influence life expectancy, even though the latter is also affected by such other determinants as genetic structure, the social and physical environment, and personal behaviors.

Activity: The second component of health status is the nature of the activity of the individual or population. Relevant qualities include those such as pertain to the kinds of disability affecting the individual and, on the population level, the proportion of the population that can carry on with normal activities.

Discomfort: This includes pain or other sensations that interfere with work and pleasure.

Perceived well-being and satisfaction: This characteristic connotes how people view their own health and the extent to which they are satisfied with it.

Disease: This involves the presence of conditions recognized as potentially or actually interfering with the well being of individuals or of the population; it includes mental as well as physical pathology.

Achievement: This reflects the positive aspects of health that must be considered in achieving what the WHO has defined as ''a state of well being.'' Achievement signifies the level of development or accomplishment and the potential for future development of better health. A common way of describing achievement relates to how normal social roles are performed.

Resilience: This characteristic of health also pertains to a state of well being. It refers to the ability to cope with adversity and is the category that measures the potential for resisting a range of possible threats to health. Ability to respond constructively to stress may be measured by physiological techniques, by psychological techniques, or by evidence that certain defenses known to increase resistance are present or have been provided. The prototype of biological re-

LONGEVITY	Normal Life Expectancy	Dead
ACTIVITY	Functional	Disabled
DISCOMFORT	Comfortable	Uncomfortable
PERCEIVED WELL-BEING	Satisfied	Dissatisfied
RESILIENCE	More Resilient	Less Resilient
VULNERABILITY	Less Vulnerable	More Vulnerable
ACHIEVEMENT	Achieving	Not Achieving
DISEASE	None Detectable	Multiple

Figure 3.2. Health status/outcome of care. Source: adapted from Starfield (1974).

silience is the state of being appropriately immunized against preventable diseases. A second measure of resilience is the attainment of certain nutritional standards. A third measure is the performance of certain health behaviors or environmental modifications known to reduce the likelihood of disease; a typical example is a definable level of physical exercise.

Vulnerability: This domain of health reflects characteristics that decrease an individual's ability to ward off threats to health. Examples of characteristics that increase risk include substance misuse and activities that heighten the likelihood of injury.

Viewing health as a composite of domains allows the development of profiles that reflect different combinations of strengths and weaknesses (Starfield, 1974; Riley et al, 1998a; Riley et al, 1998b).

An assessment of the effectiveness of a health system, whether it concerns the individual, the community, or the entire population, should take into account at least some aspects of *all* of these features of health status. (Chapters 12 and 13 consider different approaches to health status assessment in greater detail.) To achieve equity among population subgroups, it is also necessary to have information about the health status of population subgroups so as to determine whether the health of vulnerable population groups differs from that of the rest of the population and what the differences are.

References

Briggs LW, Rohrer JE, Ludke RL, Hilsenrath PE, Phillips KT. Geographic variation in primary care visits in Iowa. Health Serv Res 1995; 30:657–71.

Carmona G, Prados A, Sánchez-Cantalejo E. Los Grupos de Atención Ambulatoria. Resultados parciales del proyecto: "Evaluación del comportamiento de los Grupos de Atención Ambulatoria en nuestro entorno de Atención Primaria." Hospitalaria 1997; 1:40–5.

Clouse J, Osterhaus J. Healthcare resource use and costs associated with migraine in a managed care setting. Ann Pharmacother 1994; 28:659–64.

Densen P, Shapiro S, Einhorn M. Concerning high and low utilizers of services in a medical care plan, and the persistence of utilization levels in a three-year period. Milbank Q 1959; 37:217–50.

Diderichsen F, Varde E, Whitehead M. Resource allocation to health authorities: The quest for an equitable formula in Britain and Sweden. BMJ 1997; 315:875–8.

Ellis RP, Pope GC, Iezzoni L, Ayanian JZ, Bates DW, Burstin H, Ash AS. Diagnosis-based risk adjustment for Medicare capitation payments. Health Care Financing Rev 1996; 17: 101–28.

Fowler L, Anderson G. Capitation adjustment for pediatric populations. Pediatrics 1996; 98: 10–6.

Fowles J, Weiner J, Knutson D, Fowler E, Tucker A, Ireland M. Taking health status into account when setting capitation rates: A comparison of risk adjustment methods. JAMA 1996; 276:1316–21.

Green B, Barlow J, Newman C. Ambulatory care groups and the profiling of primary care physician resource use: Examining the application of case-mix adjustments. J Ambulatory Care Manage 1996; 19:86–9.

Harlow J. An Analysis of Primary Medical Providers, and the Influence of Primary Care on Resource Utilization. Dissertation. Baltimore: Johns Hopkins University, 1998.

Holland WW. European Community Atlas of "Avoidable Death." Commission of the European Communities Health Services Research Series, Nos. 6, 9. Vols 1, 2. 2nd Ed. Oxford: Oxford University Press, 1991, 1993.

Holtzman N. Proceed with Caution: Predicting Genetic Risks in the Recombinant DNA Era. Baltimore: Johns Hopkins University Press, 1989.

Iezzoni L (ed). Risk Adjustment for Measuring Health Care Outcomes. 2nd Ed. Chicago: Health Administration Press, 1997.

Juncosa S, Bolíbar B, Roset M, Tomś R. Performance of an ambulatory case mix system in primary care in Spain: Ambulatory Care Groups (ACGs). European J Public Health 1998 (in press).

Lamberts H, Hofmans-Okkes I. Episode of care: A core concept in family practice. J Fam Pract 1996; 42:161–7.

McDowell I, Newell C. Measuring Health: A Guide to Rating Scales and Questionnaires. New York: Oxford University Press, 1996.

Newacheck P, Stoddard J. Prevalence and impact of multiple childhood chronic illnesses. J Pediatr 1994; 124:40–8.

Orueta J, López de Munain J, Gutirrez K, Aiarzagüena JM, Aranguren J, Pedrero E. Application of the ambulatory care groups in the primary care of a European national health care system. Does it work? Manuscript submitted, 1998.

Powe N, Weiner J, Starfield B, Stuart M, Baker A, Steinwachs D. Systemwide performance in a Medicaid program: Profiling the care of patients with chronic illnesses. Med Care 1996; 34:798–810.

Reid R. Patterns of Referral for Newly Diagnosed Patients with Diabetes in Alberta. Dissertation. Baltimore: Johns Hopkins University, 1998.

Riley AW, Green, BF, Starfield B, Forrest CB, Kang M, Ensminger M. A taxonomy of adolescent health need: Development of the adolescent health profiles. Med Care. 1998a (in press).

Riley AW, Forrest CB, Starfield B, Green B, Kang M, Ensminger M. Reliability and validity of the adolescent health profile types. Med Care 1998b (in press).

Roos N, Carriere K, Friesen D. Visiting the doctor: How frequently are patients seen during the year and what do physicians have to do with it? Manuscript submitted, 1997.

Salem-Schatz S, Moore G, Rucker M, Pearson S. The case for case-mix adjustment in practice profiling: When good apples look bad. JAMA 1994; 272:871–4.

Schneeweis R, Rosenblatt R, Cherkin D, Kirkwood R, Hart G. Diagnosis clusters: A new tool for analyzing the content of medical care. Med Care 1983; 21:105–22.

Starfield B. Measurement of outcome: A proposed scheme. Milbank Q 1974; 52:39–50.

Starfield B, Hankin J, Steinwachs D, Horn S, Benson P, Katz H, Gabriel A. Utilization and morbidity: Random or tandem? Pediatrics 1985; 75:241–7.

Starfield B, Powe N, Weiner J, Stuart M, Steinwachs D, Scholle S, Gerstenberger A. Costs versus quality in different types of primary care settings. JAMA 1994; 272:1903–8.

Starfield B, Weiner J, Mumford L, Steinwachs D. Ambulatory care groups: A categorization of diagnoses for research and management. Health Serv Res 1991; 25(7):53–74.

Stein RE, Jessop DJ. A noncategorical approach to chronic childhood illness. Public Health Rep 1982; 97(4):354–62.

Tucker A, Weiner J, Honigfeld S, Parton R. Profiling primary care physician resource use: Examining the application of case-mix adjustment. J Ambulatory Care Manage 1996; 19:60–80.

Wagstaff A, Van Doorslaer E. Equity in the delivery of health care: Methods and findings. In: Equity in the Finance and Delivery of Health Care: An International Perspective. Oxford: Oxford University Press, 1993.

Weiner J, Dobson A, Maxwell A, Coleman K, Starfield B, Anderson G. Risk-adjusted Medicare capitation rates using ambulatory and inpatient diagnoses. Health Care Financing Rev 1996a; 17(3):77–99.

Weiner J, Starfield B, Steinwachs D, Mumford L. Development and application of a population-oriented measure of ambulatory care case-mix. Med Care 1991; 29:452–72.

Weiner J, Starfield B, Stuart M, Powe N, Steinwachs D. Ambulatory care practice variation within a medicaid program. Health Serv Res 1996b; 30:751–70.

White KL, Williams TF, Greenberg BG. The ecology of medical care. N Engl J Med 1961; 265:885–92.

World Health Organization. Health Promotion: A Discussion Document on the Concept and Principles. Copenhagen: WHO Regional Office for Europe, 1984.

— II —
Primary Care Practice

— 4 —

Describing
Primary Care

This chapter describes the content of primary care practice in two countries with historically different emphases on primary care as the cornerstones of their health services system. A brief discussion of family orientation in primary care follows. The last section presents a chronology of primary care and subspecialist physicians in the United States and a consideration of the future of primary care practitioners in that country.

Primary Care Practice in the United States

The major source of information about the nature of primary care in the United States is the National Ambulatory Medical Care Survey (NAMCS), a national survey of office-based practices. It was first conducted in 1974 and continued every year until the early 1980s, when it was reduced to administration once every 5 years. In 1990, it again was made annual.

Seventy percent of ambulatory care contacts with doctors in the United States are to doctors' offices or organized clinic settings; 14% are to hospital outpatient departments, 13% are by phone, and 4% are at home (National Center for Health Statistics, 1997). This represents a continuing slight decrease in office contacts and a corresponding slight increase in home contacts and organized clinic contacts. Thus, the NAMCS reflects the nature of ambulatory care for the vast majority of people in the United States. It does not, however, provide information on consultative or referral care provided within hospitals, outpatient departments, or emergency rooms, which often are located in areas where a disproportionate percentage of people who live in socioeconomically deprived areas reside. Therefore, in the early 1990s, the National Center for Health Statistics developed a comparable survey of outpatient departments and emergency departments; these data permit comparisons of care provided in these settings with those in office-based settings (Lipkind, 1996; Stussman, 1996).

The sampling frame for NAMCS is a list of physicians maintained by the

American Medical Association (which obtains the names of all medical students upon graduation from medical school and periodically requests information from them by survey questionnaire) and by the American Osteopathic Association, which keeps a roster of osteopaths.*

The sampling frame is stratified by specialty and by geographic area; about 3,000 physicians are requested to complete forms on visits made to their offices for 1 week of the year. The following 16 items of information are obtained routinely: patient's birth date, ethnicity, race, sex, presenting problem or complaint, whether the patient has been seen before, whether the patient was referred by another physician, the type of reason for the visit, diagnoses (up to three may be listed), cause of injury, diagnostic and therapeutic services, disposition, and the names of all medications administered or prescribed. Additional data may be elicited to obtain information on issues related to current national interest. Information currently derives from approximately 36,000 visits per year; about 75% of all physicians asked to participate actually do so (Woodwell, 1997).

Diagnoses are coded using the International Classification of Diseases—Clinical Modification, and drugs are coded according to a special system devised by the National Center for Health Statistics. A feature of the NAMCS is the coding of presenting problems by means of a system in which problems are categorized by "modules," as follows: symptoms; diseases; diagnostic, screening, and prevention; treatment; injuries and adverse effects; test results; or administrative. The information obtained from NAMCS provides the basis for studies to illuminate the nature of primary care, to explore reasons for differences, and to assess the impact of differences on benefits and costs of care.

Table 4.1 shows the distribution of office-based visits by age of patient and by type of physician. General and family physicians provide less then one-fourth of all care and under one-third of care for adults in each age group. Well over one-half of all visits made by children under age 15 years are to pediatricians; generalists provide care in one-fifth of children's visits; and other non-primary care physicians provide it in about 16% of visits. Internists provide relatively more care to older people, but still account for only 24% of visits for people over age 65 years. Over time, the proportion of all care delivered by family physicians has been declining, with a corresponding increase in care provided by non-primary care specialists and, for children, by pediatricians.

Table 4.2 describes the reasons for visits to primary care and non-primary care specialists by children under age 15 years. The majority of visits, both to primary care and to other types of physicians, are prompted by symptoms; this proportion has been increasing slowly over time except in the case of family physicians. It therefore is likely to reflect either an increasing proportion of first-contact visits to non-primary care physicians or greater referral of more undifferentiated problems

---

*The NAMCS data are the only routinely collected source of information that includes doctors of osteopathy—DOs—with medical doctors—MDs. Unless otherwise indicated, all other data relate only to MDs because comparable information about osteopaths is not available. In the NAMCS data, DOs are not separately distinguished so that it is not possible to determine whether and in what way their practices differ from those of MDs.

Table 4.1. Percentage of Office-Based Visits by Age and Type of Physician: United States, 1994

Age Group*	General/Family Practice	Internal Medicine	Pediatrics	Other Specialty
<15	20.8	1.5	61.6	16.1
15–24	29.7	7.5	7.7	55.1
25–44	26.4	12.0	0.8	60.8
45–64	21.4	21.1	—	57.2
65+	18.3	24.3	—	57.1
All ages	22.6	14.6	12.3	50.5

*In this and subsequent tables, children are considered as individuals less than 15 years old. Although the fields of pediatrics and maternal and child health generally include 15–17 year olds, and perhaps even those through age 20 as "children and youth," the ages of 0–14 are used to represent children in this chapter because several countries encourage or allow pediatricians to act as the primary care physician for children up to age 15.

by primary care physicians. Only about 1 in 20 visits are made specifically for a designated disease. Pediatricians also provide significantly more care prompted by diagnostic, screening, or preventive purposes than is the case for generalists. General and family physicians provide relatively more care for injuries than do pediatricians.

Table 4.3 presents the reasons for visits made by adults. Visits prompted by a need for diagnosis, screening, or prevention are consistently and significantly less common in the practice of internists than in the practice of general and family physicians. Internists provide a greater proportion of care for specific diagnoses than do general or family physicians, although the differences are not statistically significant for the different age groups separately. General or family physicians provide relatively more care for injuries experienced by adults in all age groups than do internists. Visits to non-primary care physicians (reflected in the differences

Table 4.2. Visits by Children Aged 0–15 to Office-Based Physicians, by Reason for Visit and Type of Physician: United States, 1994

Reason for Visit	Percentage of All Visits		
	General/Family Physician	Pediatrician	All Physicians
Symptoms	65.5	61.9	62.1
Disease	6.6	5.0	5.7
Diagnostic, screening, prevention	14.9	23.9	18.7
Treatment	3.5	4.3	6.5
Injury and adverse effects	5.5	2.7	4.1
Administrative purpose	0.2	0.1	0.2
Test results	3.8	0.9	1.6
Other	0	1.1	1.2

Table 4.3. Visits by Adults to Office-Based Physicians by Reason for Visit and
Type of Physician: United States, 1994

	Percent of All Visits*		
Reason for Visit	General/Family Physician	Internist	All Physicians
Ages 15–24			
Symptoms	59.6	75.3	52.4
Disease	10.0	7.0	6.3
Diagnostic, screening, prevention	18.2	9.0	23.6
Treatment	4.2	3.2	8.7
Injury and adverse effects	4.0	2.5	4.7
Administrative purpose	0	0	1.0
Ages 25–44			
Symptoms	69.2	66.2	55.6
Disease	7.1	12.4	6.7
Diagnostic, screening, prevention	12.4	9.9	20.0
Treatment	5.8	4.4	10.4
Injury and adverse effects	3.1	2.6	3.3
Administrative purposes	0.5	2.2	1..3
Ages 45–64			
Symptoms	53.2	53.7	56.5
Disease	13.5	19.6	12.7
Diagnostic, screening, prevention	17.8	12.6	11.3
Treatment	7.9	8.5	13.1
Injury and adverse effects	3.5	1.1	2.1
Administrative purpose	1.9	2.0	1.6
Test results	1.4	1.0	0.6
Ages 65+			
Symptoms	55.9	54.1	53.4
Disease	12.8	18.0	15.7
Diagnostic, screening, prevention	19.7	13.8	11.2
Treatment	5.9	10.2	14.6
Injury and adverse effects	1.8	0.8	1.6
Administrative purpose	1.5	1.3	1.3
Test results	1.0	.03	0.2

*Difference between 100% and column total includes all other reasons and unknown reasons.

between "all physicians" and the primary care physicians) are consistently more
likely to be for specific treatment.

In summary, visits to general or family physicians are more likely to focus on
patients' complaints and injuries, although the differences are being reduced over
time. Internists are more likely to focus on specific diseases and pediatricians are
more likely to focus on prevention and screening than are general or family physicians. For all types of primary care physicians, however, the majority of visits
are prompted by symptoms and complaints; only a small minority are prompted
by specific diagnoses. In general, there are neither striking nor consistent differences between primary care physicians and other specialists.

Chapter 1 indicated that primary care practice should be distinguishable from specialty practice by a greater variety of types of presenting problems and a greater variety of diagnoses. Table 4.4 shows that this is only partially the case in the United States. The table shows the similarities of family medicine, internal medicine, and general surgery when the number of the most common problems required to reach 50% of visits is considered. The number is much larger than for other specialties, including pediatrics, thus indicating more diversity among common problems in primary care practice. Over time, this diversity has been increasing in many types of subspecialty practices, again suggesting either a greater tendency of patients to directly seek care from subspecialists or increasing referrals of many common problems to subspecialists. It is only when specialties are arrayed by the percentage of problems accounted for by the top 50 problems that pediatrics, as well as family medicine and internal medicine, are separated from most traditional "specialties." Even here, however, general surgery in the United States resembles primary care rather than other specialties, and pediatrics does so only when well-baby visits are not included. There has been little change in these percentages over the past decade.

Table 4.5 presents a similar picture regarding the variety of diagnoses in primary care and other specialty practice. It shows the number of the most common diagnoses that, considering their frequencies, account for 50% of all visits to different types of physicians in the United States. Except for obstetrics/gynecology, these numbers have increased over the past decade, thus indicating a greater diversity among the most common diagnoses. If the most common diagnoses made by primary care practitioners are more varied, these practitioners should encounter *more* diagnoses in a set percentage of visits (e.g., 50%) than do other specialists. For generalists, internists, and general surgeons, at least 30 of these diagnoses must

Table 4.4. The Number of Most Frequent Problems Accounting for 50% of All Visits and the Percentage of All Presenting Problems Contributed by the 50 Most Presenting Problems, by Specialty of Physician: United States, 1994

Specialty	No. of Presenting Problems Accounting for 50% of All Visits	Percentage of All Visits Accounted for by the 50 Most Frequent Presenting Problems
Family/general practice	26	64.0
Internal medicine	22	67.0
Pediatrics	7	85.4*
Cardiovascular medicine	9	88.1
Dermatology	6	94.1
General Surgery	18	72.0
Obstetrics/gynecology	3	90.8
Ophthalmology	5	97.2
Orthopedic surgery	11	87.7
Otolaryngology	10	91.5
Urology	11	91.5
Psychiatry	2	98.5
Neurology	9	88.7

*Sixty-one percent when well-baby and well-child visits are excluded.

Table 4.5. The Number of Most Frequent Diagnoses Accounting for 50% of All Visits and the Percentage of All Diagnoses Contributed by the 50 Most Common Diagnoses, by Speciality of Physician: United States, 1994

Specialty	Routine Check-ups Included	Routine Check-ups Excluded	Percentage of All Visits Accounted for by the Most Frequent Diagnoses
Family/general pracitce	41	51	54.2
Internal medicine	34	37	57.2
Pediatrics	8	24	80.7*
Cardiovascular medicine	11	11	77.4
Dermatology	7	7	86.7
General Surgery	39	46	54.7
Obstetrics/gynecology	5	12	84.0
Ophthalmology	8	8	84.3
Orthopedic surgery†	44	44	53.5
Otolaryngology	14	14	78.6
Urology	10	10	83.1
Psychiatry	7	7	90.3
Neurology	15	16	75.9

Number of Diagnoses Accounting for 50% of All Visits

* 56.3 after eliminating well-child visits.

† The large number of categories for number of diagnoses is accounted for by the variety of types of fractures and sprains, each of which has a separate ICD code. When collapsed by Schneeweis clusters, the number of diagnoses is 4, with check-ups both included and excluded (Schneeweis et al., 1983).

be included to reach 50% of visits. For dermatologists, psychiatrists, obstetrician/gynecologists, and ophthalmologists, 10 or fewer most common diagnoses account for 50% of visits. For pediatricians, the eight most common diagnoses account for 50% of the visits, making them more like other specialists than primary care physicians. However, when the diagnoses of "well-child" or "well-person" are excluded, 24 diagnoses are required to reach 50% of the visits to pediatricians, making them appear more like primary care physicians. When the percentage of visits required to encompass the 50 most frequent diagnoses are considered (last column of Table 4.5) , surgeons resemble family physicians and internists rather than specialists, and pediatricians resemble them only when well-infants or well-children are excluded. These percentages have decreased over the past decade (except for pediatrics), indicating a larger variety of less common (although not necessarily rare) conditions in practices of all types. (It should be noted that these percentages do not necessarily reflect the total number of different diagnoses in the practices of primary care physicians versus other specialists because the differences between the percentages and 100% might be composed of *more* but very unusual diagnoses in subspecialty care than in primary care.)

It is apparent that neither variety of the most common problems nor diagnoses clearly distinguishes generalists, internists, and pediatricians, who are thought to administer primary care, from surgeons, who are not considered to be primary care providers. (This situation may change over time, however, with visits elsewhere increasingly requiring a referral from the primary care practitioner.) Furthermore, it may be true only in countries such as the United States, where most of the population has, historically, had direct access to a specialist without a referral from a primary care practitioner. This direct access to specialists may lead to a situation that makes subspecialty care resemble primary care. In this situation, it is not possible to use specific diagnoses or varieties of diagnoses as the basis for identifying primary care practice, at least with current coding schemes that cannot distinguish differences in severity of problem or diagnosis.

Primary care practices are assumed to have a larger percentage of visits classified as related to prevention, but, as is the case for variety of diagnoses and problems, the data in the United States do not uniformly support this distinction. The percentage of adult visits that are not associated with any symptom varies from 1.8 for otolaryngologists to 61.4 for obstetrician/gynecologists, with most other specialties hovering around 10% (Puskin, 1977).

Tables 4.6 and 4.7 show the referral status of patients visiting primary care and non-primary care physicians. Table 4.6 presents the percentages of specific visits that were made on referral from another physician. These percentages have greatly increased over the past decade, sometimes more than doubling. However, the percentage of such visits does not exceed one-fourth (one-third in the case of children seen by non-primary care specialists), even in the practices of non-primary care specialists. Visits to internists are more likely to be by referral than is the case for general or family physicians, but even here the percentage does not exceed 10% except for the relatively few children seen by internists. Visits to other specialists are more likely to be by referral than are visits to primary care physicians, and this difference has widened over the past decade because of a great increase over time in the percentage of visits to non-primary care specialists that are by referral.

However, the percentage of such visits is still less than 50% in all or most age groups, except in the case of neurology and neurosurgery. The percentage of visits resulting from a referral to most other non-primary care physicians ranges from 30% to 50%, whereas just a few years ago (1991) the percentage was more commonly between 10% and 20%. Among the major subspecialists, the percentage is

Table 4.6. Percentage of Visits in Which Patient Was Referred by Another Physician: United States, 1994

Physician Specialty	All Ages	Children Under Age 15	Adults			
			15–24	25–44	45–64	65+
All physicians	14.1	7.4	13.1	15.2	17.1	15.7
Primary care physicians	4.2	2.5	4.7	4.2	5.3	5.3
General/family practice	2.7	2.0	3.4	2.4	2.5	3.4
Internal medicine	7.6	25.2	10.2	7.7	7.6	6.5
Pediatrics	2.7	2.1	4.2	—	—	—
Other specialties	24.1	34.9	20.6	22.4	25.9	23.5

Table 4.7. Percentage of Visits in Which Patient Was Referred to Another Physician: United States, 1994

Physician Specialty	All Ages	Children Under Age 15	Adults			
			15–24	25–44	45–64	65+
All physicians	4.4	2.9	4.5	4.6	5.1	4.5
Primary care physicians	6.0	3.1	7.2	7.3	8.2	6.3
General/family practice	6.3	2.9	5.9	6.9	8.2	6.5
Internal medicine	7.6	9.0	8.4	8.7	8.3	6.3
Pediatrics	3.4	3.0	10.8	—	—	—
Other specialties	2.7	1.1	2.1	2.7	2.8	3.1

over 50% only for neurologists and neurosurgeons and under 20% for ophthalmologists, psychiatrists, and obstetrician/gynecologists.

In the NAMCS data, visits of patients who had been referred earlier and are returning to the specialist for continuing care are not counted as a referral. A national study of over 20 specialties in the mid-1970s used approximately the same techniques as the NAMCS but asked how the physician initially obtained the patient for the problem that prompted the specific visit and further inquired as to whether the patient had been referred just to obtain an opinion or advice or referred permanently. Physicians in all specialties had a larger proportion of patients who were referred permanently than were sent for advice or an opinion, and the percentages of patients seen on referral as a whole were, as expected, considerably greater than those found in the NAMCS. The specialists with the highest percentage of in-referrals were neurosurgeons, and the specialists with the lowest percentage of in-referrals were obstetricians/gynecologists, ophthalmologists, and dermatologists, largely due to a much smaller percentage of patients referred permanently (Robert Wood Johnson Foundation, 1982). There are no more recent data that can be used to ascertain trends over time.

However, 1994 data indicate that the vast majority of patients are not being referred back to a referring physician. Furthermore, of those patients not referred for the visit, over three-fourths (except for dermatologists, general surgeons, and ear, nose, and throat specialists) are reported as "old" patients with old problems, indicating that there is substantial continuing care in the practices of U.S. specialists. Of those patients referred in for the visit, over half are by patients seen previously for the same problem, except in the case of dermatologists and neurologists, confirming the tendency of U.S. specialists to see the same patients repeatedly for the same problem. The extent to which this pattern represents a delegation of care by primary care physicians to specialists rather than shared care with specialists serving as a consultant to the primary care physician is unknown. A recent study of patients with diabetes in Alberta, Canada, indicates that the majority of patients referred to non-primary care specialists continue to see the primary care physician also for their diabetes, suggesting the likelihood of shared care, but the generalizability of this finding to other areas and countries is unknown (Reid, 1998).

Table 4.7 presents the percentages of visits that result in a referral to another physician. This percentage is smaller for children than for adults and generally similar for family physicians (for visits by children) and pediatricians. Although the differences in referral rates of adults by the different types of primary care physicians are not striking, family physicians refer fewer adults of younger ages than do internists; as age of patients increases, the difference narrows until age 65, when family physicians refer slightly more patients than do internists. Non-primary care specialists refer a smaller percentage of both their adult and child patients than do primary care physicians, but the generally low rates of referral by all types of physicians is striking. Referral rates have been increasing over time and, contrary to the perception that HMOs inhibit referrals from primary care to specialists, HMO patients are more likely to be referred even though they have lower self-referral rates. Despite the increase in referral rates, however, about one-half of all new patients seen by specialists are self-referred in the United States (Forrest and Reid, 1997).

Another characteristic that should distinguish primary care from specialty practitioners is the distribution of patient visits by familiarity with both the patient and the patient's problems. Both primary care physicians and other specialists would be expected to see new patients and to see "old" patients with old problems. Primary care practitioners should see more old patients with new problems, since they are responsible for the patient's care over time, regardless of the particular problem. Table 4.8 shows that the practices of certain specialists and primary care physicians differ in some respects. Non-primary care specialists of all types see fewer *old* patients with new problems than do primary care physicians. However, general internists see fewer such patients than either family physicians or pediatricians. The differences are even more striking when only nonreferred visits are considered (Table 4.9). Over the past decade, these percentages have remained relatively constant, except for a decline in the proportion of old patients with new problems seen in the practices of obstetrician/gynecologists, thus suggesting a decline in the longitudinality aspects of obstetrician/gynecologist practice.

Table 4.8. Distribution of Office Visits by Familiarity With Patient or Patient's Problems by Specialty of Physician: United States, 1994

	Percentage of Office Visits		
Specialty	New Patient	Old Patient, New Problem	Old Patient, Old Problem
Family/general practice	14.3	31.3	54.4
Internal medicine	9.2	26.5	64.4
Pediatrics	5.0	28.5	66.5
Medical subspecialists	11.5	10.4	78.1
General surgery	17.3	17.1	65.6
Obstetrics/gynecology	12.2	15.6	72.2
Other surgical specialties	15.2	7.6	77.2
Psychiatry	12.0	1.3	86.7
All other specialties	25.4	17.5	57.1

Table 4.9. Percentage of Nonreferred Visits by Prior Visit Status: United States, 1994

Physician Speciality	New Patients	Old Patient, New Problem	Old Patient, Old Problem
All visits	11.2	19.6	55.1
General and family practice	14.1	32.6	50.7
Internal medicine	8.8	24.5	59.1
Pediatrics	9.1	36.6	51.4
Obstetrics and gynecology	10.9	13.7	63.6
Orthopedic surgery	12.2	5.2	49.2
Ophthalmology	10.2	7.1	69.3
Dermatology	18.8	10.6	48.0
Psychiatry	10.0	1.1	71.5
General surgery	11.7	11.1	41.4
Otolaryngology	13.9	5.9	41.6
Cardiovascular diseases	5.0	6.7	61.5
Urology	7.5	2.3	47.2
Neurology	7.9	2.0	38.2
All other speciality	10.1	7.9	57.7

Source: Schappert (1996).

Although there has been little change over the 15 year period from 1978 to 1993 in the clinical problems seen in primary care and the proportion of patients taking medications, there has been an increase in the percentage of visits that involve preventive services, changes in the specific medications that are most commonly prescribed, and an increasing duration of primary care visits (Stafford et al., 1998). Longer duration of visits is associated with greater performance of more diagnostic tests, prescribing more medications, and referring more patients to other physicians, as well as counseling. Moreover, organizational characteristics also play a role; visits are shorter when the number of part-time support personnel is less. Overall, the duration of visits in 1993 was 16.2 minutes for adults (Blumenthal et al., 1998) and 14.2 minutes for children (Ferris et al., 1998).

The NAMCS also obtains information on the proportion of visits in which the patient is referred back to the referring physician. For primary care physicians, these percentages have remained low (0–2%). With few exceptions (neurology, cardiovascular surgery, thoracic surgery), the percentage of visits in which patients are referred back to the referring physician is low (under 10%) and much lower than the percentage of visits resulting from a referral, suggesting that a substantial percentage of patients who are referred are not returned quickly to the referring physician. In fact, the percentage of all visits that are with nonreferred patients without new (for this visit) problems is above 40% for all and generally above 50% for most specialties. However, neurology seems to be relatively unique among the major non-primary care specialties in referring patients back to the referring physician and seeing them again at a later time for the same problem; they also have the lowest percentage of nonreferred patients without new (for this visit) problems (Schappert, 1996). That is, it may be that, in the United States, specialists in neurology are making better use of primary care physicians for ongoing care (with re-referral when needed) rather than keeping them for follow up themselves.

These data on the content of care in practice in the United States indicate that office-based primary care and non-primary care physicians do not differ as much as might be expected with regard to several important clinical characteristics of visits, such as the reasons for visit and referral characteristics. It is possible that inclusion of hospital-based specialists would reveal greater differences, but there are no studies that provide data for such a comparison.

The Content of Primary Care in the United Kingdom

The United States and the United Kingdom are at opposite ends of the spectrum in the strength of their orientation toward primary care (see Chapter 15). Existing data provide some interesting contrasts, primarily in the types of information that are collected in the two countries.

Because patients in the United Kingdom register to receive all their primary care from a particular physician (a general practitioner), each practitioner has a "list," although these are increasingly becoming group lists. In 1995, the average list size was 1,781, a gradual decrease from 2,098 in 1980. Of these, 7% were aged 0–4 years, 13% 5–14 years, 42% 15–44 years, 22% 45–64 years, 9% 65–74 years, and 7% over 74 years. The average duration of visits was 8.8 minutes (about half that in the United States). On average, only about 16% of patients seen within a year were referred to another physician; this increased with each successive age group from 10% among patients aged 0–4 and 6.7% at ages 5–15 to 45% of those above age 74, and the average number of referrals per referred individual increased progressively from 1.12 in the youngest age group to 1.27 in the oldest age group. One of 10 encounters was a home visit (Royal College of General Practice, 1995a).

Table 4.10 compares the 10 most frequent diagnoses in general practice in the United Kingdom with family medicine practice and general internal medicine practice in the United States. Except for upper respiratory infection, asthma, and hypertension, there is little similarity in the types of most common diagnoses, but the method of calculation differs and the general internal medicine sample in the United States does not include children.

The number of prescriptions per person varies in different countries. In the United Kingdom in 1993, an average of 8.8 prescriptions per person were written (Royal College of General Practice, 1995c), as compared with 16.6 in the United States. However, the latter figure includes all types of practices, not only primary care.

The percentage of practices that are computerized has grown; by 1993, 79% of practices were using computers, a figure that was projected to increase to 92% by 1997. In 1993, almost all of these (98%) were using computers for patient registration; 94% were using them for prescribing, 90% for at least partial clinical records, 42% for patient recall, and 84% for practice annual reports. The use of computers for practice (rather than for billing) in the United Kingdom is fostered

Table 4.10. Top 10 Diagnoses in Primary Care Practice

United Kingdom 1991–92 General Practice		United States 1992			
		Family Practice		General Internal Medicine	
Diagnosis	Rate Per 10,000 Person Years of Risk	Diagnosis	$ of Non-referred Visits	Diagnosis	% of Non-referred Visits
Upper respiratory infection	772	General medical examination	12.1	Hypertension	15.5
Bronchitis	719	Acute upper respiratory tract infection	9.0	Acute upper respiratory tract infection	6.0
Asthma	425	Hypertension	6.8	General medical examination	5.6
Conjunctival disorders	415	Lower respiratory infection	5.0	Diabetes	5.5
Essential hypertension	412	Sinusitis	4.8	Acute lower respiratory infection	3.9
External ear disorders	409	Sprains, strains	4.5	Ischemic heart disease	3.8
Acute tonsillitis	407	Otitis media	4.4	Sinusitis	3.2
Ill-defined intestinal infection	394	Depression	2.8	Depression	2.5
Other and unspecified disorders of the back	372	Lacerations/contusions	2.4	Degenerative joint disease	2.1
		Asthma	1.8	Sprains, strains	2.0

Source: NAMCS data for United States; Royal College of General Practice (1995a) for United Kingdom.

by a specific recognition by the National Health Service of the importance of information in creating a better health system and its proposals to develop minimum specifications for information systems and to support projects to enhance the electronic transfer of information from and to practices (Royal College of General Practice, 1996).

The Family in Primary Care

A 20-year-old unskilled manual worker with an obscure skin rash was referred to a dermatologist by an ophthalmologic surgeon. He was treated unsuccessfully over many weeks until seen by his general practitioner, who confirmed that the patient shared a bed with his brother. The brother also had a rash, and both itched more at night. The general practitioner was thus able to diagnose and control the underlying scabies.   A clinical experience

A family orientation has always been thought to contribute to good health services. Knowledge of the family provides not only the context for evaluating patients' problems and helping to sort out the likelihood of various possible diagnoses, but it also is important in deciding on an appropriate intervention because families may differ in their ability to carry out different treatments and management strategies. The family is likely to become even more important as knowledge about genetics increases and the possibilities for both prevention and management widen.

Although family medicine is based on a strong theoretical foundation developed during the first decade of the formation of the discipline (in the 1970s in the United States), there is a relative dearth of literature on the family orientation of primary care practitioners. A study of the content of six U.S. journals of family medicine from 1989 to 1993 divided the subject matter into six categories: care of the patient in the context of the family, the family as the patient, instruments to measure family functioning, genogram and life cycle, care of family members, and family review papers. In the 5-year period of study, only 47 papers on the family were published in the six journals; of these, at least half (and over 60% in the journal with the most articles) were limited to just two of these six categories. Thus, there appears to be little in the way of evidence, at least in the U.S. literature, that could help to judge the magnitude of special contributions to primary care made by family physicians (Smilkstein, 1994).

Many techniques are available to help practitioners consider family context as a part of their care for patients. North and colleagues (1993) examined the extent to which 10 of these were used by family physicians. Of the 10, one (the genogram) is for the specific purpose of identifying predispositions to illness in families. Eight serve the purpose of identifying the family context in which the care of patients occurs: family conferences, understanding of family life cycle, family systems theory, family charts, family APGAR (Adaptation, Partnership, Growth, Affection, Resolve), self-awareness of physician's own family dynamics, and family counseling sessions. An additional technique is specifically intended to deal with the problem of chemical dependency and families. The most formal of these techniques (the genogram, family charts, and the family APGAR) were used the least: More than one-half of the physicians (and 95% in the case of the APGAR) had never used them. Except for self-awareness of one's own family dynamics, fewer than 15% of the physicians employed any of the techniques daily. Although prior training in the specific techniques increased the likelihood of their use, this was not the case for the most formal of the tools (APGAR), suggesting that the time demands of practice may interfere with systematic attention to family-oriented care.

In the United States, where family medicine shares primary care with internal medicine and pediatrics, a substantial proportion of the population identify a family physician as their source of primary care. Data from the 1987 National Medical Expenditure survey, a household panel survey conducted in waves over a 1 year period, revealed that in one-third of families, at least one parent and one child were receiving care from the same physician. When this was the case, 85% of the parents' spouses were also receiving care from the same source. In 80%–90% of these families (depending on whether the mother, the father, or the child was considered), this physician was a family physician. When the physician seen by the parent and child differed, a family physician was likely to be identified as the primary care source for 49% of mothers, 57% of fathers, and only 18% of children. Families whose care was paid for by Medicaid (the poor) or Medicare (over age 65 or disabled) were more likely to have family-centered care, as were families living in rural areas, mothers with lower educational levels, and mother-headed families (Doescher and Franks, 1997).

The substantial proportion of primary care delivered by family physicians, undoubtedly higher in many countries other than the United States, indicates a need to better understand the special contributions that are made by a family orientation, particularly with increasing recognition of the importance of biological as well as social and environmental characteristics that cluster in families.

Primary Care Practitioners in the United States

Although the term *primary care* has a long history, it was virtually unused in the United States before the mid-1960s. Even today, it is not widely accepted by the medical profession, which uses the terms *family medicine, general internal medicine,* and *general pediatrics* to reflect the concepts that are embodied in the broader term *primary care.* It seems likely that this is a result of the emphasis on specialization that has long characterized U.S. medicine.

Specialization was well underway during the second decade of the century (Stevens, 1978). In 1915, 66% of graduates of medical schools said they eventually planned to subspecialize. Ophthalmology was the first medical specialty to be formally organized (Wechsler, 1976). In the 1930s, many specialties emerged as separate entities; by 1937 there were formal certifying boards in ophthalmology (1917), otolaryngology (1924), obstetrics/gynecology (1927), dermatology (1932), pediatrics (1933), orthopedic surgery (1934), psychiatry and neurology (1934), radiology (1934), proctology (1935)—later to become colon and rectal surgery—urology (1935), internal medicine (1936), and surgery (1937). Subsequent formalization was achieved for neurological surgery (1940), physical medicine (1947), preventive medicine and public health (1948), and thoracic surgery (1950). Several of these ''specialties'' later changed their names, and the American Board of Thoracic Surgery was not officially recognized as a separate major specialty until 1970. Thus, by 1950, there were over 15 boards to certify the competence of physicians entering specialty fields, but no specialization for family physicians (Wechsler, 1976). By 1996, there were 38 separate certifications, plus 43 in subspecialities, and over 21 other special certifications, as well as a family medicine certification (Randolph et al., 1997).

The availability of federal funds to provide assistance for education of veterans of World War II accelerated the entry of physicians into specialties, and as a result the proportion of physicians who were generalists fell rapidly from 75% in 1935 to 45% in 1957 (Knowles, 1969). By the mid-1960s, a crisis in the availability of primary care physicians was widely anticipated, and several national commissions recommended steps to reverse the trend with proposals to establish a ''specialty'' of family medicine. However, the traditional specialists actively resisted the establishment of a specialty of general/family practice. In 1965, the American College of Physicians (the internists) went only so far as to state their interest and feeling of responsibility to promote the family practice of medicine (Knowles, 1969). After repeated attempts by the Academy of General Practice to establish a certifying board in family practice, in 1969 one was finally approved. In 1971, Congress passed legislation (The Health Professions Educational Assistance Program) that for the first time authorized the expenditure of funds to support training in family medicine. Since 1968, many states, starting with New York, have enacted laws calling for the development of family practice programs in state medical schools. By 1972, 31 schools had created departments of family practice and another 30 had set up divisions of family practice; these accounted for about three-fifths of all medical schools at the time. There were 107 approved residency programs in family medicine: 63 in community hospitals, 41 in university or university-affiliated hospitals, and 3 in military hospitals, with a total of over 1,000 residency positions (Rousselot, 1973). *Family practitioner* is the designation for graduates of these approved family medicine training programs; *general practitioner* is reserved for similar physicians who graduated from medical school before these training programs were developed.

Legislation passed in 1963 and 1968 facilitated expansion in the overall supply of all physicians, including specialists, but in 1971 federal legislation to support the growth of family medicine failed to affect the supply of primary care physicians relative to that of other specialists.

In 1976, concern about the maldistribution of physicians (relatively low physician/population ratios in most nonurban areas) and the lagging supply of primary care physicians led the U.S. Congress to pass legislation that provided funding for primary care training programs in family medicine, general internal medicine, and pediatrics. The number of family physicians, internists, and pediatricians and the ratio of such physicians to the population increased, more than compensating for the decline in the number of general practitioners. The number of primary care physicians per 100,000 population increased from 69.6 in 1980 to 78.8 in 1985 and 83.7 in 1990. Despite this increase, the growth in number of primary care physicians was less than that of nonprimary care specialists so that they accounted for a smaller proportion of all physicians in 1990 than in 1985.

Table 4.11 provides the distribution of physician specialties in the United States from 1963 to 1995. In 1995, only 39% of all active physicians (and 39% of all active office-based physicians) were primary care physicians. However, this percentage includes most pediatric subspecialties as well as some internal medicine subspecialties because they are not enumerated separately. In contrast to most family medicine and general practice specialists, not all internal medicine and pediatric specialists practice primary care. In the late 1980s, for example, almost 30% of physicians who classified themselves as general pediatricians actually either had a subspecialty concentration in their practices (17%) or practiced a subspecialty exclusively (11%) (McCrindle et al., 1989). Between one-half and two-thirds of all internists in training in the 1980s pursued subspecialty training (Institute of Medicine, 1989; Barnett and Midtling, 1989). This increase in subspecialization occurred in osteopathic medicine as well; between 1980 and 1987, the number of subspecialty certificates in osteopathy doubled.

Between 1990 and 1995, the percentage growth in primary care specialists ranged from 2% for family and general practitioners to 11% for general internists

Table 4.11. Number (Per 100,000 Population) of Professionally Active Physicians, Selected Years 1963 and Following*

	1963	1970	1975	1980	1990	1995
Total active MDs†	134.8	148.3	156.1	188.0	218.3	245.8
Primary care‡	56.7	56.2	59.9	69.6	82.1	92.6
General/family practice	34.4	27.7	25.0	26.0	27.5	29.0
Internal medicine	15.7	20.0	24.9	30.9	38.3	43.8
Pediatrics‡	6.6	8.6	10.0	12.7	16.3	19.8
Other medical specialties	6.3	8.3	8.7	15.6	24.9	29.9
Surgical specialties§	34.9	41.1	44.0	47.8	53.4	56.2
Other specialties	36.9	42.8	43.4	40.8	49.8	56.1

* In addition, there were 25,479 osteopathic physicians in the United States in 1986. Osteopathy is a separate and smaller branch of medicine that is based on a different philosophy of pathology than is the case in the predominant allopathic medicine. Of all osteopathic physicians in 1986, 61% practiced primary care, mostly general practice. Osteopathic physicians comprise 3% of all physicians in the United States, but they represent 9.3% of primary care physicians and 12.2% of family physicians (Barnett and Midtling, 1989).

† Excludes unknown specialties.

‡ Includes pediatric subspecialties as well as general pediatrics.

§ Includes obstetrics/gynecology.

Sources: 1963–1990, U.S. Department of Health, Education, and Welfare; 1980, 1990, 1995, Randolph et al. (1997), as cited in Starfield B. Primary Care: Concept, Evaluation, and Policy, Oxford University Press, 1992 (2nd printing) page 93. or U.S. Department of Health, Education, and Welfare. A Report to the President and Congress on the Status of Health Professions Personnel in the United States. DHEW Publication No. (HRA) 78–93, Washington D. C. 1978.

and 21% for pediatricians, or an overall percentage increase of 9%. In contrast, the rate of increase in medical subspecialists was 80%, whereas the number of surgical specialists remained relatively constant but other subspecialists declined about 12%.

Table 4.12 shows the overall number of persons for each type of physician in the United States in 1990 and in 1995. In 1995 there was 1 active physician for every 365 people, but fewer than one-half of these were primary care physicians. On average, there was one primary care physician for every 1,080 people and only 1 family/general practitioner for every 3,448 people.

Even though medical school graduates are increasingly choosing primary care specialties, the likelihood of substantially increasing the proportion of primary care physicians appears remote. In 1996, the proportion of all physicians completing their training who were primary care physicians was less than 30% (American Medical Association, 1997).

The appropriate number of physicians of different types is difficult to specify. Although international comparisons including countries that differ in the relative proportions of different types of physicians might inform the debate, it would not provide a definitive answer due to the myriad of other differences among countries. In the United States, integrated health systems with good data on personnel provide a reasonable standard against which other health systems can be compared. Data from 106 group and staff model HMOs indicated that the proportion of primary care physicians to total physicians (expressed as full-time equivalents) varied between 45% and 49%. However, the smaller the enrollment in the plan, the smaller

Table 4.12. Population Per Physician: United States, 1990 and 1995

	1990	1995 Total	Office-Based
Total active physicians	454	365	615
Primary care physicians	1,186	1,080	1,572
General/family physicians	3,529	3,448	4,386
Internists	2,529	2,283	3,623
Pediatricians (children aged 0–14)	1,280	1,111	1,667
Other medical specialists	6,009	3,344	4,762
Obstetrician/gynecologists (per female)	—*	3,566	4,595
Surgical specialists	—*	2,387	3,155
Other specialists	1,559*	1,783	2,793

*Included with surgical specialists prior to 1995.

Source: Randolph et al. (1997).

the proportion of primary care physicians. In the HMOs with enrollments below 80,000, only 33%–37% of the full-time physicians were primary care physicians, whereas the comparable percentage for larger HMOs was about 60% (calculations from Dial et al., 1995). Smaller organizations use a much greater number of sub-specialists per 100,000 enrolled population than larger organizations. The extent to which the work of these specialists in the larger and smaller organizations differs is unknown. Although a more recent study in two large staff model HMOs suggests that these organizations continue to have more primary care physicians per population than the country as a whole, it may no longer be true that they have fewer subspecialists, especially medical subspecialists (Hart et al., 1997).

As is shown in Chapter 15, this subspecialty orientation is not universal in Western industrialized nations. Moreover, the growth in the supply of all primary care physicians combined is less than that in the supply of other specialists, thus predisposing to an increasingly specialized orientation to medical practice in the United States.

The relative proportions of primary care and non-primary care specialists is likely to have a major impact on practice patterns in both types of specialities. In the United States, the proportion of non-primary care specialists is high compared with other countries and not falling markedly, even in this era of managed care. This is reflected in practice patterns in which non-primary care physicians in the United States have a much greater role in ongoing, disease-oriented care of patients, with consequent greater costs, than is the case in many other countries. The number of subspecialists that are required to meet the needs for consultation with primary care physicians or for ongoing management of rare or uncommon conditions is not known and remains a challenge for future policy-oriented research in all countries. Countries vary in their primary care and non-primary care physician to population ratios; this variability is seen even within countries.

Thus it is clear that where there is a relative dearth of primary care physicians relative to other specialists in general (as in the United States), alterations in both governmental and nongovernmental policies might be considered. Some possibilities include (Starfield and Simpson, 1993)

1. Raising the professional earnings of primary care physicians to parity or near parity with specialists
2. Establishing a more rational basis for referral and especially for long-term management of patients (In particular, primary care physicians could care for more patients with ongoing health problems with more appropriate consultation arrangements and shared care with subspecialists, thus reducing the demand for direct services by subspecialists. That is, primary care with appropriate back-up from specialists could reduce the demand for subspecialist care.)
3. Restructuring state licensing policies to limit physician supply to areas of need
4. Providing financial incentives to programs that educate primary care physicians
5. Expanding and improving loan forgiveness programs for primary care physicians
6. Restructuring fee schedules for primary care to encourage the provision of important primary care services
7. Reducing burdensome administrative paperwork associated with billing and quality assurance activities
8. Providing bonuses for achieving important primary care objectives
9. Providing bonuses for team practice in primary care
10. Rewarding higher levels of achievement of primary care functions
11. Earmarking increased funding for primary care research to enhance the intellectual challenges of primary care and increase the scientific base for its practice
12. Involving trainees in ongoing quality of care monitoring to prepare them for critical review of their own practices

Many countries have already instituted policies directed at these objectives. As Chapter 15 shows, policy efforts are reflected in the way physicians practice, thus providing the basis for optimism about the ability of health systems to respond to the challenges to improve the provision of health care services.

References

American Medical Association. Graduate medical education. Appendix II. JAMA 1997; 273: 781.

Barnett P, Midtling J. Public policy and the supply of primary care physicians. JAMA 1989; 262:2864–88.

Blumenthal D, Chang YC, Causino N, Culpepper L, Marder W, Saglam D, Stafford R, Starfield B. The duration of ambulatory physician visits. Manuscript submitted, 1998.

Dial T, Palsbo S, Bergsten C, Gabel J, Weiner J. Clinical staffing in staff- and group-model HMOs. Health Aff 1995; 14:168–98.

Doescher M, Franks P. Family care in the United States: A national profile. Med Care 1997; 35:564–73.

Ferris T, Saglam D, Stafford R, Causino N, Starfield B, Culpepper L, Blumenthal D.

Changes in the daily practice of primary care for children. Arch Pediatr Adolesc Med 1998; 152:227–33.

Forrest C, Reid R. Passing the baton: Referral rate estimates in the United States, 1989–1994. Health Aff 1997; 16:157–62.

Hart LG, Wagner E, Pirzada S, Nelson A, Rosenblatt R. Physician staffing ratios in staff-model HMOs: A cautionary tale. Health Aff 1997; 16:55–70.

Institute of Medicine. Primary Care Physicians: Financing Their Graduate Medical Education in Ambulatory Settings. Washington, DC: National Academy Press, 1989.

Knowles J. The quantity and quality of medical manpower: A review of medicine's current efforts. J Med Educ 1969; 44:81–118.

Lipkind K. National Hospital Ambulatory Medical Care Survey: 1994 Outpatient Department Summary. Advance Data From Vital and Health Statistics, No. 276. Hyattsville: National Center for Health Statistics, 1996.

McCrindle B, DeAngelis C, Starfield B. Subspecialization within pediatrics practice: A broader spectrum. Pediatr Res 1989; 25:135A.

National Center for Health Statistics. Health US 1996–97 and Injury Chartbook. Hyattsville: National Center for Health Statistics, 1997.

North S, Marvel MK, Hendricks B, Morphew P, North D. Physicians' usefulness ratings of family-oriented clinical tools. J Fam Pract 1993; 37(1):30–4.

Puskin D. Patterns of Ambulatory Medical Care Practice in the United States: An Analysis of the National Ambulatory Medical Care Survey. Dissertation. Baltimore: Johns Hopkins University, 1977.

Randolph L, Seidman B, Pasko T. Physician Characteristics and Distribution in the U.S. Chicago: American Medical Association; 1997.

Reid R. Patterns of Referral for Newly Diagnosed Patients With Diabetes in Alberta. Dissertation. Baltimore: Johns Hopkins University, 1998.

Robert Wood Johnson Foundation. Medical Practice in the United States. Princeton, NJ: Robert Wood Johnson Foundation, 1982.

Royal College of General Practice. Information Sheet No. 4. London: Royal College of General Practice, 1995. July 1995.

Royal College of General Practice. Information Sheet No. 7. London: Royal College of General Practice, 1995b.

Royal College of General Practice. Information Sheet No. 10. London: Royal College of General Practice, May 1996.

Rousselot L. Federal efforts to influence physician education, specialization distribution projections and options. Am J Med 1973; 55:123–30.

Schappert SM. National Ambulatory Medical Care Survey: 1994 Summary. Advance Data From Vital and Health Statistics. No. 273. Hyattsville: National Center for Health Statistics, 1996.

Schneeweis R, Rosenblatt R, Cherkin D, Kirkwood R, Hart G. Diagnosis clusters: A new tool for analyzing the content of medical care. Med Care 1983; 21:105–22.

Smilkstein G. The family in family medicine, revisited, again. J Fam Pract 1994; 39:527–31.

Stafford R, Saglan D, Causino N, Starfield B, Culpepper L, Marder W, Blumenthal D. Trends in adult visits to primary care physicians in the United States. Archives of Family Medicine 1998, in press.

Starfield B. Measuring the attainment of primary care. J Med Educ 1979; 54:361–9.

Starfield B, Simpson L. Primary care as part of U.S. health services reform. JAMA 1993; 269:3136–9.

Stevens R. Graduate medical education: a continuing history. J Med Educ 1978; 53:1–18.

Stussman B. National Hospital Ambulatory Medical Care Survey: 1994 Emergency Department Summary. Advance Data From Vital and Health Statistics. No. 275. Hyattsville: National Center for Health Statistics, 1996.

Wechsler H. Handbook of Medical Specialties. New York: Human Sciences Press, 1976.

Woodwell D. National Ambulatory Medical Survey: 1995 Summary. Advance Data From Vital and Health Statistics. No. 286. Hyattsville: National Center for Health Statistics, 1997.

— 5 —

Primary Care, Subspecialists, and Non-Physician Practitioners

Since antiquity, the physician has been the officially sanctioned practitioner of medicine, with other types of practitioners assisting or complementing the physician's role in providing health services. Where physicians were (or still are) in short supply, practitioners such as nurses or medical auxiliaries substituted for physicians. Experimentation with augmented primary care roles for these other practitioners was provided impetus by the "barefoot doctor" movement in China after the 1949 revolution and by the training of nurse practitioners and "physician assistants" in the United States starting in the 1960s and 1970s.

Although the role of these non-physician practitioners has never been formally delineated, their training and involvement in primary care raise questions concerning the relative effectiveness and efficiency of different types of practitioners involved in primary care. These questions were particularly salient in the United States, where increasing specialization was producing a surfeit of subspecialists at the expense of primary care physicians. Moreover, in the United States (in contrast to most other industrialized countries), primary care services are provided not only by general practitioners and family physicians, but also by pediatricians and general internists. Responsibility for primary care may be assumed by other types of physicians even in countries where the family physician is the mainstay of primary care. For example, in Spain and Italy, pediatricians are the primary care physicians to children under age 14 years. In the United States until relatively recently, pediatricians were considered the primary care physicians to children under age 14 years; now the age has been increased to include adolescents. Obstetric services are sometimes not considered part of family medicine in some countries, where routine prenatal care is done by midwives or obstetricians. Thus, the issue of who provides primary care better, and to whom, is relevant almost everywhere because the decisions influence policy concerning educational content and organization and financing of services.

One issue concerns the relative merits of providing primary care services by family physicians compared with their "specialoid" (Fry and Horder, 1994) counterparts (i.e., general pediatricians and general internists). The growth in

75

power and influence of specialists and an increasing tendency of some segments
of populations to believe that specialist care is better than generalist care, as well
as early assertions that other specialists provide "primary care" (Aiken et al.,
1979), also lead to questions about the relative merits of specialist and generalist
care. A special case of "specialist" versus "generalist" care concerns the matter
of services to be provided to women; in particular, are obstetricians primary care
physicians if at least some women believe them to be their principal source of
care? A third issue, of particular interest in the United States, concerns non-
physician practitioners as primary care providers. Finally, the role of the team in
primary care requires consideration. The particular questions to be answered are:
Is the practice of primary care equally effective, regardless of the type of physician? Or does theoretical or practical justification exist for limiting the practice
of primary care to certain types of physicians, perhaps with the aid of other
members of a "team"?

One special note: Some primary care physicians resent the designation as "generalist," particularly when counterposed against the term "specialist" because it
connotes inferiority in the minds of some people. For the purposes of this chapter,
the term "generalist" is retained because it is the subject of expertise in "generalism" that is under consideration (Smilkstein, 1994).

The Theoretical Basis for the Primary Care Physician

Dr. S. is a well-known physician and biomedical researcher who began to lose
his vision in his early 60s. Given his background as a physician and distinguished
scientist, he had no problem in searching out the best ophthalmologists in the field.
Nor did he have trouble communicating with them. He spoke their language and
shared their knowledge. Dr. S. was diagnosed as having macular degeneration, an
irreversible and progressive cause of blindness, and was told that there was nothing
that could be done for him. Only much later, and through discussions with nonpro-
fessionals, did Dr. S. learn that there was much that could be done for him. These
are his words:

"I think it is the rare physician who has the time and energy and insight to
devote profound attention to what is happening to the rest of his patient. It may be
that my physician can do nothing for my eyeballs, but behind those eyeballs is an
anxious worried man who demands inputs but is now deprived of his accustomed
inputs, and there is lots that can be done for him. The complications of blindness
are not in the eye but elsewhere. One of them is a feeling of soreness on the anterior
surface of both tibias about 12 inches from the floor, which is about the height of
the conventional coffee table. It is a problem of a patient who is blind, but it isn't
mentioned in any of the ophthalmological textbooks. I believe that blindness to
most ophthalmologists represents failure, just as death represents failure to the internist. The internist doesn't have to deal with the patient who has died, but the
patient who is blind lives on, and the inability of the ophthalmologist to cope with
the blindness has a major impact on the patient. Ophthalmologists deny the patient
any other help because they feel defeated. Ophthalmologists are unaware of dozens
of aids that make life more tolerable for the blind patient.

Had my doctor told me about talking wristwatches and talking books, my world would have been transformed from a living hell to a roaring inferno, and sometimes to a heaven.

Dr. S. went to the "best ophthalmologist available by all professional criteria." He might have been better off being seen by a primary care physician, with consultation from the ophthalmologist.

From a theoretical viewpoint, the interests and skills involved in providing care should be different from those involved in specialist care. Physicians who practice primary care must tolerate ambiguity because many problems never reach the stage of a diagnosis that can be coded using standard diagnostic nomenclature. They must be comfortable in establishing and maintaining relationships with patients and in dealing with problems for which there is no demonstrable biological aberration. They also must be able to manage several problems at once, even though the problems may be unrelated in etiology or pathogenesis. Furthermore, over long periods of time, the problems of patients change, and specialists who are appropriate for the problem for which the patient originally sought care may be challenged beyond their skills and interests when other types of problems arise.

Medical progress and new technologies provide the impetus for an increasingly specialist orientation; the same phenomena also call for increasingly well-honed generalist skills. Better strategies for management will improve life expectancy so that the complexity of illness management will increase over time; increased survival will also result in the conglomeration of different types of illnesses. Health problems are becoming more complex, with more syndromes, handicaps, impairments, and disabilities than those with which physicians are accustomed. Both increased aging of populations and increased survival of individuals challenged by anatomical, physiological, or psychological problems are likely to heighten the need for home-based care and for knowledge about the existence of community resources.

In primary care practice, disease presents at an earlier stage than it does in specialist care because specialists usually see the problems after the patients have been referred from primary care physicians. Because the training of specialists takes place in tertiary medical centers, their exposure is to patients with problems in a more differentiated stage. As a result, specialists tend to overestimate the likelihood of serious disease in unscreened populations, a phenomenon consistent with the findings of many studies of the ways people evaluate the probability of events (Kahnemann et al., 1982). On the basis of these considerations, a theoretical viewpoint suggests that primary care should be provided by individuals trained for primary care in primary care settings rather than by those trained in tertiary medical centers.

The theoretical arguments for having primary care physicians assume responsibility for primary care is buttressed by experience in other professions, in the health systems of other industrialized nations, and in organized health care systems. As Moore (1992) noted, most other professions and industries employ specialization to deal with increasing complexity. However, when size and complexity reach a certain level, organizations employ general managers who plan, allocate resources, supervise and coordinate the work of specialists, and monitor the results. Few industrialized nations rely on specialists to provide primary care; most have systems that are based on the generalist physician with back-up from specialists (Kaprio, 1979). In the United States, all organized health service systems (such as group practice forms of health maintenance organizations [HMOs]) employ primary care physicians; by the late 1990s virtually all the graduates of primary care programs would be needed to staff the HMOs if their programs grow, as predicted, at 10% per year (Moore, 1992) .

Empirical evidence of the benefits of a primary care physician supports the theoretical notions. The higher the proportion of general physicians in a community, the lower its frequency of hospitalization. Experiences in Sweden indicate that primary care both reduces the flow of patients into specialized secondary care services such as consultants and emergency rooms and lowers age-adjusted total health care costs (Moore, 1992). Data from an international collaborative study of medical care utilization showed that areas with higher specialist to generalist ratios have higher rates of physician visits that cannot be accounted for by greater health needs (Kohn and White, 1976). Specialists may overtreat patients; for example, allergists treating children and adults with asthma use more corticosteroid than do the family physicians and pediatricians with whom they have been compared (Engel et al., 1989).

Important determinants of the quality of care are the length of postgraduate training, the extent of experience with the particular problem under consideration, and the nature of the organization in which the physician works (Palmer and Reilly, 1979). The diverse roles of the physician may heavily influence decision-making, not always in consistent directions. Eisenberg (1986) characterized these roles as "self-fulfilling practitioner," "patient's agent," and "guarantor of social good." Sometimes one role dominates, while at other times another prevails. Physicians may have needs for "self-fulfillment" in terms of an expected income because they find certain ways of practice more personally satisfying to them, because they have been trained in certain ways that are therefore more comfortable for them, because the setting in which they practice has certain expectations that may be difficult to overcome, or because their professional societies or colleagues recommend practicing in certain ways. Acting as the patient's agent may also produce differences in practice patterns because different physicians may interpret patients' needs differently, because patients may make demands for certain types of interventions, or because convenience to the patient may be considered a critical factor. As a "guarantor of social good," physicians may make decisions on the basis of their beliefs about competing priorities. For example, they may be concerned about the benefit of an intervention when the required resources might be more beneficial to other patients. All of these considerations may contribute in a major way to differences in practice patterns among different types of physicians and to determining the best approaches to reducing the variability where it seems desirable to do so.

If training specifically in primary care is important for its practice, what evidence is there that certain types of such training are superior to others? In particular, is the training of family physicians, general internists, and pediatricians equally effective? The research literature provides a wealth of data on this issue. Most studies here considered were conducted in the United States, the only western industrialized country in which both general internists and pediatricians have equal status as primary care physicians with family physicians or "generalists."

The literature contains several types of approaches to comparing the practice of family physicians with general internists in the care of adults and that of family physicians with pediatricians in the care of children. (A few studies have also included specialists of different types in their comparisons.) Diagnostic and treatment methods, referral practices, and the use of resources have been studied by a variety of methods, including medical record reviews, logs kept by physicians for several days, questionnaires sent to physicians, and programmed (simulated) patients. Some studies have been national in scope, whereas others were limited to individual clinical facilities. Some only describe differences in practice characteristics, whereas others have specifically assessed the technical quality of care, satisfaction with care on the part of patients, reductions in the utilization of services, or some aspects of the outcome or costs of care. A few studies have addressed the attainment of the unique feature of care; these are summarized in other chapters.

Family physicians, general internists, and general pediatricians: practice profiles

The National Ambulatory Medical Care Survey provides descriptive information on a variety of characteristics of patients, patient problems, and practice characteristics. This survey can be used to compare the practices of various types of physicians. For example, internists spend more time with patients (18.4 minutes) than do family/general practitioners (13.0 minutes). Internists order more laboratory tests (73% of visits) and x-ray tests (53% of visits) than the generalists (34% and 19%, respectively). Internists are also more likely to provide instructions regarding health problems (17.8% of visits) than generalists (12.4%), but there are no apparent differences in frequencies of therapy for emotional problems (3%) (Noren et al., 1980).

The same survey has been used to compare characteristics of the practices of family physicians and general practitioners with those of pediatricians. Pediatricians order more laboratory tests but prescribe fewer drugs for the major categories of illnesses (fever, sore throat, abdominal pain, diarrhea, and earache) (Fishbane and Starfield,1981).

Logs kept by physicians were the source of information in another national survey of face-to-face encounters of family physicians and pediatricians. One study from this survey examined the care provided to children having five types of visits (well-patient and skin, ear, mouth or throat, and upper respiratory conditions) and five major diagnoses (medical examination, upper respiratory infections, pneumonia, pharyngitis, otitis media) in the ambulatory setting. Pediatricians performed more diagnostic tests for all diagnoses and did more immunizations and gave more counseling about growth and development, but they provided less specific therapy than did family physicians. However, family physicians did more counseling about family and sex matters than did pediatricians. Family physicians were also more likely to provide a broader range of services, especially minor surgery, for every age group in childhood (Starfield et al., 1985).

The same national survey was used to study a sample of 132 family physicians and 102 general internists who completed questionnaires and kept log diaries on 3,737 and 2,250 adult office visits, respectively. Analysis revealed that general internists were twice as likely as family physicians to order blood tests, blood counts, chest x-rays, and electrocardiograms. They also spent more time with patients and referred and hospitalized them at a greater rate whether all patients were considered or just those with essential benign hypertension. The average charge per visit for patients of internists was about twice that for patients of family physicians even after controlling for a variety of patient, practice, and physician characteristics (Cherkin et al., 1987).

Although these data are over a decade old, similar analyses of more recent data suggest that the situation in the United States has not changed (D. Blumenthal et al., unpublished manuscript; Ferris et al., 1998).

Diagnostic methods of internists and family physicians have been compared using research assistants who are trained to present problems as if they were from real patients. For example, the diagnostic methods of nine family physicians were compared with those of nine internists, using these "programmed" patients to present three clinical problems. Family physicians asked fewer history questions, requested fewer items of data about physical examination, and ordered fewer laboratory investigations. In two of the three problems, the study revealed that family physicians asked relatively more questions about mental status and life situation. There were no significant differences in the diagnoses reached (Smith and Mc-Whinney, 1975).

In another study using simulations, the diagnostic methods of third year residents in internal medicine (n = 31) were compared with those in family practice (n = 22) using written descriptions of five patients, each with a different problem. The family practice residents targeted far fewer physical examination items. Laboratory charges were greater for the internists but only for two of the simulations. However, the two groups of physicians did not differ in their number of diagnostic hypotheses (Scherger et al., 1980).

Medical records were the source of information in other comparisons of the care provided by different types of primary care physicians. In one such study 520 patients were randomized to an internal medicine or to a family practice clinic. After about 2 years, the charts of the patients were evaluated for frequency of visits, laboratory studies ordered, number of referrals, acute care clinic visits, emergency room visits, and frequency of broken appointments. Associated costs were also ascertained. Patients seen by the internists had, on average, more frequent visits to the primary care clinic, the emergency room, and the acute care clinic. They were less likely to have kept their appointments to the primary care clinic. The median total annual cost of laboratory tests for patients in the internal medicine clinic was significantly higher because of higher referral rates to specialists and higher laboratory test charges generated by specialists (Bertakis and Robbins, 1987).

Medical records were also used to study about 2,000 inpatients of family physicians and internists with regard to their length of stay, charges generated, charges generated per day, disposition, number and type of diagnoses, and number of procedures. The only differences were in number of diagnoses; family physicians assigned fewer. Review of a random sample of 50 charts of family physicians and a matched sample of 50 charts of internists revealed no differences in severity of illness, and multivariate adjustment for differences in case mix did not change the findings (Franks and Dickinson, 1986).

A study of care provided to 10,608 adults from panels of 60 family physicians and 245 general internists indicated that patients of family physicians had lower pharmacy costs and made fewer visits to dermatologists, psychiatrists, and gynecologists, but used more urgent care (nonappointment) visits so that their total costs were no lower than were those of patients of general internists. Hospitalization rates, ambulatory visit rates, and laboratory and x-ray costs were the same for patients of family physicians and general internists (Selby et al., 1998).

A survey of family physicians, internists, and obstetrician/gynecologists in Maryland asked the physicians to report the percentage of their patients who had been referred and the percentage whom they referred. Family physicians received fewer referrals than did the other two types of physicians, but they referred the same percentage (10%–11%) of patients as did generalists (Sobal et al., 1988).

These studies indicate that care provided by pediatricians and internists differ from care provided by family physicians, at least in some ways. Is there any evidence to suggest that this is associated with less satisfaction, poorer diagnosis, management, or outcomes of care? The following categories of studies address these questions.

Patients' satisfaction with care. Satisfaction of patients with their care has been studied by follow-up telephone interviews as well as mailed questionnaires. In one study using both medical records and telephone interviews, satisfaction was greater among family practice patients than a matched group of patients seen by internists or pediatricians (Farrell et al., 1982).

Questionnaires sent to patients provided information from a national study in which patients were randomly sampled from logs kept by family physicians and internists. These patients were asked how satisfied they were with the medical care they were receiving. Two hundred thirteen adult patients of 124 family physicians and 218 patients of 98 general internists responded. Patients of both types of physicians reported similar levels of satisfaction on all four dimensions measured (access, humaneness, quality, and general satisfaction) even after controlling for a variety of patient, practice, and physician characteristics (Cherkin et al., 1988).

Technical quality of care. Physicians' recognition of patients' problems and their adherence to professionally defined standards of care for diagnosis and management in primary care have been studied with a variety of approaches, including medical record reviews, physician interviews, and auditing of claims forms.

Audits of medical records were the basis of a study that found that family physicians recorded fewer of the health supervision criteria than did pediatricians but did as well in recording items related to disease management (Thompson and Osborne, 1976).

When quality of care was judged by examining medical records to ascertain diagnosis and management for specific conditions, specialists performed better in their own area of specialized training than did family or general practitioners or specialists performing outside their specialty areas (Payne et al., 1984). This is consistent with the known relationships between volume of care and quality of care on inpatient units in hospitals; the higher the volume of care for a problem by a particular surgeon or by a hospital in general, the better the quality of care. However, the *overall* quality of care by a given practitioner or particular practice cannot be judged by assessing the care for any particular diagnosis, especially when the selected diagnosis reflects problems often seen in specialty care rather than those more characteristic of primary care.

In one survey, a representative sample of physicians in Maryland were queried about their attitudes toward patients with hypertension. Family physicians were slightly less likely to indicate that they would order certain diagnostic tests for patients. They were also more cautious in recommending antihypertensive medication at mildly increased blood pressure but were more in favor of some non-pharmacological regimens (reducing weight and smoking, increasing exercise, reducing alcohol intake, and eating a low cholesterol diet) than were either internists or other specialists. All types of physicians were equally likely to support the use of diuretics for initial therapy of patients with mild hypertension (Cloher and Whelton, 1986).

Patients have also been queried concerning their physician's practice patterns. In one such study, college freshmen were asked about the extent of health counseling they had received from their primary health care practitioners. Patients of internists had received more counseling about smoking and alcohol use than had patients of pediatricians or family physicians, received more counseling about drug abuse and heart disease prevention than did patients of pediatricians, and received more counseling about weight control and nutrition than did patients of family physicians. Pediatricians gave more counseling about weight control than did family physicians but did not exceed internists in any area mentioned above (Joffe et al., 1988).

In another study, a screening test was given to 1,452 patients attending two primary care clinics in a large comprehensive health ˆare facility to identify existing psychosocial problems. Family physicians were less likely than internists to recognize existing mental health problems, but the research design could not determine if the differences were due to other differences in practice style in the two clinics or to the difference in type of physician (Kessler et al., 1985).

In another study, both medical records and interviews of primary care physicians were used to study the attainment of a minimum set of standards (developed by consensus of physicians) for management of patients with four indicator conditions. The four conditions were care of normal infants, care of pregnant women, care of adult-onset diabetes, and care of patients with congestive heart failure. A random sample of all physicians in one county were asked to participate; the sample included 34 family physicians, 11 internists, 8 pediatricians, and 8 obstetricians with 523 infants. It involved 363 pregnant women, 244 diabetic patients, and 128 patients with congestive heart failure who visited the practices during the time of the study. Data were collected from medical records and interviews with physicians. Management scores were better for pediatricians and for obstetricians for two conditions, care of normal infant and pregnant women,. respectively, than they were for family physicians. For the other two conditions, adult-onset diabetes and congestive heart failure, there were no differences between the management scores of family physicians and internists. Neither patient nor disease characteristics explained the differences that were found (Hulka et al., 1976).

Questionnaires were also used in a study of 200 randomly chosen pediatricians and 300 family physicians in Georgia to inquire about their treatment of enuresis, their prescribing habits, and their knowledge of the side effects and toxic effects of tricyclic antidepressants. A total of 190 physicians responded. Nearly one-half of both family physicians and pediatricians reported using tricyclic antidepressants for management of enuresis. Only one-third of prescribers of these drugs were aware of the side effects or toxicity of this class of drugs. Among physicians who did *not* prescribe the drug, a greater proportion of pediatricians were aware of the side effects and toxicity than was the case for family physicians. Pediatricians were more likely to treat patients for a shorter period of time, to limit prescription refills, and to promote the availability of ipecac syrup in the home for use when a child accidentally took an overdose. (Rauber and Maroncelli, 1984).

In an evaluation of a state peer review system, Brook and Williams (1976) audited claims forms and found that general practitioners had a smaller proportion of injections denied by the peer review organization than internists but had more denied than pediatricians. However, general practitioners tended on average to give more injections per visit and had higher absolute numbers of injections denied per visit than had either internists or pediatricians. General practitioners tended to give more injections on average per visit than did other types of physicians and had slightly higher numbers of injections denied per ambulatory visit.

Several studies have compared family physicians with either pediatricians or internists by means of presenting them with hypothetical clinical scenarios. In one study, physicians were queried as to their use of antibiotic therapy for an acute episode of purulent rhinitis. Family physicians were more likely to report prescribing antibiotics, and to do so earlier in the course of illness, than pediatricians, except for children in day care (where frequency of prescribing was high and equal) (Schwartz et al., 1997).

Family physicians and pediatricians were surveyed as to their immunization practices, particularly with regard to mechanisms to identify underimmunized children and use of illness visits to provide needed immunizations. A slightly greater percentage of pediatricians reported vaccinating children during chronic illness and follow-up visits and were more likely to use tracking systems to detect underimmunization (Szilagyi et al., 1994). However, a study in a large military hospital without any financial barriers to care found that children followed up by family physicians were more likely to be up to date on immunizations than children followed by pediatricians (Weese and Krauss, 1995).

Hypothetical case studies concerning the care of a patient with diabetes, angina, or hypertension were presented to physicians, who were also asked whether they would recommend a follow-up visit for the condition. There was great variation in reported recommendations across the disease types (Petitti and Grumbach, 1993).

In some places, primary care physicians care for their patients when they are hospitalized, thus raising the question of possible differences between family physicians and other primary care specialists. In one large study of 31,321 hospital admissions in an entire state, outcome measures of morbidity, mortality, length of stay, and hospital charges were ascertained for the 10 most common diagnostic categories. The distribution of admission diagnoses was the same for both types of physicians, and there was no difference in mortality or hospital charges once relevant patient characteristics (including severity on admission) and hospital characteristics were taken into account. The patients of internists experienced slightly higher morbidity and had slightly longer hospital stays (McCann et al., 1995).

In none of these comparisons between family physicians and either pediatrician or internists were primary care characteristics of the practice examined, despite the likelihood that the strength of primary care characteristics could account for differences in the variability of care provided, both within the primary care specialities as well as across them.

Utilization, costs, and outcomes of care. Both retrospective and prospective approaches have shown few systematic differences in use of resources and outcomes of care. Some studies suggest that family physicians are more efficient and effective practitioners of primary care, whereas others show either no difference or an advantage of internists and pediatricians.

For example, there were few differences in a study of care in two clinics involving pediatricians. In one of the clinics, however, internists and allied health workers formed teams with the pediatricians so that there was a family orientation with both children and parents receiving care in the same clinic. In both clinics medical records were reviewed for (1) overall use of the center, (2) immunizations performed, (3) processes and outcomes in three conditions (dental caries, iron deficiency anemia, and respiratory infections), (4) parental perceptions of the child's health status, (5) parental perceptions of child's behavior, (6) parental view of the center's services, and (7) parental attitudes regarding the efficacy of medical care. There were few measurable differences between the two groups of children in utilization or in outcome. Where there were differences, they tended to favor the family approach: Older children stayed with the clinic rather than going elsewhere as they grew older, immunizations were somewhat more timely, and children appeared to make fewer visits over time to sources of care other than the center (San Agustin et al., 1982).

Another study involving pediatricians found differences. This study used a prospective design to assess the relative competence of pediatricians and general practitioners in managing febrile illnesses among 259 children under age 10 years, one group in an emergency room of a children's hospital, and the other group in a general hospital in Canada. Both groups of children were similar in their demographic characteristics, presenting complaints, and degree and duration of fever. A telephone interview was conducted within 2 weeks of the visit to determine out-comes based on duration of the acute illness and further physician contacts or hospitalizations. Although no significant differences in the measured outcomes of febrile illness were found, a trend in favor of the pediatricians was discernible with respect to two measures: unresolved symptoms at 2 weeks (8.3% vs. 12.5%) and subsequent hospitalization (0.8% vs. 3.0%) The overall frequency of laboratory use and antibiotic prescriptions were the same for both types of physicians, but significant differences were found in the type of test: General practitioners ordered more x-rays and fewer microbiological tests than did the pediatricians (Leduc and Pless, 1982).

Case–control studies have found little systematic advantage to the care of children by one type of physician compared with another. In one such study, pediatricians and family physicians were compared with regard to their ability to recognize severe acute illness or to avoid preventable complications. Children who had contacted a physician more than 24 hours prior to their emergency room visit were divided into two groups, one with acceptable outcomes and the other with potentially preventable complications or delayed diagnosis, treatment, or referral. Cases and controls were matched for age, socioeconomic status, and illness type. On follow-up interviews with patients, there was no evidence of better care by pediatricians than by family physicians even after taking into account other factors that might have influenced the results (Kramer et al., 1984).

Another case–control study used medical records and telephone interviews to assess utilization and costs of care in a group of 45 patients of family physicians matched with 63 patients attending medical and pediatric clinics over a 33 month period. Despite a 25% greater prevalence of significant chronic medical problems, family practice patients used specialist care less than one-half as much as did other patients (0.9 vs. 1.8 visits per year), although they made an average of one more visit per year due to higher visit rates to their family physician (4.4 vs. 2.5 visits per year). Costs for procedures did not differ (Farrell et al., 1982).

Studies of adult health care have also failed to show systematic differences between internists and generalists. In one study, charges for ambulatory and continuing patient care prescribed by residents in internal medicine were compared with those in family medicine for visits of patients with one of four diagnoses: congestive heart failure, diabetes, degenerative joint disease, or hypertension. Medical records of 4,991 encounters in internal medicine clinic and 700 encounters in the family medicine clinic were audited. The charges per encounter in the internal medicine clinic were greater than those in the family medicine clinic after accounting for differences in patient age, diagnosis, and severity of condition. However, family practitioners scheduled follow-up visits more frequently with shorter durations between visits. Because the total duration of medical care for the selected problems (maximum of 18 months) was shorter in family medicine for only two of the conditions and because the number of visits for each condition within the total study period was greater, total charges over the period of the study were similar for the two types of residents even though the charges per visit were much greater for the patients of the internists (Bennett et al., 1983).

Another study compared the effect of physician specialty and of board certification on costs and outcomes of health care for 213 patients with chronic lung disease followed for 1 year. Patients' pulmonary function, functional ability, number of medical conditions, and insurance status were predictors of outcome, but neither physician specialty nor board certification had a significant impact on outcomes or costs after controlling for the other factors (Strauss et al., 1986).

Family physicians and internists do not appear to differ in their hospitalization practices, even after controlling for several characteristics related to severity of illness. For example, one study of 523 hospitalized patients indicated that the length of stay and readmission rate in the intensive care unit and hospital, severity of illness, discharge diagnosis, proportion who died, time until death, consultation rate, and hospital charges did not differ significantly between patients cared for by the two types of physicians (Hainer and Lawler, 1988).

Another study contrasted the inpatient treatment of diabetic ketoacidosis by internists and by family physicians in a teaching hospital. Laboratory use and length of stay were studied for 12 patients cared for by internists and for 16 patients cared for by family physicians. Hospitalization was longer and the total number of laboratory and x-ray procedures per patient was greater in the internal medicine group. Serum glucose levels and urine spillage were comparable (Hamburger et al., 1982).

Many of these studies have limitations in study design, including a lack of power to detect true differences and difficulties in controlling for differences in case mix (Bowman, 1989). Nevertheless, the findings are strikingly inconsistent. This suggests that whatever differences exist among the different types of primary care physicians in profiles of care, patient satisfaction, technical quality, or utilization, the costs and outcomes of care may have more to do with factors *other* than that of the type of primary physician—family physician, internist, or pediatrician.

Primary care physicians and other specialists

In many countries, the boundaries between primary care and subspecialty care are relatively clear. In others, particularly when subspecialist practice is not limited to hospitals or where first-contact care is not highly developed so that patients may go directly to subspecialists, the relative "quality" of care provided by the two types of physicians may be an important issue. In the United States, the increasing power and influence of primary care physicians is threatening the historical dominance of subspecialists, and there have been several recent studies that have compared the two types of physicians.

Most comparisons between primary care physicians and other specialists examine care of selected conditions that are especially within the purview of the specialists in the study. Not surprisingly, they find specialist care to be superior.

For example, a national (U.S.) survey of gastroenterologists, family physicians, and general internists collected data on reported prescriptions of antibiotic therapy to eradicate *Helicobacter pylori*. The specialists adopted antibiotic therapy earlier than did the generalists, both before and after the time that efficacy of the regimen had been established. However, generalists who worked in groups with specialists were equivalent to the gastroenterologists in their adoption of this indicated therapy, suggesting that educational and promotional efforts are more likely to reach disease-oriented specialists directly; they then convey them to primary care physicians with whom they work (Hirth et al., 1996).

Perhaps the largest comparison of primary care physicians and disease-oriented specialists was carried out in three urban areas of the United States. Patients of family physicians, general internists, cardiologists, and endocrinologists were sampled from HMOs, large multispecialty groups, and solo or single-specialty groups if they had hypertension, noninsulin-dependent diabetes mellitus, recent myocardial infarction, or depression. After adjusting for patient case mix (type of disease and co-morbidity), no major differences were found except for higher utilization rates among patients of internists (Greenfield et al., 1992). An additional analysis of the care of patients with diabetes mellitus or hypertension examined mortality and health status (physiological and psychological states as well as functioning) after 2 and 4 years; mortality was followed for 7 years. The only specialty differences found were better foot–ulcer and infection status among patients of endocrinologists and higher utilization rates among patients of internists (Greenfield et al., 1995).

In the study of 10,608 adults in a group-model HMO, care provided by general internists was compared with care provided by subspecialty internists. In this HMO, subspecialty internists had to agree to function as primary care physicians as well as subspecialists in their particular area of training. Costs for pharmacy and radiologic services as well as for urgent care visits were higher among patients of subspecialty internists, even after differences in complexity of their patients' problems were taken into account (Selby et al., 1998).

Clinical scenarios concerning patients with symptoms possibly indicating syphilis were sent to board-certified internists and experts in sexually transmitted diseases; compared with internists, the sexually transmitted disease experts ordered diagnostic tests at a lower likelihood of disease, but had higher indications for performing lumbar puncture to detect evidence of neurosyphilis than the internists. Because the scenarios were hypothetical, there was no way to determine the accuracy of diagnosis in the two groups of physicians (Winkenwerder et al., 1993).

In one state, practitioners agreed to enroll consecutive patients appearing with acute low back pain in a study. The patients were contacted by phone periodically for up to 6 months to assess functional status, work status, use of health services, and satisfaction with care received. Patients of urban primary care physicians, rural primary care physicians, chiropractors, or orthopedists did not differ in time to recovery or return to work; mean costs were highest for the orthopedic surgeons and chiropractors. Satisfaction was highest among patients under the care of chiropractors (Carey et al., 1995).

In many countries (see Chapter 15), hospitalized patients are cared for by staff physicians who are specialists in the particular condition occasioning hospitalization, presumably on the assumption that hospitalized patients require the care of the disease-oriented specialist. In these countries, there is a clear and separate role for the two types of physicians. In other countries, primary care physicians care for their hospitalized patients, with consultation from disease-oriented specialists as needed. Although this generally is the case in the United States, there are proposals to replace the primary care physician/specialist model with a model that would involve the training of a "hospitalist." This type of physician would be a primary care physician trained in the care of common problems of hospitalized patients and undertake their care with appropriate consultation from the patient's own primary care physician and other appropriate specialists. Such an approach is currently used in a few managed care organizations (Wachter and Goldman, 1996). Questions about the relative effectiveness of hospital care provided by primary care physicians versus specialists are relevant in a context where there is no clear separation of their two separate roles.

Hospital care of patients with acute myocardial infarction or stroke has received considerable research attention because both types of patients are relatively common and therefore theoretically in the purview of primary care. One study showed that patients admitted to the neurology service at one hospital had better prognostic profiles and hence were likely to have better outcomes than patients of general internists (Horner et al., 1995). Hence, studies of the relative effectiveness of the two types of physicians should control for severity of problems on admission. A subsequent study by the same team of researchers indicated that patients treated by neurologists had lower mortality and better functional status on discharge, but generated one-third more costs than patients of family physicians and one-fifth greater costs than patients of internists as a result of undergoing more diagnostic tests. Neurologists also were more likely to prescribe the anticoagulant warfarin, to begin early rehabilitation, and to discharge patients to inpatient rehabilitation facilities rather than nursing homes (Mitchell et al., 1996). A survey of physicians with regard to their management of patients with extracranial carotid stenosis, who are at high risk of strokes, revealed that neurologists and internists are more likely than surgeons to prescribe platelet antiaggregants or aspirin. Differences in the use of anticoagulants were even greater: Family physicians were most likely to prescribe them, followed by internists, and then neurologists (Goldstein et al., 1996).

One large study conducted in two states found that care for patients admitted by a cardiologist for acute myocardial infarction resulted in better survival on average within the following year than patients admitted by primary care physicians, after controlling for a variety of patient and hospital characteristics, although the differences were not large. As is generally the case, the disease-oriented specialist had a much higher likelihood of using cardiac procedures and medications (Jollis et al., 1996). These findings are buttressed by those of another study conducted in two states, which found that cardiologists believed more strongly in the benefit of medication therapy and were more likely to report prescribing medications for patients with acute myocardial infarction than internists and family physicians (Ayanian et al., 1994).

Competence in dealing with a problem comes not only with training but also with practice; studies have demonstrated that the frequency with which a problem is encountered is an important determinant of quality of care. Therefore, it is not surprising that subspecialists caring for patients with diagnoses that fall within the scope of their speciality generally are found to provide care of better quality for these conditions than do primary care specialists. Would subspecialists, however, want to be evaluated according to how well they deal with vague symptoms or diseases or preventive care outside the interests of their specialty? The issue is not only how primary care physicians deal with particular diseases but also how specialists perform in carrying out the functions and tasks of primary care.

One of the challenges of primary care is deciding when to refer to a subspecialist. The frequency of problems in a practice population, not the interest of subspecialists in the care of particular diseases, should be the determinant of whether the responsibility lies with a primary care physician or a specialist. Subspecialists and primary care physicians should decide jointly who should bear the responsibility for addressing certain types of problems and at what stages a referral is indicated; sometimes shared care is appropriate. These decisions may vary from area to area, as the incidence and prevalence of the problem vary.

In the United Kingdom and Spain, for example, the response to the Saint Vincent Declaration (which set target dates for reduction of complications of diabetes) reversed, through government and professional policy, the tendency of general practitioners to refer patients with noninsulin-dependent diabetes mellitus to diabetes specialists or endocrinologists. Noninsulin-dependent diabetes mellitus has been declared a primary care problem, and general practitioners are given a small financial incentive for undertaking the care of patients with it. Many general practitioner teams have set up special clinics that follow protocols for care, which involve practice nurses as well as optometrists and podiatrists. Special community-based diabetes centers set up by hospitals and serving populations of one-fourth to one-third of a million people support the general practice teams for education as well as consultation. The shift from specialty care to primary care accompanies an increasing recognition of the seriousness of this common disease and concerted efforts to improve care through shared goals rather than competition across specialty lines (Keen, 1996).

The special case of care for women

In some places, most notably in the United States, a substantial proportion of women seek the services of an obstetrician/gynecologist rather than a family physician or general internist. Certainly, many of the health concerns of women are not as directly experienced by men: family planning, unintended pregnancy, infertility, female reproductive tract infections, screening for female reproductive tract cancers, preconception risk assessment, and uncomplicated maternity care, as well as spousal sexual abuse. In the United States, about one-third of family physicians do obstetric care. Studies that have been reported show no differences in outcomes, at least for patients without serious underlying disorders.

Several studies have compared family physicians and obstetricians for care pertaining to pregnancy. Deliveries were attributed to family physicians or obstetricians according to who provided the prenatal care. Risk scores were assigned to each of the 1,942 pregnancies to explore the likelihood of differences in biological risks in the two groups of patients; none were found. Patients of family physicians had a significantly lower incidence of cesarean section, use of forceps, diagnosis of cephalopelvic disproportion, and premature births, despite a much higher percentage of women at high risk resulting from social disadvantage (Deutchman et al., 1995).

In a retrospective review of medical records at five sites across the United States, women who had been cared for by family physicians during pregnancy were less likely to receive epidural anesthesia during labor or an episiotomy during delivery and had a lower rate of cesarean section than patients who had been cared for by obstetricians, even after adjustment for other factors that could have exerted an influence. Neonatal and maternal outcomes in the two groups of women were similar (Hueston et al., 1995a, b). These findings are consistent with those of an earlier study that consisted of a retrospective, matched pair design to compare the outcomes of management of low-risk pregnancy care delivered by family physicians or obstetricians. Family physicians had lower rates of induction of labor, external and internal fetal monitoring, narcotic analgesia use, and postpartum oxytocin use. Their patients spent less time in the hospital, both during labor and postpartum (MacDonald et al., 1993).

For many other types of health needs, studies have shown that women do not receive care equivalent to men, even when the problem is the same. For example, women (and minorities) in California were significantly less likely to receive seven of the nine procedures studied, including hip replacement, pacemaker implant, endarterectomy, angioplasty, defibrillator implant, heart transplantation, and coronary artery bypass surgery, even after controlling for other characteristics that might cause the difference (Giacomini, 1996).They also are less likely to receive indicated therapy for acute myocardial infarction (McLaughlin et al., 1996).

Thus, it may be that the general unpreparedness of many primary care physicians and disease-oriented specialists to care for problems among women calls for an approach that enhances the likelihood of their receiving equivalent care for equivalent needs. A team approach, for example, may be most appropriate (see below).

Non-Physician Providers

In some situations, largely in the developing nations, primary care providers are often not physicians. They may be nurses working in the community, or pharmacists, or personnel trained specifically for a role that does not require a traditional medical education. The tasks that are required and the available resources determine the type of personnel involved (Kaprio, 1979). In industrialized nations, nonphysician personnel do not play a significant role in delivering primary care, at least as defined as the attainment of all of the unique and essential features of primary care. However, they may play an important role in improving certain aspects of primary care.

Few physicians work alone; most have at least one other individual who is not a physician who interacts with patients in the office setting. Some of these staff members merely greet patients, make their appointments, or obtain and record administrative data. Others participate in the clinical encounter by carrying out the physician's instructions, such as taking x-rays or drawing blood for laboratory tests, administering medications or immunizations, or helping the physician to perform a surgical procedure.

In some places, non-physician staff members function more independently, even seeing patients themselves under the general guidance of the physician or as a result of training directed at enabling them to perform certain functions by themselves. In some cases, the non-physician staff member performs functions that are unlikely to be performed well or with enthusiasm by physicians. For example, nurses may make home visits to help assess a patient's problem, to help a patient with a medical regimen, or to resolve some social problem that is interfering with the medical treatment.

Thus there are three types of functions for non-physician personnel. One type performs a "supplementary" function, which extends the efficiency of the physician by assuming part of the tasks, generally those that are technical in nature and usually under the direction of the physician. The second type exists when the non-physicians provide services that are often provided by physicians; they function as "substitutes." The third type of role is "complementary" wherein such personnel extend the effectiveness of physicians by doing things that physicians do not do at all, do poorly, or do reluctantly (Starfield, 1993).

Most evaluations of the roles and effectiveness of non-physician personnel as substitutes for physicians were conducted during an era when there was a perceived physician shortage and an effort to train non-physician personnel to compensate for this shortage. These evaluations were consistent in supporting a role for such personnel in primary care, although the role has never been specified precisely enough to distinguish the supplementary, the substitute, and the complementary functions. The few evaluations that have been conducted demonstrated that trained non-physician personnel could provide care for many acute and chronic conditions, as well as preventive care, at a level of quality that equaled or exceeded that provided by physicians (LeRoy, 1981; Record, 1981). There are some functions that non-physician personnel perform better than physicians: They identify more symptoms and signs in their patients and prescribe more non-drug therapies than do physicians (Simborg et al., 1978). They also perform effectively in helping patients to implement sustained and difficult regimens where therapeutic effects are often delayed (Starfield and Sharp, 1968).

A review of 155 studies concerning nurse practitioners conducted in Canada and the United States (Canadian Medical Association, 1995) found only a handful that were considered methodologically sound and achieved results for a sufficiently broad sample of practices to be considered generally applicable. Relatively consistent findings were that employment of nurse-practitioners or physician assistants in primary care provided the potential for an increase in practice size, with no adverse impact on quality of care or overall costs. Time spent by such practitioners was much greater than time spent by physicians; about one-third of patients were referred to the physician for some aspect of care (Scherer, 1977). Thus, it might be inferred that these practitioners could make a considerable contribution to primary care particularly in areas where there are not enough primary care physicians to provide needed services.

Unfortunately, no studies have examined the potential of non-physician practitioners to carry out or contribute to the functions of primary care. In theory, it might be inferred that such practitioners could enhance the delivery of its four features. First contact could be enhanced if increased availability of services led people to increase their seeking of care from primary care rather than from emergency services or hospital outpatient units. Longitudinality could be improved for at least some patients if a personal relationship is established more easily than with the physician. Contributions to comprehensiveness could accrue if these practitioners complement the current focus of physician-provided services. As coordinators of care, nurse-practitioners may be superior to physicians. However, the one study that examines recognition of information about patients that was generated outside the primary care facility indicated that nurses functioned equally poorly to physicians (Simborg et al., 1978).

It is apparent that the literature does not strongly support a substitute role for nurse-practitioners or physician assistants, at least as long as primary care physicians are willing to undertake to provide such services. However, primary care probably could not function well without the participation of non-physician practitioners functioning either in supplementary or complementary roles. An extensive review of the potential role of "physician assistants" in the United States, who are in a separate category than nurse-practitioners, revealed that such professionals are, at least until recently, increasingly employed in institutional and inpatient settings rather than in primary care for which they were originally intended. Even when employed in outpatient settings, they are more likely to be working with medical and surgical specialist physicians than with primary care physicians. Studies show that task delegation and supervision of physicians is a major determinant of physician assistant productivity; the roles of the physician assistant are clearly more in the area of supplementation rather than substitution or complementarity (Jones and Cawley, 1994).

Little is known about the extent to which health services or outcomes of care are improved by teamwork or under what conditions teams function most effectively. The next section addresses this issue.

The Team in Primary Care Practice

Support for "team practice" in primary care is widespread, particularly in the United Kingdom, where primary care practice is most highly developed. In that country as well as many others (e.g., Finland, Spain, Portugal), teamwork is actively encouraged by national policy, which even provides additional financial support for it (Pearson and Spencer, 1995). Composition of the primary care team varies. General practitioners, practice nurses, and community nursing staff (many of whom also have social work training) are invariably included; midwives and pharmacists, who usually work in the community but outside the practice, are often but not always included. Relationships with community-based mental health care teams and with social care workers have been less clearly defined.

A framework (Table 5.1) for considering the operation of the team could help to characterize the potential as well as the actual contributions of team workers and facilitate evaluation of their effectiveness in contributing to improved effectiveness and efficiency of services. This framework poses three models of teamwork:

Table 5.1. Three Types of Teams

Delegated Model	*Collaborator Model*	*Clinical Consultative Model*
Has team leader	No team leader	No pre-specified team leader
Splits tasks (complementary and supplementary roles)	Shared tasks (substitute roles)	Role defined by clinical area (variable across sites and settings depending on mix of personnel interests and skills
Responsibility for primary care functions assumed by team leader	Each member focused on all primary care functions	Assumption of responsibilities for primary care functions unclear and unstable (similar to disease management)
Financial role assumed by team leader	Financial risk shared	Tendency toward clinical specialization predisposing to hierarchy
Clear locus of legal responsibility (team leader)	Locus of legal responsibility is team Longitudinality and coordination functions require special attention Allows choice by patient of primary practitioner	Locus of legal responsibility unclear

the Delegated model, the Collaborative model, and the Clinical Consultative model. Probably the most common is the Delegated model in which the physician is the team "leader." Roles are defined according to tasks that need to be performed; tasks are relatively formally split so that the non-physicians are assigned a largely supplementary role (although some tasks may be complementary) , and primary care functions as well as financial responsibility are assumed by the team leader. In this model, legal responsibility is clearly the physician's.

The second model is Collaborative. There is no designated leader. Tasks are shared; each member of the team focuses on primary care functions. Both financial risks and legal responsibility are shared. There is, however, an agreed-upon "key worker" (Stott, 1995), who might be any member of the team, for individual patients; this person would serve as the locus of personal longitudinality for these patients (Freeman and Hjortdahl, 1997). Thus, each member of the practice population would choose the individual most suited by virtue of interests and interpersonal skills to the patient's own expectations. This model forms the basis for health services delivered in many community health centers, such as the CLSC (Centre Locaux de Services Communautaires) in Quebec, and in at least some HMOs (particularly group and staff model) in the United States. This type of model may be especially appropriate for women's health care.

The third model is the Clinical Consultative. Roles are nonstandard and vary from site to site depending on the personal interests and skills of team members who decide to affiliate. This model fosters clinical subspecialization, with the individual specialists functioning to provide care for problems in their area of interest regardless of whether those problems actually require the services of the subspecialist. The model may tend toward greater hierarchy over time as one specialist becomes dominant over another, as through providing services that command more resources. The assumption of responsibility for the four primary care functions is unclear and unstable, similar to the situation under disease case-management schemes (see chapter 8). The locus of both financial and legal responsibility also may be unclear.

The growth in use of alternative medicine clinicians (such as chiropractors, naturopaths, and practitioners of Oriental medicine) as well as traditional non-physician clinicians who practice in fields overlapping those of physicians (such as podiatrists, psychologists, optometrists, and midwives) may make the third model increasingly common. Furthermore, government policy in many places (including Medicare in the United States and Medicaid in many states) allows reimbursement specifically for some of these types of practitioners. Health plans in the United States are offering increased access to these clinicians (Cooper and Stoflet, 1996).

A special case of "teamwork" is found in disease management clinics that are part of primary care practices. For example, six general practices in the south of London, England, used a randomized controlled trial in which adult patients with epilepsy were assigned to a nurse-run clinic, whereas the others continued with their physician care. The nurse-run clinics took place in the physician's own practice under defined protocols of activity. An initial and 3 month follow-up visit were held, and patients were sent a questionnaire after 6 months. Better management of appropriate blood levels of medication were achieved in the nurse-run clinics, which often resulted in a change in management that had been previously set by the physician (Ridsdale et al., 1997). Thus, in this example of teamwork, the different professionals who are involved complement each other's particular skills.

Effective teamwork is not easy to achieve. The most salient of the problems is the challenge to the communication and information transfer that is needed for coordination of care. The number of lines of communication required is nonlinear and described by the equation $(n^2 - n) \div 2$, where n = the number of team members (Stott, 1995). A rule of thumb is that decision-making is optimal with six team members; teamwork is highly unlikely with more than 12 members (Stott, 1993).

Although the initial impetus for teamwork (at least in the United States) was to stretch the potential of primary care physicians who were in short supply, other imperatives are now at the forefront. An aging population and an increase in illnesses that last longer or recur more frequently have created the need for a primary care approach that is broader. It is meeting these two new needs as well as improving the provision of primary care that will sustain the movement toward teamwork everywhere.

Implications: The Training of Primary Care Physicians

Primary care should be provided by clinicians best trained and most skilled in its practice. The evidence summarized in this and in Chapters 7 through 11 indicates that family physicians, general internists, and pediatricians are more effective and more efficient in providing the functions of primary care than are specialists. Whether this superiority will continue depends on the ability of all primary care physicians to respond to the challenges posed by changes in illness patterns and to use new technology appropriately to prevent, cure, or ameliorate illness. With improvements in survival, the complexity of illness will increase. Illnesses with multisystem manifestations and multifactorial etiology will change the ways in which practitioners deal with patients' needs and how they relate to the community.

The primary care physicians of the future will become medical managers and team collaborators to a much greater extent than in the past. This will require skills in resource allocation, integration and coordination, and performance monitoring and quality assurance. Home care services will become more important, not for purposes of management of acute illness, but rather for the appropriate assessment of social factors complicating diagnosis and management and for the care of patients who are home-bound as a result of a functional disability. Advances in information technology can assist in diagnosis and in management. They can also provide a better mechanism to obtain advice from consultants as well as to coordinate care. The skills to adapt and use these systems for primary care will have to be developed. Clinical epidemiology, decision-making, economics, and training in the social and behavioral sciences related to health and health care will become part of the basic armamentarium in the education of the primary care physician. The success of primary care depends on the adoption by society of the importance of primary care and mechanisms for its improvement as central in its health policies for primary care training and delivery.

References

Aiken L, Lewis C, Craig J, Mendenhall R, Blendon R, Rogers D. The contribution of specialists to the delivery of primary care: A new perspective. N Engl J Med 1979; 300: 1363–70.

Ayanian JZ, Hauptman PJ, Guadagnoli E, Antman EM, Pashos CL, McLeil BJ. Knowledge and practices of generalist and specialist physicians regarding drug therapy for acute myocardial infarction. N Engl J Med 1994; 331(17):1136–42.

Bennett MD, Applegate WB, Chilton LA, Skipper BJ, White RE. Comparison of family medicine and internal medicine: Charges for continuing ambulatory care. Med Care 1983; 21(8):830–9.

Bertakis K, Robbins J. Gatekeepers in primary care: A comparison of internal medicine and family practice. J Fam Pract 1987; 24:305–9.

Bowman MA. The quality of care provided by family physicians. J Fam Pract 1989; 28(3): 346–55.

Brook R, Williams K. Evaluation of the New Mexico peer review system 1971 to 1973. Med Care 1976; a4(suppl):1–122.

Canadian Medical Association. Cost-Effectiveness of Primary Health Care Providers: A Systematic Review. Working Paper (95-04). Ottawa: Canadian Medical Association, April 25, 1995.

Carey TS, Garrett J, Jackman A, McLaughlin C, Fryer J, Smucker DR (and the North

Carolina Back Pain Project). The outcomes and costs of care for acute low back pain among patients seen by primary care practitioners, chiropractors, and orthopedic surgeons. N Engl J Med 1995; 339(14):913–7.

Cherkin DC, Hart G, Rosenblatt RA. Patient satisfaction with family physicians and general internists: Is there a difference? J Fam Pract 1988; 26(5):543–51.

Cherkin DC, Rosenblatt RA, Hart LG, Schneeweiss R, LeGerfo J. The use of medical resources by residency-trained family physicians and general internists. Med Care 1987; 25(6):455–69.

Cloher TP, Whelton MD. Physician approach to the recognition and initial management of hypertension. Arch Intern Med 1986; 146:529–33.

Cooper RA, Stoflet SJ. Trends in the education and practice of alternative medicine clinicians. Health Aff 1996; 15(3):226–38.

Deutchman M, Sills D, Connor PD. Perinatal outcomes: A comparison between family physicians and obstetricians. J Am Board Fam Pract 1995; 8:440–7.

Eisenberg J. Doctors' Decisions and The Cost of Medical Care. Ann Arbor, MI: Health Administration Press Perspectives, 1986.

Engel W, Freund D, Stein J, Fletcher R. The treatment of patients with asthma by specialists and generalist. Med Care 1989; 27:306–14.

Farrell Dl, Worth RM, Mishina K. Utilization and cost effectiveness of a family practice center. J Fam Pract 1982; 15(5):957–62.

Ferris T, Saglam D, Stafford R, Causino N, Starfield B, Culpepper L, Blumenthal D. Changes in the daily practice of primary care for children. Arch Pediatr Adolesc Med 1998; 152:227–33.

Fishbane M, Starfield B. Child health care in the United States: A comparison of pediatricians and general practitioners. N Engl J Med 1981; 305:552–6.

Franks P, Dickinson JC. Comparisons of family physicians and internists: Process and outcome in adult patients at a community hospital. Med Care 1986; 24:941–8.

Freeman G, Hjortdahl P. What future for continuity of care in general practice? BMJ 1997; 314:1870–3.

Fry J, Horder J. Primary Health Care in an International Context. London: The Nuffield Provincial Hospital Trust, 1994.

Giacomini MK. Gender and ethnic differences in hospital-based procedures utilization in California. Arch Intern Med 1996; 156:1217–24.

Goldstein L, Bonito AJ, Matchar DB, Duncan PW, Samsa GP. U.S. national survey of physician practices for the secondary and tertiary prevention of ischemic stroke. Stroke 1996; 27(9):1473–8.

Greenfield S, Nelson EC, Zubkoff M, Manning W, Rogers W, Kravitz RL, Keller A, Tarlov AR, Ware JE Jr. Variations in resource utilization among medical specialties and systems of care. Results from the medical outcomes study. JAMA. 1992; 267(12):1624–30.

Greenfield S, Rogers W, Mangotich M, Carney M, Tarlov A. Outcomes of patients with hypertension and non-insulin–dependent diabetes mellitus treated by different systems and specialities. Results from the medical outcomes study. JAMA 1995; 274(18):1436–44.

Hainer BJ, Lawler FH. Comparison of critical care provided by family physicians and general internists. JAMA 1988; 260(3):354–8 .

Hamburger S, Barjenbruch P, Soffer A. Treatment of diabetic ketoacidosis by internists and family physicians: A comparative study. J Fam Pract 1982; 14(4):719–22.

Hirth RA, Fendrick AM, Chernew ME. Specialist and generalist physicians' adoption of antibiotic therapy to eradicate *Helicobacter pylori* infection. Med Care 1996; 34(12)1199–204.

Horner RD, Matchar DB, Divine GW, Feussner JR. Relationship between physician specialty and the selection and outcome of ischemic stroke patients. Health Serv Res 1995; 30(2): 275–87.

Hueston WJ, Applegate JA, Mansfield CJ, King DE, McClaflin RR. Practice variations between family physicians and obstetricians in the management of low-risk pregnancies. J Fam Pract 1995a; 40:345–51.

Hueston WJ, Rudy M. Differences in labor and delivery experience in family physician- and obstetrician-supervised teaching services. Fam Med 1995b; 27(3):182–7.

Hulka BS, Kupper LL, Cassel JC. Physician management in primary care. Am J Public Health 1976; 66(12):1173–9.

Joffe A, Radius S, Gall M. Health counseling for adolescents: What they want, what they get, and who gives it. Pediatrics 1988; 82:481–5.

Jones E, Cawley J. Physician assistants and health system reform. JAMA 1994; 271:1266–72.

Jollis JG, DeLong ER, Peterson ED, Muhlbaier LH, Fortin DF, Califf RM, Mark DB. Outcomes of acute myocardial infarction according to the specialty of the admitting physician. N Engl J Med 1996; 335(25):1880–7.

Kahnemann D, Slovig P, Tversky A. Judgement Under Uncertainty: Heuristics and Biases. Cambridge: Cambridge University Press, 1982.

Kaprio L. Primary Health Care in Europe. Copenhagen: Regional Office for Europe. World Health Organization, 1979.

Keen H. Management of non-insulin–dependent diabetes mellitus. The United Kingdom experience. Ann Intern Med 1996; 123(1 pt 2):156–9.

Kessler L, Amick B, Thompson J. Factors influencing the diagnosis of mental disorder among primary care patients. Med Care 1985; 23:50–62.

Kohn R, White KL. Health Care: An International Study. London: Oxford University Press, 1976.

Kramer MS, Arsenault L, Pless IB. The use of preventable adverse outcomes to study the quality of child health care. Med Care 1984; 22(3):223–30.

Leduc DG, Pless IB. Pediatricians and general practitioners: A comparison of the management of children with febrile illness. Pediatrics 1982; 70(4):511–5.

LeRoy L. The costs and effectiveness of nurse practitioners. Case Study 16. Washington, DC: U.S. Congress, Office of Technology Assessment, 1981.

MacDonald SE, Voaklander K, Birtwhistle RV. A comparison of family physicians' and obstetricians' intrapartum management of low-risk pregnancies. J Fam Pract 1993; 37: 457–2.

McCann KP, Bowman MA, Davis SW. Morbidity, mortality, and charges for hospital care of the elderly: A comparison of internists' and family physicians' admissions. J Fam Pract 1995; 40(5):443–8.

McLaughlin TJ, Soumerai SB, Willison DJ, Gurwitz JH, Borbas C, Guadagnoli E, McLaughlin B, Morris N, Cheng SU, Hauptman P, Antman E, Casey L, Asinger R, Gobel F. Adherence to national guidelines for drug treatment of suspected acute myocardial infraction: Evidence for under treatment in women and the elderly. Arch Intern Med 1996; 156(7):799–805.

Mitchell JB, Ballard DJ, Whisnant JP, Ammering CJ, Samsa GP, Matchar DB. What role do neurologists play in determining the costs and outcomes of stroke patients. Stroke 1996; 27(11):1937–43.

Moore G. The case of the disappearing generalist: Does it need to be solved? Milbank Q 1992; 70(2):361–79.

Noren J, Frazier T, Altman I, DeLozier J. Ambulatory medical care: A comparison of internists and family-general practitioners. N Engl J Med 1980; 301(1):11–6.

Palmer RH, Reilly M. Individual and institutional variables which may serve as indicators of quality of medical care. Med Care 1979; 18:693–717.

Payne B, Lyons T, Newhaus E. Relationships of physician characteristics to performance quality and improvement. Health Serv Res 1984; 19:307–32.

Pearson P, Spencer J. Pointers to effective teamwork: exploring primary care. J Interprofessional Care 1995; 9(2):131–38.

Petitti DB, Grumbach K. Variation in physicians' recommendations about revisit interval for three common conditions. J Fam Pract 1993; 37(3):235–40.

Rauber A, Maroncelli R. Prescribing practices and knowledge of tricyclic antidepressants among physicians caring for children. Pediatrics 1984; 73(1):107–9.

Record J. Staffing Primary Care in 1990. New York: Springer, 1981.

Ridsdale L, Robins D, Cryer C, Williams H. Feasibility and effects of nurse run clinics for patients with epilepsy in general practice; randomized controlled trial . BMJ 1997; 314: 120–2.

San Agustin M, Siedel VW, Drosness DL, Kelman H, Levine H, Stevens E. A controlled clinical trial of "family care" compared with "child only care" in the comprehensive primary care of children. Med Care 1982; 19(2):202–22.

Scherer K, Fortin F, Spitzer WO, Kergin DJ. Nurse practitioners in primary care. VII. A cohort study of 99 nurses and 79 associated physicians. Can Med Assoc J 1977; 116(8): 856–62.

Scherger JE, Gordon MJ, Phillips TJ, LoGerfo JP. Comparison of diagnostic methods of family practice and internal medicine residents. J Fam Pract 1980; 10(1):95–101.

Schwartz R, Freij BJ, Ziai M, Sheridan MJ. Antimicrobial prescribing for acute purulent rhinitis in children: A survey of pediatricians and family practitioners. Pediatr Infect Dis J 1997; 16(2):185–90.

Selby J, Grumbach K, Quesenberry C, Schmittdiel J, Truman A. Differences in patterns and costs of primary care in a large HMO according to physician specialty. Manuscript submitted, 1998.

Simborg D, Starfield B, Horn S. Physicians and non-physician health practitioners: The characteristics of their practice and their relationships. Am J Public Health 1978; 68: 44–8.

Smilkstein G. The family in family medicine revisited, again. J Fam Pract 1994; 39:527–31.

Smith DH, McWhinney IR. Comparison of the diagnostic methods of family physicians and internists. J Med Educ 1975; 50:264–70.

Sobal J, Muncie Jr HI, Valente CM, Levine DM, DeForge BR. Self-reported referral patterns in practices of family/general practitioners, internists, and obstetricians/gynecologists. J Community Health 1988; 13(3):171.

Starfield B. Roles and functions of non-physician practitioners in primary care. In: Clawson D, Osterweis M (eds): The Roles of Physician Assistants and Nurse Practitioners. Washington, D.C.: Association of Academic Health Centers, 1993, pp. 11–20.

Starfield B, Sharp E. Ambulatory pediatric care: The role of the nurse. Med Care 1968; VI: 507–15.

Starfield B, Hoekelman RA, McCormick M, Mendenhall RD, Moynihan C, Benson P, DeChant H. Styles of care provided to children in the United States: A comparison by physician specialty. J Fam Pract 1985; 21(2):133–8.

Stott NC. William Pickles Lecture 1993. When something is good, more of the same is not always better. Br J Gen Pract 1993; 43(371):254–8.

Stott NCH. Personal care and teamwork: Implications for the general practice-based primary health care team. J Interprofessional Care 1995; 9(2):95–9.

Strauss MJ, Conrad D, LoGerfo JP, Hudson LD, Bergner M. Cost and outcome of care for patients with chronic obstructive lung disease. Med Care 1986; 24(10):915–24.

Szilagyi P G, Rodewald LE, Humiston SG, Hager J, Roghmann KJ, Doane C, Cove L, Gleming GV, Hall CB. Immunization practices of pediatricians and family physicians in the United States. Pediatrics 1994; 94(4):517–23.

Thompson H, Osborne C. Office records in the evaluation of quality of care. Med Care 1976; XIV:294–314.

Wachter R, Goldman L. The emerging role of the "hospitalist" in the American health care system. N Engl J Med 1996; 335:514–7.

Weese CB, Krauss MR. A "barrier-free" health care system does not ensure adequate vaccination of 2-year-old children. Arch Pediatr Adolesc Med 1995; 149:1130–5.

Winkenwerder W, Levy BD, Eisenberg JM, Williams SV, Young MJ, Hershey JC. Variation in physicians' decision-making thresholds in management of a sexually transmitted disease. J Gen Intern Med 1993; 8(7):369–73.

— 6 —

Primary Care in the Context of Health Systems

In a talk at a major professional meeting, a colleague who was asked to speculate about how medical care would be organized five years hence replied that he wasn't sure what it would be like when he returned to his office that afternoon!

Reported by JK (1997)

Many different characteristics determine the way that health service systems appear and how they operate. The multiplicity of these characteristics provides the opportunity for innumerable permutations and combinations, so that no two health systems look alike or perform in the same way. This is the case when countries are compared as well as when subsystems within countries are examined. Nevertheless, all health service systems face similar challenges: to provide health services in an effective, efficient, and equitable manner.

Rapidly accumulating knowledge about the determinants of health and development of complex technology are leading to a heightened capacity to detect and manage disease, to prevent illness, and to promote health, even in the face of changing demographic profiles such as aging of populations and changing patterns of disease and risks of disease. All countries are facing the imperative to alter their health systems to better meet these challenges without bankrupting their economies by expenditures on health services.

Thus, health care reform involving major changes in the characteristics of health service systems are underway in many countries. Some of these changes are truly innovative; others are modifications based on experiences elsewhere. This chapter considers the basic features of health care systems, the major approaches that are being taken to reform them, the likely impact of these reforms on primary care, and the special case of "managed care." Because there is a trend toward convergence of certain characteristics of health systems, this discussion will take advantage of an international literature derived primarily from the experiences of western industrialized nations.

101

Types of Health Services Systems

The major defining features of health service systems in the most recent century consist of the types of health insurance coverage, the characteristics of the insurer (government, government-regulated private, and largely private organizations), and the mechanisms and types of reimbursement to practitioners (Organization for Economic Cooperation and Development, 1992). Practitioners (health professionals) may be paid directly by patients (with reimbursement to the patient for services covered by insurance) or by the insurer, either in full or in part in both cases. Three major types of payment are salary (fixed compensation paid regularly), capitation (fixed payment per individual identified as eligible for care), or a fee for each service, set according to what is usual and customary in the community, negotiated with professional groups based on relative costs of the services or skills required or based on historical charges (Table 6.1). In the early parts of the twentieth century, fee-for-service dominated as the method of reimbursement; with the passage of time, this form of payment has diminished everywhere. Countries have always differed, however, in the commitment of government to involvement in financing and organization of health services.

Figure 6.1 shows the large number of possibilities for financing primary care services. The letters A–F characterize the payers. Governments may pay practitioners directly, with funds obtained from taxes (A) or from designated social security funds (B), as in the case of the Medicare fund, built from employer–employee contributions. Employer–employee contributions may also be paid into a nongovernmental and nonprofit fund (C), often called a "sick-fund"; these are usually heavily regulated by governments. Alternatively, employer–employee contributions may be paid to a for-profit private insurance company (D), such as is commonly the case in the United States. Individuals themselves sometimes pay for services (F) (particularly when their basic insurance does not cover all services or when there is a co-payment) and sometimes purchase insurance from insurance companies; the latter generally is to supplement coverage obtained through other

Table 6.1. Three Methods of Payment

Fee-for-Service: Practitioners are reimbursed for each service or procedure provided to patients. The more the services and the greater the number and complexity of services, the higher the payment. Sometimes patients must pay the physician at the time of service or in response to subsequent billing. The patient may be reimbursed by insurance companies (indemnity plans). In other arrangements, physicians may be paid directly by insurance companies or by governmental agencies

Salary: In this method of payment, physicians receive a fixed sum of money based on the amount of time they devote to their professional work.

Capitation: In this method of payment, practitioners are paid according to the number of patients assigned to receive services from them. With this form of remuneration, patients must be enrolled for a defined period of time, which may vary from 1 month to 1 year. Practitioners can receive no more than a set sum of money for providing services unless the insuring or managing agents provide for added payments under predetermined circumstances or for services they wish to encourage.

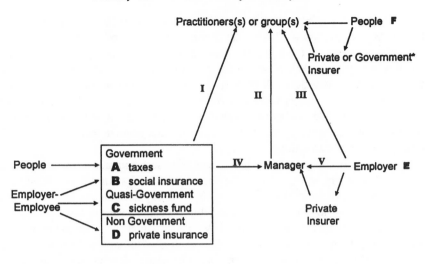

Figure 6.1. Financing and reimbursement for primary care services.

Examples from Different Countries*

United States
  Medicaid   **A** I a, **A** I c, A (IVc II a,b,c)
  Medicare (Part B)   **A** I a, **A** IV c, II a,b,c
  Community Health Ctrs **A** I b
  Managed Care   **D** (IV a,c; II a,b,c); **E** (Va,c II a,b,c); **E** (III a b c)
United Kingdom   **A** I c
Spain   **A** I b
Netherlands   **C** I c
Germany   **C** (IV c II a)
France   **C** I a
Finland   **A** I b
Denmark   **A** I c
Canada   **A** I a
Australia   **A** I a
Everywhere (Private Insurance) **F** a

Legend
I-V *See Figure Above*
Reimbursement
  a *fee-for-service*
  b *salary*
  c *capitation*

* In almost every country, additional, combination, and even some experimental forms exist, e.g. employer-employee contributions to the purchase of private insurance (D I a); premium contributions by people covering about 25% of Medicare Part B charges (Path F).

mechanisms. Employers themselves (E) may be the financers of health services either to practitioners directly or through private insurance companies.

Until recently, payers either paid for services directly (by hiring and managing the clinical facilities themselves) or paid independent practitioners to organize services (path I). The former was common in countries in which the government both paid for and provided the services. The introduction of another tier, interposed between payers and practitioners, has become common in many places and is known as *managed care*. Government, nongovernment agencies (path IV) , and employers themselves (path V) may pay organizations, whose function is to pay practitioners (path II). When employers themselves pay for health services for their employees, they may do so directly (path III) or through private insurance companies or management organizations (path V). The mechanism by which practitioners are paid need not bear any relationship to the mode of financing; fee-for-service reimbursement, capitation, or salary may characterize most if not all of the different financing arrangements.

The bottom of Figure 6.1 characterizes the most common form of financing and reimbursement arrangement in several different Western industrialized countries, at least as of the mid-1990s, using the Pathway designation. Each country is characterized by the main form of financing arrangement (A–E), whether practitioners are paid directly or indirectly (I–V), and whether the most common mechanism of payment is by fee-for-service, capitation, or salary (a–c). In many cases, there are different arrangements even within countries, depending on the place or circumstances.

Types of Health Care Reform

Approaches to health care reform are as diverse as the possibilities presented by the different characteristics of the health services system. Health care reforms, although they may be catalogued in diverse ways (Office of Economic Cooperation and Development, 1996; Defever, 1995; Etheredge et al., 1996), are of two main types: demand-side approaches and supply-side approaches. The former depend on instituting disincentives to seeking services whereas the latter limit the resources that are made available to support a system of services.

Demand-side approaches

Many countries have or are considering user charges and other barriers to care. User charges take the form of deductibles (wherein the first defined amount of payment in a year is assumed by the patient) or co-payments (wherein a certain proportion or certain dollar amount of the charges for services provided are paid by the patient). Deductibles are particularly regressive. They constitute a major barrier to access to care for low income individuals and are not used or are used very minimally in most Western industrialized countries (except for Switzerland and the United States) (Organization for Economic Cooperation and Development, 1995). In some places, co-payments are imposed, or are higher, only for some services. Such is the case in the point-of-service option of many health care plans in the United States: requirements for payment by the patient are greater if the individual chooses to seek care from a physician or facility not affiliated with the health plan in which the patient is enrolled. Other barriers designed to decrease demand for services include organizational characteristics, such as making facilities less accessible; usually these take the form of requiring appointments for acute care services, increasing waiting times for appointments, or reducing the number of telephone lines available for making appointments quickly. Barriers in the latter category are generally instituted by individual health plans or facilities rather than through large-scale policy decisions. Co-payments, however, are increasingly being adopted by policy-makers as a way of reducing demand for primary care services. As of 1995, the only Organization for Economic Cooperation and Development countries that did not have co-payments for primary care services were Germany, the United Kingdom, Canada, Greece, Spain, and Turkey (Organization for Economic Cooperation and Development, 1995). In the United Kingdom, general practitioners have gone on record as opposing cost-sharing for their services.

Supply-side approaches

In supply-side approaches, policy decisions are intended to change incentives to provide services.

Global caps. During the 1980s and early 1990s, global budget caps were instituted in many countries to reduce the increasing rate of growth of health expenditures. In some countries these caps were instituted at the national level; negotiations for reimbursement for services or contracts for providing services have to fit within the set global budget. In other places, these budgets are set at local levels (in the case of services that are budgeted by region) or at the health plan level. Since these budgets have to cover all services (not only primary care services), they are likely to affect all levels of health services, although not necessarily equally.

Physician reimbursement strategies. In the most recent 50 years, forms of payment other than fee-for-service have been used in different countries and even within countries in different types of organizations. Commonly, specialists have been paid by salary, particularly in places where they primarily work in hospitals. Payment by fee-for-service encourages the performance of tests and procedures, as well as the use of services through shorter waiting lists, and return for follow up. Capitation discourages the use of unnecessary tests and procedures (but runs the risk of underservice relative to patients' needs). However, it facilitates the establishment of good relationships with patients (because there is an implied contract between physicians and their panel of patients) and encourages early care to avoid the later expenditure of more resources. Salary tends to remove incentives for productivity. Moreover, because it implies an employer–employee relationship between the payer of the salary and the physician, it predisposes to a bureaucratic structure within the health services system. Without other compensating incentives, it also lacks the constructive elements of competition to produce better services. It does, however, remove any financial incentives to provide excess services or to underprovide services.

Scott and Hall (1995) reviewed 18 studies concerning remuneration of primary care physicians; seven of the studies evaluated the impact of different modes of reimbursement on physician behavior, taking quality of the study into consideration. (The remaining 11 concerned differences in level of reimbursement.) Despite differences in study design, the evaluations were consistent in showing an increased use of all types of services (number of office visits and home visits, laboratory tests) with change from capitation to fee-for-services reimbursement. None of the studies, however, examined the impact of patient characteristics on the nature of the effect or the impact of the change on aspects of patients' health.

Although common in some countries for decades, capitation has taken on a wider life in other places, primarily for the payment of primary care physicians. (Specialists are generally paid by salary in most countries, where they work primarily in hospitals and under the hospital's budget.) Recent changes in the United States have led to rapid increases in the proportion of primary care physicians who are paid by capitation and by salary (as employees of large corporate health care organizations rather than the government, as in the United Kingdom). In an attempt to find a compromise between the relative advantages and disadvantages of the different payment modes, many countries and health care organizations are combining them in different circumstances. For example, where capitation is the mode, incentives may be provided through fee-for-service, for care of conditions that tend to be neglected, or for accomplishing preventive care objectives. More extensive "experiments" (usually without formal evaluation) are underway in many places, including novel schemes such as resumption of fee-for-service for primary care physicians (to discourage their referral of patients to specialists) and assumption of capitation for other specialists (to reduce the tendency to order tests and carry out procedures).

"Management" of care by physicians. Even in countries where primary care physicians have served as the link to other specialty services, there has been little control over either costs of care or the nature of care provided because, once patients are referred, the primary care physician has little influence on content or extent of care provided. In many places, this situation is changing. A typical example of this is "fund holding," wherein general practitioners in the United Kingdom are given budgets to pay for services (except for those covered by special incentive payments). These primary care practitioners then contract for services to be provided by other specialists. Because hospitals no longer receive completely open-ended budgets, the payments made by general practitioners are important to the hospitals and to the specialists who work within them; competition for general practitioner contracts is intended to both improve care and to decrease overall costs of care. In the United States, where there has been little historical experience with having the primary care physician act as a filter to specialty care, except for staff or group model organizations where they have been paid either by salary or capitation, this form of physician control is relatively new and most often combined with managerial control to ensure that these physicians maintain a relatively low rate of referral.

Management of physicians by managers. A range of options are available to managers whose aim is control of health practitioner behavior. As a result of improved (and often electronic) data collection, it is possible to profile the practice of physicians and to compare them with each other to determine rates of use of various types of services (visits per patient or per time; laboratory tests per patient or per illness episode; referral rates per patient population, per patient, or per illness) and costs of services in different categories or total. Physicians who appear to be outliers may not have their contracts renewed, or they may have their earnings reduced for failure to reach pre-set targets. Alternatively, they may be rewarded for keeping utilization or costs low among the patients for whom they have responsibility; these rewards may take various forms, including sharing in the profits accumulated by profit-generating managed care organizations. (Note: The European Union forbids such profit-making schemes in its member countries.) Another form of control is the imposition of guidelines for practice. When these guidelines are based on appropriate evidence of effectiveness, they may improve practice (although not necessarily decrease its cost). When based on inappropriate or inadequate evidence, they become mere agents of control over physician discretion and judgment.

Restrictions on scope of practice. In some places, practitioners are restricted from managing certain kinds of conditions and problems experienced by their patients. In some cases, this is a result of limitations in the kinds of problems covered by the patient's insurance; in others, the restriction is a result of "carve outs" by the health plan or organization. In the United States, for example, it is common for certain types of problems to be financed separately, usually by capitation, and managed by a group of practitioners (often non-physicians) who are completely separate from the primary care practitioner. Although this is most common in the case of mental and behavioral problems, it is also increasingly common for certain common chronic conditions such as asthma and diabetes.

There are a number of trends in the organization and financing that appear to be common throughout western industrialized nations, if not in the world in general (Defever, 1995). Among them is a trend toward making competition more operative in health services. Under competition, practitioners and practice organizations are less subject to public regulation in deciding how they will provide services and with whom. In many countries, practice organizations are provided with a defined level of funding (sometimes including deprivation allowances to compensate for the increased costs of elderly, poor, or sicker populations) and charged with the responsibility to provide services. Purchasers of services (patients or, more commonly, agents of people or employers) are then free to choose practitioners or practice organizations whose characteristics are most to their liking.

Another pervasive trend is privatization. Many countries that formerly relied on government to provide services at least to some segments of the population are now turning to private organizations and contracting for the provision of services. These approaches are intended to decrease bureaucratization and increase the likelihood of responsiveness to consumers. However, lower costs (a key rationale for competition) have often not materialized in the case of health services, largely because the market often imposes its own demands on competitors, with a resulting increase in the costs of care (Defever, 1995).

A third trend consists of the imposition of a management structure between the payer and the practitioner of health services. Although intended to reduce costs by means of stimulating innovation and monitoring unnecessary utilization of services, an increase in nonmedical management has its own costs that often more than compensate for the intended reductions. Large amounts of documentation are required for the micromanagement of utilization; the costs of both obtaining (from practitioners) and analyzing and maintaining information systems can be considerable (Defever, 1995).

Increased decentralization to regions is also a feature of many health system reforms. It is especially strong where tax funds from central governments (as in Denmark, Finland, Norway, Spain, and Sweden) or from public insurers (as in Germany, the Netherlands, and Switzerland) flow to regional governments. In some of these countries (Finland and Spain), the region both pays for and organizes the primary care services, whereas in others the services are provided separately (Germany) or there is experimentation with contracting separately for them (such as in Denmark, Sweden, the United Kingdom, and Catalonia, Spain (Gérvas, 1996).

Some of these aspects of reform strengthen the position of the primary care practitioner. Others, however, weaken various aspects of primary care practice and compromise the achievement of some or all of the cardinal features of primary care.

Health Care Reform And Managed Care

Managed care is an attempt to control costs and the provision of services by means of an array of externally imposed incentives and disincentives designed to alter utilization of services. Although initially imposed most selectively on the primary care sector of health services systems, it has indirect effects on other levels of the health system through its effect on primary care. Thus, health care reform and managed care have led to new types of linkages among the different levels of health systems, with a general thrust toward greater integration among them. Four types of models are found in different degrees in different places. Integrated health enterprises, which are becoming common in the private sector in the United States, pull together insurance and health care delivery under one aegis. Thus, they replicate the older government-financed and government-operated health systems (as were common in health systems of socialist countries), but this time under private aegis. Integrated delivery systems, which are less formal arrangements, generally involve contracts between different levels of the health system (such as primary care physician services, other specialty services, and hospital care) under joint management rather than joint ownership. Linkages between teaching hospitals and health maintenance organizations (or physician groups) in the United States can form integrated health systems. Little is known about the way in which they operate, their permanence in a shifting health system, or their impact on costs or quality of care. An even less formal mechanism of integration consists of improving the mechanism for achieving information flow and coordination within primary care as part of a management structure.

> That any sane nation, having observed that you could provide for the supply of
> bread by giving bakers a pecuniary interest in baking for you, should go on to give

a surgeon a pecuniary interest in cutting off your leg, is enough to despair of political
humanity.   George Bernard Shaw (1911)

Reform efforts in many countries of the world long ago did away with the
pecuniary interests of physicians who stood to gain from performing as many procedures as possible, even inappropriate ones. Even in the United States, where fee-
for-service practice lasted longer than elsewhere in the Western industrialized
world, this aspect of "profit" is on its way out only to be replaced by a corporate
health system management structure based on private gain rather than community
health improvement. Among its Western industrialized nation peers, the United
States remains the only country that still lacks assurance of financial coverage for
all of its citizens.

Organizational arrangements that are assuming increasing importance elsewhere
have had their protypes in the United States. These are characterized by various
combinations and permutations of organizational format and reimbursement. The
conventional typology divides these combinations into three major types: health
maintenance organizations (HMOs), preferred provider organizations (PPOs), and
managed indemnity plans (MIPs). The following section describes these forms of
care.

Health maintenance organizations

In the past 40 years, prepayment for services has been gradually increasing in
frequency. In this form of reimbursement, third party payers contract with physicians or physician groups. In return for prepayment, the practitioners agree to furnish a package of services as defined in a contract. In some forms of prepayment,
these physicians are also at least at some financial risk of costs of care that result
from referrals or hospitalizations, although most arrangements exempt certain "catastrophic" costs over which the physician has no control. These arrangements are
known as HMOs.

In 1932, the Commission on the Costs of Medical Care in the United States
recommended that health care be provided by organized groups of health professionals, preferably in a hospital setting, on a prepayment basis. Although care
provided by such organized groups is a feature of many health care systems, it is
only in the United States that they are organized primarily within the private sector
and reimbursed largely through private insurance plans.

In HMOs, payment to physicians or groups is either fixed in advance depending
on the number (and sometimes type) of enrolled patients or is subject to some risk-
sharing. Physicians who work in the HMO must control health care expenditures;
if more care is provided than the HMO anticipates, the HMO will incur a deficit.
On the other hand, if too little care is provided, the HMO may be suspected of not
providing necessary care.

Originally, HMOs were not-for-profit service organizations that provided clinical services. In current terminology, however, the HMO is often the fiscal agent
that contracts either with a management tier or directly with a medical care group
to provide services for its defined population. The physicians or physician groups
within an HMO are of several types:

Staff model: The physicians work directly for the HMO, on salary but sometimes with a bonus depending on the HMO's earnings or their productivity.

Group model: The HMO contracts with a separate physician group to provide its services. These are also known as *prepaid group practices*, and physicians may be paid a salary or a capitation. In network model HMOs, the contract is with multiple physicians or group practices instead of just one.

Individual practice association (IPA): The HMO contracts with individual physicians who are in independent practice or with a collective of physicians whose members work independently, usually in solo practice or single-specialty groups. As is the case with other types of HMOs, IPA plans typically require primary care physicians to act as gatekeepers for their patients. This role requires them to approve referrals, admissions, and high-cost procedures and tests. A capitation fee is paid to the HMO for each person enrolled. Physicians may be paid a capitation for primary care services or may be reimbursed according to a fixed fee schedule for services rendered; the fees are typically based on a percentage of the physician's usual fee. Primary care physicians may receive additional capitation for referral and ancillary services arranged by the primary care physician and paid for by fee-for-service or by a prearranged payment schedule. Usually a portion of the fee or the capitation payment is withheld by the IPA. If utilization and costs are in line with expectations, the withheld amount is returned to the physicians.

All forms of HMO plans may have a *point-of-service* arrangement in which patients are free to seek care from non-HMO physicians but pay considerably more for doing so.

Except in staff or group model HMOs, practitioners may contract with HMOs to care for enrolled patients. They typically retain the right to provide services for several HMOs and/or fee-for-service patients.

Managed indemnity plans and preferred provider organizations

Although often not included under the rubric of *managed care* because they lack capitation or salary arrangements, at least two other forms of micromanagement are common, primarily in the United States. A managed indemnity plan is a conventional (indemnity) fee-for-service arrangement in which the use of services and procedures is carefully monitored.

A PPO is an administrative entity that contracts with employers or insurers to provide services to individuals for a negotiated fee, usually discounted below the prevailing level. In a PPO, patients may choose a physician, regardless of whether the physician participates in the PPO. If they use a non-PPO physician, they must pay a higher out-of-pocket fee. In an EPO (exclusive provider organization), use of non-PPO physicians is not covered except in emergency situations. The EPO, therefore, is similar to the IPA except that EPO pays its physicians a negotiated fee-for-service whereas the IPA usually shares risk with its physicians (and always with its primary care physicians) by withholding a portion of the capitation or fee-for-service until all expenditures are tallied. This portion is not returned unless financial targets are met.

Integral to PPOs is a managing organization that provides certain administrative functions to monitor the use of services. These may include pre-admission certification (i.e., approval of elective admissions), second opinions before surgery, certification of treatment plans for certain nonemergency services such as mental health services, and review of the medical care that is provided.

Many features of managed care are common in different nations, although to different degrees and extent. These include capitation, gatekeepers (primary care physician as the point of first contact for each new need), user fees, consumer education, medical practice guidelines, greater use of non-physicians when they can substitute for physicians, better clinical information systems, and telemedicine as an extension of primary care services (Smith, 1997).

In Europe, managed care tends to be defined as "a process to maximize health gain of a community within limited resources by ensuring an appropriate range and level of services are provided and by monitoring on a case by case basis to ensure continuous improvement to meet national targets for health and individual needs" (Fairfield et al., 1997a). This view focuses on community health gains through the integration of policy, decentralization of management, and individual patient care management, including disease management that is never "carved out" but rather an extension of the relationship between primary care and specialists. National policy (lacking in comparable form in the United States but existing in some degree in only a very few U.S. states) takes the form of defining health needs, evaluating treatment effectiveness and cost effectiveness, and setting priorities (Fairfield et al., 1997b). Setting of local priorities (replaced in the United States by private organizations) focuses on contracting with hospitals, specialists, and different types of practitioners to provide services extending from primary care; clinical practice is increasingly encouraged by guidelines rather than medical profiling, which often is used punitively against physicians in the United States. Membership in the European Community carries with it the requirement that health services be provided under not-for-profit arrangements—the opposite of the increasing trend toward profit-making in the United States. Moreover, the concept of equity in the provision of health services, as reflected in the term *solidarity*, ensures that the underlying values that have guided the development of European health service systems for decades is not being sacrificed in health care reforms directed at containing costs and improving quality of care.

Managed Care and Primary Care

Despite its almost universal inclusion of "gatekeeping," managed care is not necessarily conducive to the achievement of primary care. Where the focus is on empowerment of the primary care physician to make decisions about the care received by populations of patients, it is likely to facilitate all four features of primary care. First-contact care will be enhanced by not only having the primary care physician be the point of contact for all new needs but also by placing responsibility in the hands of primary care physicians for making informed referrals when they are needed. Longitudinality will be fostered by formally linking populations with an identifiable source of primary care and, if that physician is freely chosen by people, by enhancing the likelihood that long-term relationships will develop. Comprehensiveness will be encouraged by the development of integrated systems in which the needs of populations are documented and services planned so that the most appropriate level of care takes responsibility for providing appropriate services. Coordination will also be facilitated by more formal linkages between the levels of care and better lines of communication and enhanced by electronic mechanisms of information flow to better integrate care across different levels and types of practitioners. In the United States, for example, the older nonprofit staff and group model HMOs generally performed well on these characteristics.

However, the directions taken by managed care in health care systems where its main goals are cost containment and competition are likely to be inimical to the achievement of the features of primary care (Reid et al., 1996; Starfield, 1997).

> J.A. is a middle-class hairdresser who developed calcaneal spurs that caused her to discontinue her daily exercise of walking on a track. She is scheduled for outpatient surgery but reported that she was required to see her "preliminary physician" to obtain the referral. When asked whether she really meant "preliminary care" rather than "primary care," she said, "Oh yes, primary care; that's the right word."
>
> J.A. (1997), United States

Instead of viewing first-contact care as a strategy to empower patients and their physicians to come to agreement on the most appropriate clinical management strategy, managed care may view it as a barrier (the necessary "preliminary") to other services. Thus, first-contact access is endangered by a profit motive that imposes barriers to the seeking of primary care in the interests of reducing costs in the short term. Managed care that focuses on the enrollment of healthier populations (such as the gainfully employed) can selectively draw resources away from the least healthy segments of the population (the unemployed, the poor, the elderly), thus reducing their access to needed services. Furthermore, "point of service" plans, which allow patients to seek care elsewhere without discussion with their primary care physicians, may enhance consumer satisfaction in the short run while actively interfering with the benefits of first-contact care.

Although managed care in theory fosters longitudinality by linking patients with a source of primary care, a lack of appreciation of the essence of longitudinality actively interferes with its attainment.

> A recent comparison of the relative benefits of care provided by primary care physicians and specialists used a controlled trial in which very ill elderly men being discharged from the hospital were randomly assigned to receive ongoing care from a primary care physician–nurse team or from the specialty clinic from which they had been receiving care prior to hospitalization. *Individuals who already had an identifiable source of primary care were excluded from the trial.* Follow-up six

months later failed to find any difference in costs or outcomes of care for individuals in the two study groups.

A study reported in a prestigious U.S. medical journal (1996).

When there is little familiarity with the concept or meaning of primary care, there is a tendency to equate it with the type of physician who provides it rather than with the concept itself. Longitudinality cannot be achieved without time to provide the knowledge needed to achieve person-focused care. The benefits of longitudinality cannot be achieved in periods of time shorter than 1 year, and, when utilization is infrequent, it often takes several years. Many managed care organizations not only limit the free choice of physician; they also actively break physician–patient relationships by means of periodic contract negotiations between employers and managed care organizations, or employers and physician groups, which change the roster of groups and physicians who are eligible to participate in the plan that is chosen for patients. Because competition, by definition, carries with it the expectation that these changes will indeed occur as more attractive "packages" are made available in the market, it actively interferes with the achievement of longitudinality. A variety of studies demonstrate that maintenance of relationships with particular physicians is often disrupted by this process (Commonwealth Fund, 1995; National Committe for Quality Assurance, 1995; Kerstein et al., 1994; Commonwealth Quarterly, 1992). For example, in one study of patients in a network of 138 community-based physicians in an urban U.S. area, one of four patients with IPA or PPO health insurance experienced an involuntary change of physicians in a 2-year period (Flocke et al., 1997).

Market-oriented health systems compromise comprehensiveness by focusing on providing services that save money in the short term. Since there is no incentive for them to retain particular panels of patients over the long term, they have no incentive to provide services early in the course of development of ill health or to provide preventive services with only long-term returns on the investment.

Coordination of care is not necessarily compromised by market-driven health systems; to the extent that they are part of integrated health systems with common information systems, coordination may even be enhanced. However, certain aspects of these systems act against the achievement of coordinated care. Limited panels of subspecialists reduce the likelihood that the most appropriate one can be chosen in instances of special need. Furthermore, it restricts the ability of primary care physicians to choose the most appropriate one because they must often refer to subspecialists with whom they are unfamiliar. Written summaries are substituting for personal discussions about patients (Roulidis and Schulman, 1994).

The natural history of managed care in the United States, with its focus on short-term gain, does not bode well for future improvements in primary care. There is little incentive for managers to work with physician and consumer groups to adapt modes of delivering services that have been demonstrated to enhance care. Many managed care organizations are allowing patients to chose specialists, especially obstetrician/gynecologists, as their primary care physician or to chose both a generalist and a specialist as dual primary care physicians, thus negating all of the advantages of the four features of primary care. Thus, managed care as it is implemented in the United States, is assuming many of the characteristics of conventional primary care, leaving only the difference in reduced physician autonomy and discretion in the care of patients.

> As managed care invaded my limited practice, the logistics of competing to stay in medicine became impractical because the system required so much more wrangling with insurance companies. I finally sold my practice to the community hospital. The staff increased to three employees, plus a "practice management team" in control of all operations. Office hours were theoretically expanded, but the doctor was available less and less of the time.   Dr. R.M., a New Jersey physician

The Future of Health Care Reform

Imperatives for reform stem from perceived inadequacies in organization and financing of services that have been in place for decades. These imperatives include cost containment; bureaucratic management practices in highly controlled systems; an absence of responsiveness to consumers in an era of rising consumer information, knowledge, and expectation; and absent competition. Although not all systems have been equally exposed to all of these inadequacies, all are experienced in some degree by all countries. The imposition of reform strategies, in the absence of adequate prior research and evaluation (and with little likelihood of systematic collection of data to monitor their impact), is bound to lead to its own inefficiencies and deficits. Where reform is taking place in the private sector with little public involvement or oversight from a publically accountable body, the only remedy for inadequate performance is legal or social remedy for identified deficits. In the United States, such microregulation is already in evidence. Restrictions on access to services have resulted in alternative means of providing services where they are perceived as needed. The fastest growing form of health plan is the "point of service" plan in which individuals may opt out of care from the designated primary care physician or specialist by paying an extra fee to seek care outside the plan from a physician of their own choosing. Because only those who can afford these extra payments will use this option, this strategy is primarily directed at attracting higher income individuals to the health plan.

Other remedies are more equitable in their effect. Severe restrictions on use of services, including mandatory maximum stays in the hospital for a variety of conditions (including postpartum newborn stays) have been perceived widely as compromising the quality of care and particularly interfering with physician autonomy to judge individual patient's particular needs. In response, many states have passed laws in response to professional as well as consumer advocacy to overturn these plan practices. Many state regulations now mandate the coverage of specific services such as mental health, drug and alcohol abuse, mammograms, and prenatal care. Some states mandate that health plans allow people to seek care directly from specialists; several others have such direct-access laws for obstetrician/gynecologist services. Many states have set minimum lengths of stay in the hospital to prevent health plans from refusing to pay for hospital care, particularly for newborns (Hellinger, 1996). Unfortunately, not all health plans are subject to state regulations, thus making these remedies inapplicable to everyone. Futhermore, many of these "remedies," which are directed at limiting the abuses of managed care, are themselves antithetical to the attainment of good primary care.

Health care reform (in the form of managed care in the United States) is generally credited with reducing the rate of increases in health care costs, but not in reducing such costs or redistributing them. Evidence of its impact on quality of care is mixed, but assessment is compromised by the plethora of organizational types and a consequent inability to attribute performance to specific organizational and financial arrangements (Miller and Luft, 1997). Perhaps its main effect has been to de-professionalize physicians, particularly primary care physicians, whose autonomy over medical decision-making has been greatly reduced as a result of managerial strategies in the private sector. Similar effects threaten Europe, although the magnitude of their effect will depend on the specific policies taken by national governments. The lesson to be drawn from both the successes and the failures of the U.S. experience is the importance of developing, introducing, and using scientific professional standards of quality not only for the technical aspects of care but also for health service delivery aspects. Sharing responsibility for the development of these standards with consumer groups runs a risk of compounding the process of de-professionalization (Groenewegen and Calnan, 1995), but this is likely to be far preferable to the loss of autonomy based on managerial control with the main aim of cost containment.

The future of various aspects of managed care is uncertain. New Zealand abandoned competition in favor of collaboration just a few years after its implementation (Ham, 1997). A brake on the vigorous expansion of competitive fund-holding in the United Kingdom was instituted with the return of the Labor government to power in 1997. Even in the United States, the future of managed care is under question. Governmental efforts to place the elderly population (for whom it has financial responsibility in the form of Medicare) and socially disadvantaged populations (for whom states bear financial responsibility in the form of Medicaid) in managed care organizations is likely to lead to the increasing enrollment of sicker individuals into managed care organizations, thus threatening the profitability that has accrued from the heretofore preferential enrollment of less sick individuals. Physician groups have shown increasing interest in competing with managed care organizations for contracts with hospitals and employers. Public concern about perceived inadequacies of managed care is also likely to broaden and further threaten the relative freedom of the private managed care sector in determining the way in which health services are delivered. Furthermore, rapid growth in enrollment in managed care organizations has not prevented large increases in health care costs, which quadrupled from 1980 to 1995. As managed care becomes less profitable, it is unlikely that it will continue to attract the capital that is necessary for its further expansion (Ginzburg and Ostow, 1997).

The multiplicity of possible arrangements for financing and organizing health care systems leaves considerable room for experimentation by different health systems by nations and within nations. In the past, reform efforts have not been accompanied by systematic efforts to evaluate their impact. Greater attention to the need for such evaluations, and with a specific emphasis on the impact on primary care, should provide a better basis for choosing among the alternative approaches.

References

Commonwealth Fund. Report on the Results of a 1994 Survey of Patients' Experiences With Managed Care. New York: Commonwealth Fund, 1995.

Commonwealth Quarterly. New York: Commonwealth Fund, 1992, Vol 2, p. 1.

Defever M. Health care reforms: The unfinished agenda. Health Policy 1995; 34:1–7.

Etheredge L, Jones SB, Lewin L. What is driving health system change? Health Aff 1996; 15(4):93–104.

Fairfield G, Hunter DJ, Mechanic D, Rosleff F. Managed Care: Origins, principles, and evolution. BMJ 1997a; 314:1823–6.

Fairfield G, Hunter DJ, Mechanic D, Rosleff F. Managed Care: Implications of managed care for health systems clinicians and patients. BMJ 1997b; 314:1895–8.

Flocke S, Stange K, Zyzanski S. The impact of insurance type and forced discontinuity on the delivery of primary care. J Fam Pract 1997; 45:129–35.

Gérvas J. Health Care Reform in Europe: The Case of Primary Health Care. In: Goicoechea J, (ed). Primary Health Care Reforms. Copenhagen: World Health Organization, European Region, 1996, pp. 17–37.

Ginzburg E, Ostow M. Managed Care—A look back and a look ahead. N Engl J Med 1997; 336(14):1018–20.

Groenewegen PP, Calnan M. Changes in the control of health care systems in Europe. Eur J Public Health 1995; 5(4)240–4.

Ham C. Reforming the New Zealand health reforms. BMJ 1997; 314:1844–5.

Hellinger F. The expanding scope of state legislation. JAMA 1996; 276(13):1065–70.

Kerstein J, Pauly MV, Hillman A. Primary care physicians turnover in HMOs. Health Serv Res 1994; 29:17–37.

Miller R, Luft H. Does managed care lead to better or worse quality of care? Health Aff 1997; 16:7–25.

National Committee for Quality Assurance. Report Care Pilot Project: Technical Report. Washington, D.C.: National Committee on Quality Assurance, 1995.

Organization for Economic Cooperation and Development. Health Care Reform: The Will to Change. Health Policy Studies No. 8. Paris: Organization for Economic Cooperation and Development, 1996.

Organization for Economic Cooperation and Development. The Reform of Health Care: A Comparative Analysis of Seven OECD Countries. Health Policy Studies No.2. Paris: Organization for Economic Cooperation and Development, 1992.

Organization for Economic Cooperation and Development. New Directions in Health Policy. Health Policy Studies No. 7. Paris: Organization for Economic Cooperation and Development, 1995.

Reid RJ, Hurtado MP, Starfield B. Managed care, primary care and quality for children. Curr Opin Pediatr 1996; 8(2):164–70.

Roulidis Z, Schulman K. Physician communication in managed care organizations: Opinions of primary care physicians. J Fam Pract 1994; 39:446–51.

Scott A, Hall J. Evaluating the effects of GP remuneration: Problems and prospects. Health Policy 1995; 31:183–95.

Smith R. The future of healthcare systems. Information technology and consumerism will transform health care worldwide. BMJ 1997; 314:1495–6.

Starfield B. The future of primary care in a managed care era. Int J Health Serv 1997; 27(4): 687–96.

— III —
Accountability
in Primary Care

— 7 —

Accessibility and First Contact: The "Gate"

When I was a resident, I had an experience that changed my career. I started in surgery and often patients would come to the clinic with aches and pains and they didn't have any surgical problem, so I would refer them to the appropriate clinic and give them the phone number to call. I assumed that I'd taken care of the problem. But one day I called the phone number just to see what patients were experiencing. The first time I called I got cut off. So I tried again and I got cut off again, and the next time I was put on hold and the next time they told me they were going to transfer the call. It ended up taking me 14 phone calls to make an appointment. And I speak English. So I started worrying about how I was referring my patients, where they are going and what we are doing to them. We function ok because we know the system, but most folks go home and they run into barriers right away and don't know how to handle them. I switched from surgery to family medicine and now I do as much for them as I can. Only when I feel I can't do any more do I refer them, and I don't let them go until the appointment is made. I'm available to take care of diseases, but that's not all I do. My patients are much larger than their diseases. Now I feel that I am really doing something for patients— that there's really something to practicing medicine. The best thing we can do for patients is to understand what they say, and a prerequisite is listening. Obviously I take care of their diseases—I'm available to do that in ways that they need me to do that—but that's a small part of what I do.
Dr. C., a physician

Inherent in the organization of health services by level of care (primary, secondary, tertiary) is the idea that there is a point of entry each new time care is needed for a health problem and that this point of entry must be easily accessible. In current parlance, this point of first contact is known as the *gatekeeper*.

The idea of a "gate" make sense. First, most people do not know enough about the technical details of medical care to make informed judgments about the appropriate source and timing of care for many of their problems. Individuals who believe they have a health problem should be able to consult a professional who can help them to understand whether the problem is serious enough to require additional care or whether it is a self-limited problem that needs no further care. Lacking an easily accessible point of entry, adequate care may not be obtained or may be delayed and additional expense incurred. Advice and guidance from a primary care physician could be expected to facilitate the selection of the best source of care.

Not every physician can be equally skilled in all facets of medical care, and the entry level of care provides special challenges. Problems brought by patients are often vague and unrelated to particular organ systems. Because of varying thresholds for seeking care, some patients seek care earlier in the course of their disease than other patients. Therefore, primary care physicians confront a much greater variety of presentations of illness than do specialists, who generally see patients in later and more differentiated stages of illness. Primary care physicians work in the community where the manifestations of illness are heavily influenced by their social context. In contrast, other specialists, especially those who work in hospitals, deal with problems more removed from their social context.

Evidence for the benefits of successful first contact is important in supporting its inclusion as a key characteristic of primary care. The following section considers these benefits.

Benefits of First-Contact Care

The importance of easy access to care to lower mortality and morbidity has been known for many years. The nature of the evidence was summarized for child health (Starfield, 1985); similar types of evidence are available for adults. For example, because of budget deficits, many individuals were no longer permitted to receive outpatient services from the Veterans Administration Hospital, which they had previously used as a source of care. When questioned, they were much less likely to report that they had access to needed medical care and that they actually had been receiving care. They also were more likely to report that they were in poor health and were more likely to have poor blood pressure control 1 year later than those individuals who were kept in treatment, even though the latter were initially more sick (Fihn and Wicher, 1988). When California terminated health care benefits for many indigent adults, there was a decline in use of services and a deterioration of health status that persisted for at least 1 year thereafter (Lurie et al., 1986).

Maximization of access to a *primary care source* is also important. Several studies indicate that patients should see a generalist before consulting a specialist.

> Evan R. is a 15-year-old boy who came home from school one day with a swollen foot, having spent several hours playing basketball with his friends. Evan's mother took him to an orthopedist she knows, who took an x-ray that showed a possible hairline fracture. The orthopedist decided to send Evan to a rheumatologist, who saw him immediately and mentioned the possibility of sarcoidosis. Evan had a chest x-ray (normal), and blood was drawn for a variety of tests including angiotensin-converting enzyme (ACE), a test used to diagnose sarcoidosis in adults. The level of ACE was elevated. It was suggested that Evan be followed for 6 months to confirm or rule out the diagnosis of sarcoidosis. Evan's mother was terrified that this was a fatal condition. Evan underwent a bone scan to rule out bone cancer. Before he went home, he returned to the orthopedist to have his ankle set in a cast.

A week later, his uncle (a pediatrician) visited and found him shooting baskets in the driveway of his home, with the cast on his foot. The pediatrician mentioned to his mother that sarcoid rarely presents this way and that the ACE test is nonspecific and highly sensitive to the hormonal changes of puberty. Evan was going through puberty. The disease that should have been treated with an ice pack and elevation resulted in a bill for several thousand dollars for unneeded diagnostic tests. A week later, the pediatrician convinced the orthopedist to remove the cast.   B.G. (1994)

Using data from a panel survey involving a national sample of individuals in the United States, Forrest and Starfield (1998) demonstrated that better accessibility of services was associated with a higher likelihood of first-contact care and continuity with the primary care physician. Accessibility was measured by responses to one question about geographic barriers (travel time of more than 30 minutes), one question on financial barriers (no insurance for all or part of the year), and three questions concerning organizational barriers (availability of after-hours care at the primary care site, 5 or more days wait to get an appointment, and more than a 30 minute wait in the office). The after-hours care component itself had five components: emergency hours, house calls, evening hours, Saturday morning hours, other weekend hours). First contact was assessed by the proportion of visits in a year for any of 24 types of acute conditions in which the first visit in the episode was with the self-identified "particular doctor that is usually seen at the primary care site." Continuity was assessed by measuring the proportion of *all* visits in the year, regardless of where they occurred, that were with the physician. An increasing number of barriers to access was associated with less first-contact care and lower continuity, even after control for a variety of influential patient characteristics, types of primary site, and types of primary care practitioner.

One experiment required those enrolled in a health insurance program to first receive care from a generalist physician; no hospitalizations or visits to a specialist were allowed without a referral from the primary care physician. After a year of enrollment, those in the program spent fewer days in the hospital than did those whose insurance permitted them to seek initial care anywhere (Moore, 1979). However, a subsequent evaluation failed to show any differences in costs of either inpatient or outpatient services, largely because the primary care "gatekeeper" was not able to control the practices of other specialists who were paid on a fee-for-service basis with no financial risk. In fact, 70% of the hospitalizations were controlled by specialists other than the primary care physician (Moore, 1983).

Studies in Canada showed that appropriate indications for tonsillectomy and/or adenoidectomy were more often present in children who had been referred from a pediatrician or who had some pediatric contact than in those children who had visited only an ear, nose, and throat specialist. The outcomes of care were also better for the children seen initially by a pediatrician; such children had fewer postoperative complications, a greater decrease in respiratory episodes following surgery, and a greater decrease in episodes of otitis media following surgery (Roos, 1979).

In a study comparing visit rates in two prepaid group practices (Starfield, 1983), children in the group practice plan who required a referral from a primary care provider before visits to other specialists had fewer visits to these specialists than did children in the plan not requiring referral. There is no evidence that the additional visits in the latter plan led to better health of the children.

Requiring a visit to a "gatekeeper" before a visit can be made elsewhere is associated with reduced utilization of both other specialty services and emergency room visits. In a study in which new enrollees were randomized either to a system that required visits to a gatekeeper or to one with equal benefits but no gatekeeper requirement, patients in the plan with a gatekeeper requirement had an average of 0.3 fewer visits to a specialist over a 1 year period than did patients in the other group (Martin et al., 1989). In another study of stratified random samples of patients enrolled in four Medicaid demonstration programs that required a gatekeeper, patients had large reductions in the proportion of patients with at least one emergency room visit, ranging from 27% to 37% for children and 30% to 45% for adults (Hurley et al., 1989).

A national panel study of illness experiences and medical care utilization provided a good basis for estimating the cost savings of first-contact care with a primary care physician. All episodes of care for 24 prevention and acute illness visits were studied with regard to the place from which care was first sought. Episodes that began with visits to the individual's self-identified primary care provider were 53% less costly overall: 62% for acute illnesses and 20% for preventive care after controlling for many other characteristics associated with costs of care. The savings were almost as great even after visits to emergency rooms (which are expensive) were excluded (Forrest and Starfield, 1996).

The relationship between first-contact care and a lower percentage of the gross domestic product spent on health services was confirmed using data from a large international study. European countries were ranked according to the percentage of medical specialists who were directly accessible to people in the country (Crombie et al., 1990). Countries with a higher percentage devoted a larger proportion of the gross domestic product to health then did countries with lower percentages (i.e., those requiring referral from a primary care practitioner) (Fry and Horder, 1994).

A small study in one large urban children's hospital confirmed the benefits of first-contact care in children with acute illness (appendicitis). Those children whose parents contacted their primary care provider before arrival at the hospital were less likely to have appendiceal perforation than those who did not, irrespective of insurance coverage or type of insurance. If they presented on a weekend they also were more likely to be operated on promptly. Phone consultations were equally effective as personal examination by the physician in achieving these benefits (Chande and Kinnane, 1996).

Another study of children with appendicitis showed the same general findings. Children belonging to a health maintenance organization (with requirements that patients consult their primary care physician before seeking care elsewhere) had a shorter duration of symptoms before presenting to the hospital and shorter hospital stays than children in health arrangements without a required consultation with a primary care clinician. The consultation not only did not delay care, but it facilitated it (O'Toole et al., 1996).

Why do such benefits accrue from first-contact care?

Once upon a time there lived a Gatekeeper and a Wizard. The Gatekeeper's job was to decide who should see the Wizard. Most of the people who saw the Gatekeeper didn't see the Wizard. They were usually only a little sick or worried about being sick and the Gatekeeper was very good at deciding who needed to see the Wizard. Most of the people who saw the Wizard were pretty sick and the Wizard could cast her spells to make them better. The Wizard and the Gatekeeper needed each other. The problem was that as more people heard about the Wizard's magic potions, they wanted to see her and the waiting lines got longer and longer. Sometimes the Gatekeeper had to send people back to the Wizard because they didn't get enough of the magic potions. The people got very angry and told the Queen. The Queen said, "Let the people who want to see the Wizard go there directly and pay the Wizard themselves. The people who could pay were very happy. The problem was that the waiting lines got longer because the Wizard spent longer and longer seeing the patients who could pay. In fact, the marvelous crystal ball began to give more and more wrong answers. "Find out what is going on," cried the Queen. The Gatekeeper dialed DataSpell on his crystal ball and there appeared the message: "The value of a diagnostic test depends on the prevalence of the condition in the population tested. The Wizard is very good at deciding who is very sick but not at all good at deciding who is well. The Gatekeeper is very good at deciding who is well, but not quite as good at deciding who is very sick. Gatekeepers use examinations and tests to determine if people are normal or not whereas Wizards use tests to detect illness. If the Wizard's crystal ball is to work properly, the Wizard should only see the people who the Gatekeeper suspects are sick enough to need more care. And the Gatekeeper should see the people who think they may be sick and try to find out if they are. Then the system will work. Far from being an arrangement to deprive people of choice and access to the Wizard, it is the most efficient way of looking after sick people." The Queen found, however, that persuading the people of this was much harder—a taste for direct access to the crystal ball and magic potions once acquired is not easily forgotten.   Adapted from Mathers and Hodgkin (1989)

The reason that first contact is important is that the training of primary care physicians takes place with patients who have a low probability of being ill with a rare or serious condition. The training of other specialists, however, is with people who have a high probability of having a rare or serious condition in their area of specialization. The likelihood that a given diagnostic test will correctly diagnosis a condition in any given patient depends on the likely frequency of that illness in the patients that the physician sees. If the condition is uncommon, the test will give many false-positive results relative to the correct results. The tests that subspecialists use are calibrated to perform well with patients who have a high likelihood of having the disease. If many people with a low likelihood of the disease (such as those not referred by primary care physicians) are subjected to the test, it will not be accurate most of the time. Thus, people will be subjected unnecessarily to a chain of diagnostic tests, each of them with a finite probability of producing an adverse effect, and the costs will not be justifiable given the low yield from them.

Dr. G. is a surgeon who first sought care from an ear, nose, and throat (ENT) specialist because of bad headaches and self-diagnosed sinusitis. The ENT physician ordered a CT scan and then steroids for sinusitis, but Dr. G.'s headaches worsened to the point where she was unable to operate. Incidentally, she sought a routine check-up from her gynecologist, who advised her to stop taking her birth control pills and sent her to a neurologist who diagnosed migraine and put her on medication for this disorder. She soon developed fainting spells, which led the neurologist to increase the dose. Failure of the symptoms to abate led to a visit to her general internist who ordered a test for thyroid function. Diagnosis: Hyperthyroism. Dr. G. is now asymptomatic and back to work on medication for her disorder.

For any given presenting symptom or complaint, the probability of true disease will be lower in primary care populations than in other specialists' practices because of the higher frequency of the disease in the latter practices (Sox, 1996). Thus, faced with the same patient problems as specialists, primary care physicians will order fewer tests and procedures yet obtain the same or better outcomes in terms of accurate diagnoses of the range of conditions in primary care (Rosser, 1996).

Steven C. is a 5-year-old boy who developed joint pains in several joints. His parents took him to see his physician, who also was an academic pediatrician specializing in hematology. Concerned about the presence of rheumatoid arthritis, the pediatrician did a full battery of blood tests and x-rays; all of them reported as normal several days later. Steven needn't have had this expensive workup, which was uncomfortable for him and anxiety producing for his parents; he had received a German measles immunization the week before, but this specialist pediatrician was not aware of the reasonably common occurrence of migratory joint pains in children after this immunization.

In Western medicine, judging a sick person well is thought to be more egregious than judging a well person sick. Thus, the higher "false-positive" characteristics of diagnoses in subspecialty care are thought more acceptable than the higher "false-negative" characteristics of diagnoses in primary care. Many years ago, Scheff (1964) described the adverse impact of these assumptions on the health of patients. His warnings have received little attention in the intervening years, at least partly because the overwhelming tendency of physicians to accept overdiagnosing in preference to underdiagnosing is highly compatible with economic incentives for the use of increasingly sophisticated and expensive technology. Yet the compelling arguments of Scheff, the vast amount of evidence for a large burden of iatrogenic disease, and the preponderance of medical harm resulting from errors of commission rather than errors of omission provide the theoretical justification for the benefits of first-contact care with primary care practitioners.

The definition of a healthy person is someone who has not had enough tests.

Anonymous.

Policy and Research Implications of First-Contact Care: Cost Sharing and Gatekeepers

When costs of care appear to be out of control, policy-makers often resort to the idea that they can be reduced by imposing cost-sharing requirements on users of services. This is an approach that appears to have appeal worldwide because many countries are imposing increasingly greater requirements on patients to contribute toward supporting the costs of their own care. Cost-sharing has two forms: requiring payment of a portion of insurance premium costs and cost-sharing in the form of co-payments or deductibles. The latter type is the one that presents the most immediate access barrier because it is imposed at the point that the decision is made to seek services. Ample experience shows that co-payments or deductibles reduce use of services (Rasell, 1995) without reducing the cost (Saltman and Figueras, 1997). As a result, they might be warranted in situations where utilization is thought to be frivolous or unnecessary. In a country where utilization rates are already relatively low and where there are known barriers to access, their utility might be questioned (Table 7.1).

The crux of the matter is that cost-sharing at the point of decision to seek service reduces needed visits as much as unnecessary ones (Rasell, 1995). Accompanying this reduction in services, physicians in fee-for-service systems appear to compensate for reductions in income by increasing the level of services for those who receive them; as a result, overall costs increase (Fahs, 1992), while health outcomes, including persistence of symptoms of disease among low-income individuals, worsen (Shapiro et al., 1986). In a situation where excess costs are associated more with the high intensity of services provided by physicians rather than excessive seeking of care by patients, imposition of financial barriers to the seeking of care is a blunt and indirect instrument for cost control. Such a situation exists in the United States, where cost-sharing is common. Table 7.1 shows that the numbers of hospital beds, hospitalizations, length of stay, number of physicians, and number of physician contacts per capita are generally lower in the United States than in many countries. Imposition of additional cost controls are unlikely to further reduce costs without compromising health. A better strategy is to devise mecha-

Table 7.1. Physicians and Hospitals, Early 1990s

	Hospital Beds		Hospitalizations		Physician Contacts	
	Beds per 1,000	Ratio Long-Term to Acute Care Beds	Admissions as % of Populations	Average Stay in Days	Available Physicians per 1,000	Actual Contacts per Capita
Australia	9.8	0.8	23.0	12.7	2.2	8.8
Belgium	6.5	0.8	19.1	13.0	3.2	7.9
Canada	6.3	0.5	14.1	13.9	2.2	6.9
Denmark	5.4	0.2	21.2	7.8	2.8	4.4
Finland	11.2	1.8	22.8	19.0	2.5	3.3
Germany (West)	10.3	0.4	21.1	16.1	3.2	11.5
Netherlands	11.4	1.6	20.9	33.8	2.5	5.4
Spain	4.2	0.3	9.9	11.9	3.9	6.2
Sweden	11.9	2.0	19.9	16.8	2.9	2.8
United Kingdom	5.9	1.3	19.3	14.0	1.4	5.7
United States	4.7	0.2	13.7	9.1	2.2	5.6
OECD average	8.4		16.2	14.4	2.5	6.1

Source: Schieber et al. (1994).

nisms to identify unnecessary services, on the part of both practitioners and patients, and institute quality improvement practices to reduce unnecessary diagnostic and therapeutic interventions.

> In January 1996, over 80 percent of surveyed Canadians approved of registering with a family physician for necessary medical care, referrals to specialists and other providers, and after hours care.   Canada Health Monitor, Survey 13, January 1996

Even in the United States, the idea of a "gatekeeper" is not new. From 1953 to 1978 at the Hunterdon Medical Center in New Jersey patients were not permitted to see other specialists unless referred by primary care physicians. The gatekeeper is also often used in the military to control access to specialists. By the late 1980s, over 85% of health maintenance organizations restricted direct consultation of subspecialists by patients, and over 50% required patients to visit the primary care provider before they could see another specialist (Reagan, 1987).

In systems where there traditionally has been free choice of physician and unimpeded access by patients to any type of physician, the benefit of a gatekeeper may not be intuitively obvious. If people believe that a subspecialist has greater expertise and skill, and they believe they are competent to decide on an appropriate one for their problem, they will feel deprived of the "best" care if they have to seek care elsewhere first. If they are correct in their assessment of their problem, unimpeded access to a specialist might be more efficient, because it saves the cost of an intermediary visit. Unimpeded access also provides greater convenience in that patients do not have to make time for two visits instead of one, thus getting patients under care more quickly.

On the other hand, the training of primary care physicians makes them more familiar with how problems present in early stages, and hence they are better able to assess the relative importance of various symptoms and signs at the early stages of illness. Their knowledge of patients makes it easier for them to evaluate the nature of changes in symptoms and signs, and they are therefore likely to be more efficient in their use of resources to assess the significance of the changes. Primary care physicians might also facilitate access to other specialists and direct the patient to a more appropriate one, which can also shorten the time to appropriate care rather than lengthen it.

Thus the issue of gatekeepers is controversial and is becoming increasingly so as more types of health care organizations adopt it. In an international context, countries with gatekeeping, in which patients do not seek care from specialists before consulting with their primary care physician, are not necessarily countries whose populations are less satisfied with their health services systems (Gérvas et al., 1994). However, in the United States, there is widespread suspicion that the basis for gatekeepers is cost containment rather than rationality of organization, which is historically the case in many countries in Europe. Gatekeepers are increasingly used to deter utilization of specialists, thus raising the possibility that needed care will be denied. Failure of the gatekeeper to refer might even lead to inappropriate care; if the gatekeeper is not sufficiently knowledgeable or skilled in the diagnosis or management of the problem, necessary care is delayed. When the client enrolls in the health system, he or she may choose a physician (at least from a panel of physicians), but each subsequent contact must be through this physician. Choice of subspecialist might even be maintained at the point of each referral, but it is likely that this choice would be restricted to a relatively small group of sub-specialists. There are major concerns about equity with the imposition of gate-keepers when responsibility for payment lies with payers who have a major finan-cial interest in reducing use of specialty services. Patients whose care is paid for by employers or insurers who stand to gain financially from low levels of such services are at special risk of not being referred appropriately.

The impact of gatekeeping also depends on the financial incentives of the pri-mary care practitioners. Studies of managed care in the 1980s indicated that gate-keeping reduced patients' likelihood of seeing another specialist, with a consequent increase in primary care visits if the primary care physician was paid by fee for service. Moreover, patients visited fewer different places than they had before en-rollment in the plan (Hurley et al., 1991).

Gatekeeping involves some ethical considerations. When restriction in access to specialists is linked to financial incentives for the primary care physician, there is a potential conflict of interest between physicians' concerns about their income and concern about the welfare of patients. The right of patients to know about potential conflicts needs protection.

Most of these considerations concerning gatekeepers do not arise in countries where the concept of a point of first contact has a long tradition. In all of these countries, free choice of primary care physician and maintenance of long-term relationships with them (see Chapter 8) enhance the likelihood that patients will trust their primary care physician to choose the appropriate place to refer. In Den-mark, all people have the right to chose one of two plans. In the first, they are entitled to services free of charge from one chosen primary care physician and from other specialists on referral from this physician. In the second, they may consult any physician but have to pay part of the fee. Only 3% of the people choose the second plan. They are generally older, have higher incomes, are health-ier, and use more subspecialty care. What makes the situation different in the United States is the linkage of the referral process with a cost-containment imper-ative and consequent interference with physician autonomy in decision-making, which raises the specter of rationing rather than rational organization. As of the mid-1990s, an increasing number of U.S. states are passing laws to allow direct access to subspecialists, particularly but not only to obstetrician/gynecologists, thus potentially jeopardizing the benefits of first-contact care. These laws are part of a more extensive legislative assault prompted by a general reaction against many of the perceived abuses of managed care (Hellinger, 1996). By 1996, however, there were signs that this piecemeal approach to regulation of these abuses was being replaced by a more comprehensive requirement for mechanisms to ensure account-ability for health care practices and outcomes.

If the purpose of gatekeepers is to provide more rational use of resources, there should be a scientific rationale for the belief that primary care practitioners can efficiently and effectively judge who should be referred to a specialist and who should not. Without a clear rationale for what should be retained in primary care and what should be referred, there will always be suspicion that factors such as cost-savings are controlling the decisions.

Rates of referral from primary care physicians to other specialists vary considerably, although, on average, about 5% of visits in general practice result in a referral to a specialist (Christensen et al., 1989; Wilkin and Smith, 1987). Some variations are due to differences in patients' characteristics, especially age (Penchansky and Fox, 1970), and some are associated with types of organization. For example, physicians in prepaid group practices (including health maintenance organizations) refer less than do physicians in other types of practices, and family physicians refer less than do internists (Perkoff, 1978). More recent data indicate that this continues to be the case at least for adult patients (Franks and Clancy, 1997). However, variability remains even after taking these characteristics into account. For example, Penchansky and Fox (1970) found a degree of variation from 2% to 18% of patients referred among internists and from 2% to 10% of patients referred among pediatricians. More recent studies find up to fourfold variations in referrals by primary care practitioners in both the United States and England (Wilkin and Dornan, 1990).

One important determinant of referral rates is the availability of subspecialists in the community. For example, the number of outpatients seen in the specialty clinics in the different regions of Great Britain is strongly associated with the number of consultants and is only weakly associated with illness rates as measured by standardized mortality ratios and by the mean number of prescriptions per patient written by general practitioners (Roland and Morris, 1988). In Denmark, the rate of referrals among all 141 general practitioners in one county was most highly related to the number of specialists in different areas within the county (Christensen et al., 1989).

In the United States, where many people can seek care from other specialists without a referral from a primary care physician, rates of visits to these other specialists is directly proportional to people's ability to go to or to return to a specialist without the advice or guidance of a primary care physician (Perkoff, 1978; Starfield, 1983).

The increasing attention to and use of gatekeepers compels attention to the nature of subspecialty care as well as primary care. Research will provide planners with the basis for formalizing criteria for referrals so that reasons other than medical need should be reduced. Specification of justifiable criteria for referral will also facilitate the development of systems to enhance the ability of primary care physicians to coordinate care—a major corollary of a rational gatekeeper role. The issues involved in improving coordination of care are pursued in Chapter 11.

Measurement of First Contact Care

Inherent in the concept of "first contact" is the idea that there should be one particular place or health care provider serving as a point of entry into the health system each time a new problem is experienced. Despite misgivings about the widespread adoption of "gatekeepers," the concept of a place or person of first contact has become well accepted as a desirable approach to organizing services. Moreover, there is general agreement that the gatekeeper be a generalist physician, usually a family/general practitioner, a general internist, or a general pediatrician. This source should be accessible to the population who should use it whenever new problems arise.

The terms *access* and *accessibility* have been used interchangeably and often ambiguously. One definition (Millman, 1993) went so far as to define access as "the timely use of personal health services to achieve the best possible health outcomes," thereby implying that access is unimportant in the absence of demonstrated effectiveness of services. Because the effectiveness of most specific health services is unknown, such a definition lacks usefulness.

"Accessibility" makes it possible for people to reach services. That is, it is one aspect of the structure of a health system or facility and the one that is necessary to achieve first-contact care. "Access" is the way in which people experience that characteristic of their health service. Accessibility is not a feature of primary care only, as all levels of health services should be accessible. However, the specific requirements for accessibility differ in primary care because it is the point of entry into the health services system. As noted earlier, uncertainty regarding the urgency and severity of newly appearing or recurring problems makes easy access to advice an important aspect of people's care.

Figure 7.1, which is based on the components of the heath system as presented in Chapter 2, shows those aspects of the health care system that are involved in the attainment of first contact: the structural characteristic of accessibility and the behavioral characteristic of use of services at the point of each perceived need.

The following section reviews ways of measuring the structural ("capacity") component of first-contact care—accessibility. The subsequent section addresses measurement of the performance component—utilization.

Measuring accessibility and access

Accessibility is the "structural" element necessary for first care. To provide it, the place of care must be easily accessible and available; if not, care will be delayed, perhaps to the point of adversely affecting the diagnosis and management of the problem.

There are various types of "accessibility." Donabedian (1973) distinguished socio-organizational access from geographic access. The former includes those characteristics of resources that either facilitate or hinder efforts of people to reach care. An example is the requirement that patients pay a visit fee before receiving service, which may provide a barrier to access. Less explicit social prejudices such as age, race, or social class are also examples. Geographic access, on the other hand, involves characteristics related to distance and time required to reach and obtain the services.

Accessibility and access can be measured from the vantage of both the population and the health care facility.

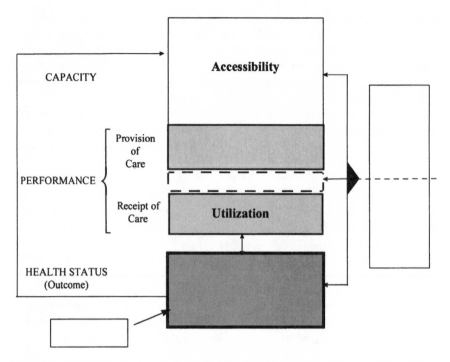

Figure 7.1. The health services system: First Contact Components. Abstracted from Figure 2.1.

Assessment of access for populations

Surveys of barriers to the use of services. Health surveys often ascertain information about the existence of various impediments to the use of services (such as the absence of insurance or other third party coverage of the costs of services) as well as information on the extent to which needed services are not received and the reasons why. Questions such as the following have been asked:

Do you have to take time off from work to go to the doctor?
About how long does it take for you to get to the doctor?
Does the doctor speak your native language (Edwards and Berlin, 1989)?

Several other surveys in the United States contain questions on access to health services (Kovar, 1989).

Surveys of people's perceptions about accessibility of care. Penchansky and Thomas (1981) described a survey in which people were asked 16 questions about accessibility to care. Accessibility was divided into five types: availability, accessibility, accommodation, affordability, and acceptability. The questions were as follows:

Availability

- All things considered, how much confidence do you have in being able to get good medical care for you and your family when you need it?
- How satisfied are you with your ability to find one good doctor to treat the whole family?
- How satisfied are you with your knowledge of where to get health care?
- How satisfied are you with your ability to get medical care in an emergency?

Accessibility

- How satisfied are you with how convenient your physician's office is to your home?
- How difficult is it for you to get to your physician's office?

Accommodation

- How satisfied are you with how long you have to wait to get an appointment?
- How satisfied are you with how convenient your physician's office hours are?
- How satisfied are you with how long you have to wait in the waiting room?
- How satisfied are you with how easy it is to get in touch with your physician?

Affordability

- How satisfied are you with your health insurance?
- How satisfied are you with the doctor's prices?
- How satisfied are you with how soon you need to pay the doctor's bill?

Acceptability

- How satisfied are you with the appearance of the doctor's office?
- How satisfied are you with the neighborhoods the offices are in?
- How satisfied are you with the other patients you usually see at the doctor's office?

To the extent that people's thresholds for adequacy are similar, responses to surveys such as these could provide a basis for judging the adequacy of accessibility or for comparing the adequacy of accessibility in different areas. If, however, different groups of people differ in standards, such a survey may conclude that there are no differences when, in fact, they are considerable.

The remaining methods (use/disability ratio, symptoms/response ratio, and episode of illness analysis) are not directed as much at the actual barriers to access as to reflections of the likely existence of barriers as manifested by lower use of services than might be expected. Moreover, none of them are specific to primary care services and would have to be significantly adapted to be useful in that context.

The use/disability ratio. This measure of accessibility (Aday et al., 1980), like the previous one, is applied in population surveys. Respondents are asked whether there were days in which they were unable to perform their normal activities because of a health problem and whether they sought medical care. The lower the use/disability ratio, the lower the access to care. Obviously, the measure is useful only for comparative purposes because there is no "correct" answer. Groups of the population that differ in their average use/disability ratio are presumed to differ in their access to care. The major problems with the measure are that both the numerator and the denominator depend on recall by the respondent and that it assumes that all disabilities are similar in their need for medical care or that different populations are similar in the nature of their disabilities. Both assumptions may be incorrect. Another problem with the use of the use/disability ratio is that the number of physician visits used in the numerator may not be linked to the number of disabilities in the denominator (Yergan et al., 1981).

The symptoms/response ratio. This measure, also used in population surveys (Andersen, 1978), elicits information as to whether respondents have had particular symptoms that are generally judged by professionals to require medical care. A panel of physicians provided the proportion of patients who should have sought care for the symptoms. The "response" is whether they actually sought medical care. The ratio is derived as follows:

$$\frac{(\text{Persons contacting}) - (\text{Those needing contact})}{\text{Those needing contact}}$$

As is the case with the use/disability ratio, the measure is useful only for comparative purposes; population groups with different ratios presumably differ in their access to care. The major limitation of the measure is that the judgments of physicians regarding the need for care are based on opinion rather than on data. Furthermore, the frequency of symptom complexes that are elicited is low (Yergan et al., 1981) so that large samples are required for stable estimates. Another problem is that all symptom complexes are counted rather than just one per patient.

The episode of illness analysis. As originally used (Richardson, 1970), individuals are asked whether they were ill during a defined period, the number of days associated with disability, and the number of days associated with use of medical care. Aday et al. (1980) expanded on the approach by asking about the results of care and by categorizing the type of illness as either requiring care or not requiring care (according to professional judgment) and the degree of worry by the patient about the problem. The major disadvantage of the method is that it is cumbersome for respondents with complex illnesses. Although there is no validated method for deriving a summary index of appropriate response, Yergan et al. (1981) suggested a mechanism for categorizing the data in order to devise one. When outcome is included in the analyses, access is considered inadequate even if the outcome was good but care was not provided for problems that engendered a great deal of patient worry.

It should be noted that the last three methods described (use/disability, symptoms/response, episode of illness) make inferences about access from measures that involve utilization. In the terminology of Aday et al. (1980, p. 35), these measures reflect "realized access." It is important to recognize that these measures of access do not relate specifically to the source of primary care, although they could be adapted to do so.

Access to care may also be assessed at the facilities (provider) level. All of the methods used at the population level can also be applied to patients coming to the health care facility. In the interpretation of findings, however, these methods will underestimate the extent of difficulty in access to services because patients with access problems that limit their use will be under-represented among the patients available for interview.

Assessment of accessibility and access in facilities or among patients

In one method of assessing accessibility (Weiner and Starfield, 1983), professionals are asked a series of questions about features of their office arrangements associated with accessibility. These include

- The availability of emergency appointment slots
- The time lags from request to appointment for acute but nonemergency problems and for nonacute problems
- The average duration of time in the waiting room
- The availability of house calls
- The use of an answering service when the office is closed
- Provision for after-hours coverage
- The availability of a sliding fee schedule related to ability to pay
- The acceptance of payment from Medicare for eligible individuals

The assumption of the method is that all these features of access ought be provided, but its major use is comparative: to assess differences in accessibility to care across different types of physicians and physician groups. When aggregated for an area, however, it could be used to compare access of the system in different areas.

In another approach to assessing accessibility, standards are set for each of its several aspects, and then a facility or practice is evaluated (or evaluates itself) against the standards (Institute of Medicine, 1978). For accessibility, 16 questions are posed. The first six relate to accessibility directly, the next three address convenience, and the remaining seven address acceptability. The questions are

Is access to primary care services provided 24 hours a day, 7 days a week?

Is there an opportunity for a patient to schedule an appointment?

Are scheduled office hours compatible with the work and way of life of most of the patients?

Can most (90%) of medically urgent cases be seen within 1 hour?

Can most patients (90%) with acute but not urgent problems be seen within 1 day?

Can most (90%) appropriate requests for routine appointments, such as preventive examinations, be met within 1 week?

Is the practice unit conveniently located so that most patients can reach it by public or private transportation?

Is the practice unit so designed that handicapped or elderly patients are not inconvenienced?

Does the practice unit accept patients who have a means of payment, regardless of source (Medicare, Medicaid)?

Is the waiting time for most (90%) of the scheduled patients less than one-half hour?

If a substantial minority (25%) of patients have a special language or other communication barrier, does the office staff include people who can deal with this problem?

Are waiting accommodations comfortable and uncrowded?

Does the practice staff consistently demonstrate an interest in and appreciation of the culture, background, socioeconomic status, work environment, and living status of patients?

Is simple, understandable information provided to patients about fees, billing procedures, scheduling of appointments, contacting the unit after hours, and grievance procedures?

Are patients encouraged to ask questions about their illness and their care, to discuss their health problems freely, and to review their records, if desired?

Does the practice unit accept patients without regard to their race, religion, or ethnic identity?

Access as measured from the viewpoint of patients can be assessed by using "simulated patients." In this approach, individuals are trained to make an appointment by phone and then are observed in their visit to the facility. Two types of measures are used, the urgency ratio and the frustration ratio. To determine urgency ratio, a panel of individuals consisting of health professionals, administrators of the facility, and patients decides ahead of time whether particular complaints are critical, serious, chronic, or routine. These designations are based on the maximum time that should elapse before the patient is seen for each category of symptoms. Then, for each simulated patient with the problem, a ratio of time to the appointment divided by appropriate time to the appointment is calculated for patients in each category of condition.

The frustration index has three components: time spent on the telephone to make the appointment, time from arrival in facility to time being seen, and time spent waiting for common laboratory tests. The appropriate time (in minutes) for each of these components was also set by the panel, and data from actual patients, regardless of their condition, are monitored and compared with the standards.

Facilities may set their own standards for performance on either of these indices. Alternatively, facilities may be compared with each other to determine which performs better.

Increasing interest in assessing all of the important aspects of primary care has led to the development of instruments that address multiple components of care including accessibility and access. These are presented in Chapter 13 in the context of instruments that measure all four features of primary care together.

Measuring use of the facility when care is first believed to be needed

Use of services is an aspect of the processes of care for two of its unique features: first contact and longitudinality. The feature of utilization relevant to first-contact care is the extent to which the *first* visit for a new problem is made to the regular source of care. It is distinguished from utilization in the case of longitudinal care in which utilization should *always* occur (except for referral visits) at the source of primary care regardless of the stage of the particular problem or of the problem type.

Measurement of first contact is best made at the population level rather than at a facility level. The reason for this is that measurements at the facility level will systematically exclude individuals who do not seek services because they have poor access or because of some other reason. Individuals with *few* visits to the facility will also be under-represented in data collected by taking a random sample of its users. Conclusions about access or utilization that derive from interviews of patients do not necessarily reflect the experiences of those who are most likely to have poor access or underutilization unless the facility uses a roster of its patients to select samples for interviewing. For this reason, population-based studies of first-contact care are preferred to facility-based ones.

Measurement of the behavioral component of first-contact care involves eliciting information concerning the place at which care has been sought. This information might be obtained from such sources as medical records, claims forms, or billing data, but one cannot be sure that they encompass all use of services. Another drawback to this technique is that these types of records usually do not indicate whether the visit was at the patient's initiative or resulted from a referral. Because first-contact care pertains only to visits that patients initiate, the absence of this information fails to accurately indicate the extent to which first-contact care is achieved.

One alternative is to ask individuals where they received care when they last sought it for a new problem and whether the visit was made on the advice of another physician. Another alternative is to explore both accessibility and use of services at the same time, through questions such as the following:

What is your regular source of care, that is, the place you usually go when you have a new problem that you think requires a doctor's attention?

Where did you go the last time you had a new problem that you thought needed a doctor's attention?

How easy was it to obtain help from the doctor to whom you went? (Various aspects of access might be explored through branching of this question.)

What was the reason you did not go to your regular source of care for this last visit? (A choice of reasons would include several that clearly relate to features that enhance accessibility to services and facilitate utilization.)

Table 7.2. Summary of First Contact

	Capacity	*Performance*
Description: Primary care is the place where care is sought for each new perceived need		
Involves	Access to services	Seeking of care from *primary care source* for each new need
Problem related	All problems	All problems
Personal relationship required	No	No
Time dependent	No	No
Specific methods of measurement	Population/patient survey Simulated patients Provider survey Observation of facility	Population survey

More recent adaptations of methods to assess use of primary care services for first contact are presented in Chapter 13, in the context of evaluation of all primary care characteristics. Table 7.2 summarizes the approach to measurement of first-contact care.

What Is Known About the Attainment of First-Contact Care?

Access and accessibility to primary care

There are several examples of how the measures previously described have been used to provide information on access to care and the adequacy of first contact in primary care.

There was a marked improvement in access to care in the United States in the 1970s as a result of the passage of the War on Poverty legislation in the mid-1960s. However, in the early 1980s there were reductions in third party coverage for care, especially for those with low incomes. A national telephone survey conducted in the mid-1980s showed how access to services changed as a result of these reductions in insurance coverage. There was a marked increase in the number of people who reported that they had no regular source of care and consequently had many fewer visits to physicians and fewer hospitalizations (Freeman et al., 1987). The situation was especially marked among individuals who had no insurance; 31% lacked any regular source of care in 1986 (Robert Wood Johnson Foundation, 1987). Although the reductions in use of care were not necessarily restricted to first-contact care, the decrease in number of individuals who reported no regular source of care suggests that first-contact care from a primary care source was seriously compromised as a result of reductions in insurance coverage.

Physicians of different specialties differ in the degree to which their practices are accessible. Studies (Weiner, 1981; Starfield et al., 1973; Cherkin et al., 1986) indicate that

• Family physicians are less likely to require appointments for visits than are other physicians.

- Family physicians are more likely to have regular office hours during weekends than are general internists.
- Family physicians and internists are more likely to report that they make house calls or special visits to emergency rooms and nursing homes and that they make more of these visits than do other types of physicians.
- Patients of family physicians wait less time for nonurgent appointments than do patients of other types of physicians.
- The offices of generalists and non-board-certified pediatricians or internists are more accessible than are those of board-certified pediatricians or internists or other specialists.

National surveys indicated that people who report no regular source of care had substantially fewer visits than they needed, as measured by the symptoms/response ratio. People who had subspecialists as their regular source of care report making more visits that experts judged to be unnecessary. In contrast, those with a clinic or a primary care physician as their source of care had approximately the same number of visits overall as experts judged to be needed (Taylor et al., 1975).

A more recent study of care provided by 60 family physicians, 245 general internists, and 55 subspecialty internists working in an organized health plan (Grumbach et al., 1998) indicated that there were few differences in patients' reporting of accessibility, with general internists doing slightly better. However, the internists had smaller patient panels and saw fewer patients per unit of work time than did the family physicians. There were no differences between general internists and subspecialty internists, but in this health plan subspecialty internists had to agree to devote a major portion of their time to primary care rather than to subspecialty care.

Use of primary care for first contact

The rate of visits to specialists in some organizational settings is much greater than in others largely because the plans (including some types of health maintenance organizations) allow patients to make appointments directly with subspecialists whereas others require patients to have a referral from a primary care physician (Perkoff, 1978; Starfield, 1986). Thus, in at least some facilities, first-contact care is not achieved by primary care physicians. Whether the situation is a result of patient choice to go directly to the subspecialist when permitted to do so or is a result of a lack of accessibility or lack of interest of the primary care physician cannot be determined from the data; only subsequent study would elucidate the reason for the failure of first contact in these primary care settings.

In a multisite study of use of services, people who reported a generalist as their source of care were much more likely to see that physician first when they had an acute illness than were people who reported that a specialist was their regular source of care (Spiegel et al., 1983).

A national study of a representative sample of office-based physicians showed that general and family physicians had a higher proportion of first visits (in which the patient was not seen before) than pediatricians. Pediatricians, in contrast, had a higher proportion of patients who had been seen previously but for other problems than the one occasioning the visit (Fishbane and Starfield, 1981). The same was the case for generalists as compared with other types of physicians, although the differences between generalists and internists, ophthalmologists, and otolaryngologists were not large (Puskin, 1977). These findings suggest that generalists may serve more as the point of first contact for new problems than pediatricians, internists, or other specialists, at least historically.

In some places in the United States, attainment of first-contact care occurs less in the 1990s than in the 1970s. For example, parents of children being seen in an urban emergency room in 1976 and in 1993 were queried as to the presence of a regular source of care (where they take their children most often for either well or sick visits). Although the percentage of children with a regular source was greater in 1993 than in 1976, a smaller proportion had contacted their regular source before coming to the emergency room (Shah-Canning et al., 1996). Thus, people not enrolled in managed care organizations with institutionalized first-contact care may be less likely to be receiving it now than previously.

Thus the few studies that have examined the extent of first-contact care indicate that individuals whose regular source of care is a primary care physician are more likely to be receiving first-contact care from that physician than are individuals who have other types of physicians as their regular source of care.

Summary

There are important theoretical as well as empirical justifications for the "gate" function of primary care.

First-contact care involves the provision of services that are accessible (a structural or capacity feature of care) and the utilization of those services when a need for care arises (a process or performance feature of care)

Information regarding the accessibility of care should be ascertained at both the population level and at the facilities level.

The best way to elicit information concerning the attainment of first-contact care is either by asking individuals in a population or by analyzing data on *all* visits made by the individuals in the population to determine where individuals went when they first sought care for a new problem or need for care.

Accessibility of care varies with the type of physician. In general, primary care physicians, especially family physicians, are more accessible than are other types of physicians, particularly with regard to flexibility in providing care without appointments and times for appointments.

Access to care is important in reducing mortality and morbidity. The use of primary care practitioners rather than other specialists for first-contact care is likely to lead to more appropriate care, better health outcomes, and lower total costs.

The increasing focus on "gatekeepers" should be accompanied by a strategy to obtain information concerning the nature and extent of referrals, the development of better criteria for referral, and the appropriate roles of subspecialists in the care of patients.

References

Aday LL, Andersen R, Fleming G. Health Care in the U.S. Equitable for Whom? Beverly Hills: Sage Publications, 1980.

Andersen R. Health status indices and access to medical care. Am J Public Health 1978; 68:458–63.

Chande V, Kinnane J. Role of the primary care provider in expediting care of children with acute appendicitis. Arch Pediatr Adolesc Med 1996; 150:703–6.

Cherkin D, Rosenblatt R, Hart L, Schleiter M. A comparison of the patients and practices of recent graduates of family practice and general internal medicine residency programs. Med Care 1986; 24:1136–50.

Christensen B, Sorensen H, Mabeck C. Differences in referral rates from general practice. Fam Pract 1989; 6:19–22.

Crombie D, van der Lee J, Backer P. The Interface Study. Occasional Paper 48. London: Royal College of General Practitioners, 1990.

Donabedian A. Aspects of Medical Care Administration. Specifying Requirements for Health Care. Cambridge, MA: Harvard University Press, 1973., pp 419–73.

Edwards WS, Berlin M. Questionnaires and data collection methods for the household survey and the survey of American Indians and Alaska Natives. Washington, DC: Department of Health and Human Services, Public Health Service. DHHS Pub. No. PHS89–3450. National Center for Health Services Research and Health Care Technology Assessment, 1989.

Fahs M. Physician response to the United Mine Workers' cost-sharing program: The other side of the coin. Health Serv Res 1992; 27:25–45.

Fihn S, Wicher J. Withdrawing routine outpatient medical services: Effects on access and health. J Gen Intern Med 1988; 3:356–62.

Fishbane M, Starfield B. Child health care in the United States: A comparison of pediatricians and general practitioners. N Engl J Med 1981; 305:552–6.

Forrest CB, Starfield B. The effect of first-contact with primary care clinicians on ambulatory health care expenditures. J Fam Pract 1996; 43:40–8.

Forrest C, Starfield B. Entry to primary care and continuity: The impact of access. Am J Public Health (In press), 1998.

Franks P, Clancy C. Referral of adult patients from primary care: Demographic disparities and their relationship to HMO insurance. J Fam Pract 1997; 45:47–53.

Freeman H, Blendon R, Aiken L, Sudman S, Mullinix C, Corey C. Americans report on their access to health care. Health Aff 1987; 6:6–18.

Fry J, Horder J. Primary Health Care in an International Context. London: The Nuffield Provincial Hospitals Trust, 1994.

Gérvas J, Pérez-Fernández M, Starfield B. Primary care, financing and gatekeeping in western Europe. Fam Pract 1994; 11(3):307–17.

Grumbach K, Selby J, Schmittdiel J, Quesenberry C. Quality of primary care practice in a large HMO according to physician specialty. Manuscript submitted, 1998.

Hellinger F. The expanding scope of state legislation. JAMA 1996; 276:1065–70.

Hurley R, Freund D, Gage B. Gatekeepers' effects on patterns of physician use. J Fam Pract 1991; 32:167–74.

Hurley R, Freund D, Taylor D. Emergency room use and primary care case management: Evidence from four Medicaid demonstration programs. Am J Public Health 1989; 79(7): 843–7.

Institute of Medicine. A Manpower Policy for Primary Health Care: Report of a Study. IOM Pub. No. 78–02. Washington, DC: National Academy of Sciences, 1978.

Kovar MG. Data systems of the National Center for Health Statistics. National Center for Health Statistics. Vital and Health Statistics 1(23); DHHS Pub. No. (PHS)89-1325, 1989.

Lurie N, Ward N, Shapiro M, Gallego C, Vahaiwalla R, Brook R. Termination of medical benefits. A follow-up study one year later. N Engl J Med 1986; 314:1266–8.

Martin D, Dieher P, Price K, Richardson W. Effect of a gatekeeper plan on health services use and charges: A randomized trial. Am J Public Health 1989; 79(12):1628–32.

Mathers N, Hodgkin P. The gatekeeper and the wizard: A fairytale. BMJ 1989; 298:172–4.

Millman M (ed). Access to Health Care in America. Washington, DC: National Academy Press, 1993.

Moore S. Cost containment through risk-sharing by primary care physicians. N Engl J Med 1979; 300:1359–62.

Moore S, Martin D, Richardson W. Does the primary-care gatekeeper control the costs of health care? N Engl J Med 1983; 309:1400–4.

O'Toole SJ, Karamanoukian HL, Allen JE, Caty MG, O'Toole D, Azizkhan RG, Glick PL. Insurance-related differences in the presentation of pediatric appendicitis. J Pediatr Surg 1996; 31(8):1032–4.

Penchansky R, Fox D. Frequency of referral and patient characteristics in group practice. Med Care 1970; 8:368–85.

Penchansky R, Thomas JW. The concept of access: Definitions and relationship to consumer satisfaction. Med Care 1981; 19:127–40.

Perkoff G. An effect of organization of medical care upon health manpower distribution. Med Care 1978; 16:628–37.

Puskin D. Patterns of Ambulatory Medical Care Practice in the United States: An Analysis of the National Ambulatory Medical Care Survey. Dissertation. Baltimore: Johns Hopkins University, 1977, p 57.

Rasell M. Cost sharing in health insurance—A reexamination. N Engl J Med 1995; 332: 1164–8.

Reagan M. Physicians as gatekeepers: A complex challenge. N Engl J Med 1987; 317:1731–4.

Richardson W. Measuring the Urban Poor's Use of Physician Services in Response to Illness Episodes. Med Care 1970; 8:132–42.

Robert Wood Johnson Foundation. Access to Health Care in the United States: Results of a 1986 Survey. Special Report No. 2. Princeton, NJ: Robert Wood Johnson Foundation, 1987.

Roland M, Morris R. Are referrals by general practitioners influenced by the availability of consultants? BMJ 1988; 297:599–600.

Roos N. Who should do the surgery? Tonsillectomy and adenoidectomy in one Canadian province. Inquiry 1979; 16:73–83.

Rosser W. Approach to diagnosis by primary care clinicians and specialists: Is there a difference? J Fam Pract 1996; 2:139–44.

Saltman R, Figueras J. European Health Care Reform. Analysis of Current Strategies. Copenhagen: World Health Organization, 1997.

Scheff T. Preferred errors in diagnosis. Med Care 1964; 2:166–72.

Schieber GJ, Poullier JP, Greenwald LM. Health system performance in OECD countries, 1980–1992. Health Aff 1994; 13(4):100–12.

Shah-Canning D, Alpert J, Bauchner H. Care seeking patterns of inner-city families using an emergency room: A three decade comparison. Med Care 1996; 34:1171–9.

Shapiro M, Ware J, Sherourne C. Effects of cost sharing on seeking care for serious and minor symptoms: Results of a randomized controlled trial. Ann Intern Med 1986; 104: 246–51.

Sox H. Decision-making: A comparison of referral practice and primary care. J Fam Pract 1996; 2:155–60.

Spiegel J, Rubenstein L, Scott B, Brook R. Who is the primary physician? N Engl J Med 1983; 308:1208–12.

Starfield B. Special responsibilities: The role of the pediatrician and goals of pediatric education. Pediatrics 1983; 71:433–40.

Starfield B. Effectiveness of Medical Care: Validating Clinical Wisdom. Baltimore: Johns Hopkins University Press, 1985.

Starfield B. Primary care in the United States. Int J Health Serv 1986; 16:179–98.

Starfield B, Bice T, Schach E, Rabin D, White KL. How "regular" is the "regular source of medical care?" Pediatrics 1973; 51:822–32.

Taylor D, Aday L, Andersen R. A social indicator of access to medical care. J Health Soc Behav 1975; 16:39–49.

Weiner J. An Analysis of Office-Based Primary Care in Baltimore City. Dissertation. Baltimore: Johns Hopkins University, 1981.

Weiner J, Starfield B. Measurement of the primary care roles of office-based physicians. Am J Public Health 1983; 73:666–71.

Wilkin D, Dornan C. GP Referrals to Hospital: A Review of Research and Its Implications for Policy and Practice. Center for Primary Care Research, University of Manchester, July 1990.

Wilkin D, Smith A. Explaining variation in general practitioner referrals to hospital. Fam Pract 1987; 4:160–9.

Yergan J, LoGerfo J, Shortell S, Bergner M, Diehr P, Richardson W. Health status as a measure of need for medical care: A critique. Med Care 1981; 19 (suppl):57–68.

— 8 —

Patient Lists and Patient-Focused Care Over Time

I wish my own doctor could have been the one that took charge of everything. He knows me and we can talk together and understand each other.

Mrs. P, after the birth of her baby who was normal but
had an extensive workup for transient symptoms.

Longitudinality is not a word that appears in any dictionary. It is derived from *longitudinal*, which is defined as "dealing with the growth and change of individuals or groups over a period of years." Although the word *continuity* is usually used instead of *longitudinality*, the latter conveys the spirit better than the former. Longitudinality, in the context of primary care, is a long-term personal relationship between practitioners and the patients in their practice. Continuity is not necessary for this relationship to be present; interruptions in the continuity of care for whatever reason need not disrupt this relationship. Therefore, the term "longitudinality," coined by Alpert and Charney in 1974, provides a much better sense of the characteristic that is a critical part of primary care.

The achievement of primary care implies that there is one place, one individual, or one team of associated individuals that serves as the source of care over a defined period of time regardless of the presence or absence of particular health-related problems or the type of problem. Having longitudinal care means that individuals in the population identify with a source of care as "theirs," that the provider or groups of providers at least implicitly recognize the existence of a formal or informal contract to be the regular source of person-focused (not disease-focused) care and that this relationship exists for a defined period of time or indefinitely until explicitly changed.

There is a distinction between identification of one physician, one team of physicians, or a particular place of care as the locus of longitudinality. When a team or a place is the source of longitudinality, the burden of coordination is likely to be greater than if a particular individual is the source because patients are likely to be seen by a greater number of practitioners. Conversely, when an individual is the source of longitudinality, the challenges of providing first contact care and comprehensiveness are greater because it is more difficult for an individual than for a team or medical organization always to be available and to provide or arrange for a range of needed services.

The essence of longitudinality (Alpert and Charney, 1974) is a personal relationship over time, regardless of the type of health problems or even the presence of a health problem, between a patient and a physician or a team of physicians and nonphysician personnel. Through this relationship, practitioners come to know patients over time, and patients come to know their practitioners. This is captured in the Institute of Medicine's Report on Primary Care as a "sustained partnership" in which "the patient is treated as a whole person whose values and preferences are taken into account" (Institute of Medicine, 1997). The benefits of this knowledge would be expected to accrue in a variety of ways. For example, patients should have fewer visits because many problems can be managed on the phone rather than requiring a visit to ascertain information that is already known. Fewer hospitalizations should also result because practitioners are more likely to be able to ascertain whether the problem could be managed at home.

"Continuity of care" is a phrase that is often used to describe the extent to which patients see the same practitioner or visit the same facility from one visit to another or even over a period of time. In this sense, continuity could be a characteristic of specialty care as well as of primary care but it would be focused on management of problems rather than on care of people regardless of what problems they may have. Chapter 11 discusses more fully these differences between longitudinality and continuity.

> I've just been going from hospital to doctors' offices over and over again and I've been asking questions. The pains started after I had my operation. The doctors all take me from test to test—any test they can find, they give it to me, from a barium enema to an upper GI series to whatever. And I just keep asking questions, and they just kept writing me prescription after prescription, telling me to take the medicines, which to this day haven't stopped the pain. I ask them "Why are you giving me all of these prescriptions when I'm so allergic to medicines?" When I asked them all these questions, they just tell me to trust them. So, at the beginning I took all the prescriptions, which haven't helped. I got tired of those doctors who were "helping me" and who were telling me what I was feeling and not listening to how I said I was feeling. You just have to tell them to "hold it a minute." So I changed doctors because I wanted a second opinion. When I went to this other doctor, he examined me and then he just shook his head, and he said "I don't know, but take this medicine." He wrote me a prescription to take the medicine and told me to come back in two weeks. The pain wasn't getting any better and the medicine wasn't doing any good. So I went back to him, and he examined me again, and I asked him for the results of the tests he had taken, but he said he hadn't gotten them yet. He just sat there about five minutes, shaking his head, and then he writes me five prescriptions! And when I asked him what they were for, he said "Just take them. Trust me and take them, and we'll get to the bottom of this." I said "ok" and then he said that he was going to send in another gentleman to examine me, and that I should come back in about five weeks. So I sat there about five minutes until the other doctor came in. He took out his stethoscope and listened to one side—my right side—and he turned around to the desk and wrote me two more

prescriptions. When I asked him what they were for, he said to just trust him and come back in two weeks. I told him that I wasn't a guinea pig and I wasn't going to take all of the prescriptions. I tore up all the prescriptions and left the office.

Finally I went back to the family doctor who has been taking care of me for twenty years. She knows me really well and she was wonderful. She listened to me and didn't try to tell me what I was feeling. She took me off all the medications and the pains started going away.   Mrs. M., a 50-year-old waitress

As is the case with each of the four attributes of primary care, longitudinality is related to the others. The relationship with a regular source of care implies that that place will be the place of first-contact care. It also implies, as is noted in the next two chapters, that the regular source of care will ensure that care is comprehensive and that it is coordinated.

The Benefits of Longitudinality

The benefits of association with a regular source of care have been documented in a wide variety of studies. Although having a place (e.g., a clinic or a neighborhood health center) as the regular source of care is not equivalent to having a physician as the regular source of care, until recently there was little evidence on the point because most studies of the benefits of longitudinality were carried out using either the place or the physician as the basis for study, and there were few comparisons of the two. However, at least half of the patients in several group practices in England (where patients generally register with specific practitioners) valued an affiliation with a particular doctor sufficiently highly to wait longer for an appointment and to wait longer in the office to see the doctor (Freeman and Richards, 1994). Patients on a doctor's own list were much more likely to have seen that doctor in consultations over a 6-year period than patients who related to a group of physicians rather than an individual physician (Freeman and Richards, 1990). Another study involving more than 2,000 patients in 89 British general practices found that patients in practices with "personal" lists (rather than "group" lists) were significantly more satisfied with their care regardless of the way in which satisfaction was assessed (Baker and Streatfield, 1995; Baker, 1996).

A national survey of patients conducted in the United States in 1988 found that individuals with a specific doctor as their regular source of care had better receipt of recommended immunizations, better screening for breast cancer, better use of services by those in poor health, and lower hospitalizations for ambulatory sensitive conditions (see Chapter 13) than individuals who reported only a place as their regular source. However, these findings were confined to those who reported a nontraditional site (e.g., a hospital outpatient clinic or other type of clinic) as their source. Furthermore, the study made no distinction between having a specialist as a regular source of care and having a primary care physician as that source (Lambrew et al., 1996).

However, a study that rated the adequacy of primary care received in urban areas of one U.S. state found that patients who had optimal adequacy of primary care (a combination of availability, continuity, comprehensiveness, and communication with providers) were no more likely to report having a particular provider at their regular source of care than those who reported the place as their source (Stewart et al., 1997). That is, when a place achieves high levels of primary care attributes, the benefits may be as great as having a particular physician. Thus, the crux of the issue is whether a place or a particular person is more likely to achieve the attributes of primary care. Unfortunately, the absence (until very recently) of tools to measure these attributes and the general lack of appreciation of the importance of studying them has prevented the accumulation of evidence on this issue.

Because the literature on the benefit of longitudinality sometimes addresses affiliation with a particular place and sometimes with a particular person, the following examples of benefit are divided according to whether the source was a particular practitioner or place. In most of the examples, actual association with a regular source of care (rather than the mere reporting of the presence of a regular source of care) was present.

Studies in which the regular source of care was an individual practitioner

Longitudinality facilitates compliance with prescribed medication. In an early study in upstate New York, Charney et al. (1967) demonstrated that the taking of medication was greater among children whose own physician prescribed it. Becker et al. (1972) demonstrated a similar effect for children being treated for otitis media.

Patients who had a regular source of care but did not see that physician were more likely to be judged as not needing care by the physician who saw them for a problem than if their own physician had made the judgment. This finding suggests that physicians who have developed a relationship with patients are more able to appreciate the needs of patients than are physicians who are not familiar with the patient (Steinwachs and Yaffe, 1978).

Longitudinality of care facilitates the recognition of certain types of problems. For example, Becker et al. (1974) demonstrated that children randomly assigned to receive care by a team, consisting of a physician, nurse, and registrar, which remained constant over time, were more likely to have their behavior problems recognized than were children seen in the same facility by the next provider available.

A Norwegian study of 1,401 adults attending 89 general practitioners found that the physician's report of how well they knew the patient was associated with better recognition of most of the types of psychosocial problems that patients independently recorded on questionnaires after the visit, even after controlling for other influential factors such as sociodemographic characteristics of the patient and doctor (Gulbrandsen et al., 1997).

Corroboration of the impact of having a personal physician comes from a large national study of 10,250 children in 172 primary care practices. By far the most salient determinant of physicians' recognition of children's psychosocial problems was familiarity with the patient, as determined by whether the practitioner seeing the patient reported that the patient was their personal patient rather than their group's patient or not a primary care patient for their practice (Kelleher et al., 1997).

Preventive care of some types, particularly for children, is better if the individual has a practitioner who serves as their source of primary care. Thus, children already affiliated with a particular place where they receive their care are more likely to receive an indicated immunization if they previously indicated a relationship with a particular doctor or nurse practitioner (Lieu et al., 1994).

Physicians have also been found to make more accurate diagnoses (among women presenting with urinary tract symptoms) and prescribe no treatment (appropriately) if they know the patient better (Nazareth and King, 1993).

Patients seen for consultation in a medical center are more likely to return to the referring physician if they consider that physician to be their regular source of care (Lawrence and Dorsey, 1976). That is, identification of a source of longitudinality improves the extent to which patients complete the referral process by returning to the referring physician.

When patients visit the same practitioner rather than different practitioners, care is more efficient. A population-based study involving review of all claims of a random sample of Medicaid patients (aged 0–21 years) for 3 years revealed that longitudinality was associated with a reduction in hospital admissions and overall costs (Flint, 1987).

Lower hospitalization rates and lower overall costs may require an even longer duration of physician–patient relationships in some population groups. In a national study of the elderly, ties of at least 5 years, and particularly those of at least 10 years, were required to achieve these benefits. No influence of duration of ties on preventive procedures, smoking, or obesity were found (Weiss and Blustein, 1996).

Longitudinality is associated with increased satisfaction on the part of patients, as shown in several studies (Wasson et al., 1984; Becker et al., 1972, 1974). The longer the duration of the doctor–patient relationship, the higher the satisfaction, even when factors such as number of consultations; age and sex of patient; age, sex, location, and type of practice and reimbursement of provider; and type of consultation, illness, and duration of problem are taken into account. For example, patients in 133 Norwegian general practices who had a duration of relationship of more than 5 years were over one-third more likely to report being very satisfied as those with relationships of 1–5 years (Hjortdahl and Laerum, 1992).

Of course, satisfaction is not a good measure of the benefits of longitudinality because dissatisfied individuals are more likely to change their practitioner if they are able to do so. However, there is independent corroboration of the benefits of longitudinality from a related study in the same 133 Norwegian practices. The patients' physicians reported knowing more about their medical history, personality, and social network when the duration of the relationship was longer; it took at least 1 and often 5 years for doctors to achieve a good knowledge base about patients (Hjortdahl, 1992). They also are more likely to manage expectantly rather than to prescribe medication (Hjortdahl and Borchgrevink, 1991).

What accounts for the beneficial effects of longitudinality? Although the specific mechanisms have not been explored, there are several possibilities. Through time, a sense of trust in the physician may make patients more comfortable in divulging relevant information and more responsive to their physician's recommendations. Similarly, physicians involved in longitudinal care may be more sensitive to relatively subtle cues that help to elucidate the nature of the patient's problem. Accumulated knowledge about the patient's background and illness experiences may aid the physician in arriving at a more accurate assessment of the patient's problem.

> My son is an 18-year-old camper, skier, swimmer, and student at the local rural high school. He is dependent on a computer for speech, a power chair for movement around the house and school, and his parents for most of his physical needs. He has an undiagnosed neurologic disease that seems to be progressive; he is adopted and his disorder is probably genetic. Our family physician takes care of immunizations and sore throats and those sorts of things, but for some special needs, Nick continues to see a specialist. The two physicians work very closely together, but our family physician is the one who can best explain to Nick what is going on, such as when Nick started having seizures.   Ms. A., a mother

The physician as a "repository of information" is the basis for the idea that continuity of care is a useful aspect of health services. This subject is addressed in Chapter 11.

In the past, concern has been expressed that longitudinality may delay the recognition of serious problems (Evang, 1960; Miller, 1973) but this has never been adequately documented as a systematic problem.

Studies where the source of care was a particular place

Children who receive their care from an identifiable regular source are more likely to receive preventive care than other children. Alpert et al. (1976) showed that children assigned randomly to a particular facility for all of their care had much higher rates of visits for health supervision and lower rates of visits for illness care than had patients not enrolled in the facility, even though their prior visit rates for both types of visits were similar. McDaniel et al. (1975) showed that children receiving all of their care from a pediatric practice were more likely to have complete immunizations than were children receiving care from both a private pediatrician and a health department clinic. (However, the findings were not consistent across the four groups of pediatricians studied, indicating that the finding is not generalizable to all practices.)

A national study of children reporting community health centers (CHCs) as their regular source of care found those who used the CHCs for both sick and routine care were more likely to have received age-appropriate preventive care than children who used a CHC only for routine care. If there was also a relationship with a particular physician at the CHC, the likelihood of having received age-appropriate routine care was even greater (O'Malley and Forrest, 1996).

Having a regular source of care was the most potent determinant (even more so than the presence of insurance) of receipt of preventive services among women in California. Moreover, if that source of care provided optimal attainment of primary care characteristics as reported by respondents in this community-based study, receipt of preventive care was even higher. The most salient component of the primary care assessment was a feature of longitudinality: reported adequacy of the extent and ease of communicating with the doctors at the place (Bindman et al., 1996).

Patients who make more visits to a facility during a period of time are more likely to receive indicated preventive care. This has been shown to be the case for children (Benson et al., 1984) and for adults, who benefitted more from computerized reminder systems for preventive care if they had more rather than fewer visits (Chambers et al., 1989).

People who have a source of primary care are more likely to keep their follow-up appointments. Spivak et al., (1980) showed that children who had a source of primary care were twice as likely to keep follow-up appointments than were children without such a source. They were at least 50% more likely to do so than children whose primary care source was used for routine care and minor illnesses but who were taken to the emergency room for more serious problems or children who used more than one primary care source, with or without emergency room use.

People whose care is longitudinal have fewer emergency hospitalizations and shorter hospitalizations, as demonstrated by a study in which men over the age of 55 years were randomly assigned to two different groups for care, one longitudinal and the other not (Wasson et al., 1984).

A more recent study, which included children as well as non-elderly adults, showed that individuals with better longitudinality in 1 year had significantly lower rates of hospitalization in the subsequent year (Gill and Mainous, 1998).

Socially disadvantaged people (i.e., those receiving public assistance for medical care in the form of Medicaid in two areas of the United States [California and New York City]) were less likely to require hospitalizations and more likely to have shorter hospital stays if they were regular users of a community health center than if a majority of visits were to other sources of care. The total costs of care for these patients were less, even though they made more ambulatory care visits. Moreover, the same was the case among the subset of patients with asthma or diabetes; that is, hospitalizations and costs were lower if they more consistently sought care at the community health center than if they did not (Duggar et al., 1994).

Inner-city children were more likely to receive care for undifferentiated episodes of illness and for earaches and to be under regular care for asthma if they had a longitudinal source of care than if they did not have such a source (German et al., 1976; Salkever et al., 1976).

People whose care is provided longitudinally are less likely to contract preventable illnesses, as was demonstrated in a study of the occurrence of acute rheumatic fever in children in Baltimore (Gordis, 1973). Longitudinality of care also may reduce the likelihood of poor birth outcomes, especially low birth weight. When prenatal care is a continuation of ongoing care, infants are more likely to be of normal birth weight than if their prenatal care was not part of a program of care that antedated pregnancy (Starfield, 1985).

Costs of care are reduced for individuals receiving longitudinal care. An analysis of national data by Butler et al. (1985) showed that children who reported a regular source of care had approximately 25% lower total costs of care than children with no regular source of care; costs for the latter group of children had a much larger standard error (indicating greater heterogeneity of experiences) than was the case for the children with a regular source of care.

In many studies it is impossible to determine whether the presence of a usual source of care causes the beneficial effect or is merely associated with it. For example, Ettner (1996) used a technique ("instrumental variables") to determine whether the presence of a regular source of care led to or resulted from differences in receipt of preventive services. For routine check-ups in children and for certain preventive procedures (e.g., recency of last blood pressure check) in adults, there was no impact of having a regular source of care; the presence of a regular source of care improved receipt for others (Pap smears, breast examinations, and mammograms). Therefore, the relationship between longitudinality of care and use of services depends on the way the issue is investigated. Those studies in which the regular source of care is identified retrospectively (i.e., after the period under study) indicate that the presence of a regular source of care is associated with an increased number of visits (Andersen and Aday, 1978; Scitovsky et al., 1979; Marcus and Stone, 1984). Studies in which the regular source of care is identified prospectively (i.e., before the patterns of use are examined) indicate that having a regular source of care reduces use (Breslau and Reeb, 1975; Alpert et al., 1976). The reason for this is that relatively recent use of services is likely to generate a perception of a regular relationship; individuals with greater use are more likely to report that the physician who provided the care is the regular source of care. Prospective studies, therefore, provide a more accurate assessment of the beneficial impact of longitudinality on use of services; they show that frequency of services, especially for illness care, is reduced.

Table 8.1 summarizes the nature of the evidence of benefit from an association with a particular place or particular provider. The benefits of association with a particular place are more extensive and consistent with the idea that increased knowledge about people that derives from a personal association confers additional benefits in the form of better recognition of needs and more accurate diagnoses. In contrast, some benefits may accrue from having a repository of stored information (as in a medical record) about individuals; this could account for the better preventive care that is associated merely with having a particular place of association rather than no such place or better coordination of care leading to lower costs.

Thus, evidence on the benefits of longitudinality indicate that its utility derives from knowledge gained over time. These benefits are most consistently found in the recognition of patients' problems rather than in aspects of technical care such as the performance of preventive procedures. When practitioners know patients, they are better able to judge the need for diagnostic interventions and to assess the relative merits of different modes of intervention. These advantages are best achieved when the relationship is with a particular practitioner rather than a particular place. The advantages that accrue from associating with a particular place rather than no identifiable place most likely derive from the increased likelihood of seeing the same practitioner or group of practitioners at that place and from the

Table 8.1. Benefits of Longitudinality, Based on Evidence from
the Literature

	Identification with a Person	*Identification with a Place*
Better problem/needs recognition	+ +	
More accurate diagnosis	+ +	
Better concordance		
Appointment keeping	+ +	+ +
Treatment advice	+ +	
Fewer hospitalizations	+ +	+
Lower costs	+ +	+
Better prevention (some types)	+ +	+ +
Increased satisfaction (Satisfaction and longitudinality are reciprocal; either influences the other, as noted in the text)	+ +	

+ +, Evidence good; +, evidence moderate (effect may be a result of greater likelihood of having a particular provider at a particular place)

other attributes of primary care that are associated with the place, in particular, the existence of a record that facilitates the recognition of certain needs such as preventive services.

Policy and Research Implications of Longitudinality: Free Choice, Managed Care, and Disease Case-Management

Free choice of primary care physician is the norm in most industrialized countries. Corroboration of the importance of free choice of primary care physicians comes from a very large study of 10,205 patients enrolled in a group-model HMO. The 47% of patients who had chosen their primary care physician were much more likely to rate their satisfaction with care as excellent or very good than the 53% of patients who were assigned to a primary care physician because they did not choose one (Schmittdiel et al., 1997)

The advent of managed care (see Chapter 6) was designed, at least in concept, on the principle of longitudinality. In theory, managed care should foster the achievement of longitudinality because it generally requires identification with a primary care practitioner. In reality, it appears to hinder the achievement of longitudinality. Many managed care organizations in the United States not only limit the free choice of primary care provider; they also often break established relationships between patients and doctors because the doctor is not on the organization's provider panel. Nearly half of all Americans who receive health insurance through their employers have their health plan chosen for them; about half of the remainder are given a choice of only two plans (Institute of Medicine, 1996; Angell and Kassirer, 1996). Absence of free choice of physician interferes with the establishment of a good relationship with a primary care provider. Moreover, because market mechanisms imply the existence of competition among health plans and perpetual free choice for purchasers, a managed care system based on market mechanisms will foster frequent changes in plans and providers as new and apparently more attractive "packages" of services are offered to enhance market position. A recent national survey found that nearly half of all physicians reported losing 10% of their patients in markets with high managed care penetration as a result of changes in patients' insurance plans (Commonwealth Fund Quarterly, 1996). The advent of point-of-service managed care plans, while theoretically increasing "free choice," actually nulls the benefits of longitudinality by increasing the ability of patients to seek care elsewhere without discussions with the primary care clinician. Virtually all studies of the impact of profit-driven managed care on long-term relationships between providers and patients indicate that long-term relationships are hindered as employers and other purchasers periodically shift to other health plans and hence move patients away from plans in which their regular provider of care lacks an affiliation (Sturm et al., 1996; Davis et al., 1995). Twenty percent of Medicare HMO enrollees drop out of their HMO within 12 months after joining (Brown et al., 1993). In Medicaid HMOs, about 5% disenroll each month, usually from losing eligibility (Woolhandler and Himmelstein, 1996). Forty percent of all women in the United States change providers each year in search of a more satisfying relationship (Commonwealth Fund, 1993). Among enrollees of individual practice associations and preferred provider organizations managed care programs (see Chapter 6), individuals who were forced to change their primary care physician had significantly lower scores for various aspects of longitudinality (including quality of interpersonal communications, reports of physician knowledge of their patients, and patients' perceptions that they can go to their physicians for almost all of their problems) than individuals who were able to remain with their physician (Flocke et al., 1997).

The term *case management* has a long history, originating in social work. It has varied meanings depending on its professional context, with the only common thread being the idea of a mechanism to find and coordinate diverse services where care must be received from a myriad of sources. Some services may be clinical, whereas others may be managerial (Hurley, 1986). However, the use of the word *case* is not consistent with the concept of longitudinality, which regards people as more than the sum of needed services.

Because case management may encompass so many different types of functions, someone other than a physician may be required to fulfill the role. Liptak and Revell (1989) surveyed family physicians and pediatricians working in medical center specialty clinics and parents of patients with chronic illness from the same clinics. About 60% of the physicians thought the primary care physician should be the case-manager, 20% thought parents were more appropriate for the role, 15% suggested a specialty clinic or physician, and 5% suggested a community health nurse. Physicians were unsure who was providing case management for 51% of their own chronically ill patients. Specific considerations that physicians thought would be most important in their own role as case manager were diagnosis, severity of the illness, and resources available in the specialty area. Parents, however, rated specialty clinics and primary care physicians almost equally knowledgeable about their child's health as well as equally accessible.

The approach taken by the New York State Department of Social Services and Health (Child Health Financing Report, 1990), which paid physicians to undertake ongoing care for low-income children, paved the way for many state Medicaid agencies to adopt primary care case management (PCCM) in which patients elect or are assigned to a particular physician. Physicians generally must provide for 24-hour coverage of the practice, must arrange for hospital admissions, specialty consultations, and ancillary services, and must adhere to guidelines for preventive care. Specialists must also provide summaries of consultations to the primary care physician and inform the latter when arranging hospital admissions. Thus, "managed care" in this context includes integration (coordination) of care as well as first-contact care by means of encouraging longitudinality.

Financing for case management was incorporated into U.S. public policy with the passage of Section 9508 of the Consolidated Omnibus Budget Reconciliation Act of 1985, which provided funds for the provision of case management within the Social Security Act (Medicaid). Similarly, Public Law 99-457 (the Early Intervention Program for Infants and Toddlers with Handicaps) mandates case-management services for children who are part of the program.

The theory of case management, as well as cost considerations, provides the basis for the current vogue of disease case management, in which the care of certain diseases is "carved out" of primary care and given to a separate disease-oriented team. "Carve out" care is carried out by means of separate contracts with companies, usually for profit and often under the aegis of pharmaceutical companies, to provide services for a specific disease, or, even more commonly, for mental health and substance abuse problems. Services are usually provided by nurses, social workers, or other non-physician practitioners. People with these diseases go directly to these identified practitioners rather than to their primary care practitioner when their problem is in the purview of the "carve-out." Disease case management, like case management in general, is not compatible with the principles of longitudinality if it indeed focuses on management of the disease rather than a partnership for care of the whole patient over time.

> At a large national meeting, the medical director of a large for-profit managed care organization was lauding disease case management as a strategy for improving care and containing costs. He showed data from such a program to care for children with asthma. His data demonstrated clearly that costs of care were lower for these children than was the case prior to the institution of the program. However, when costs of care were divided into those associated with asthma care and those associated with the remainder of care, the savings were all in the category of non-asthma care. When asked by a member of the audience to explain this he commented: "The nurse case manager took care not only of the asthma but of all the children's needs." Morale of the story: to achieve cost savings from a disease management program, it is necessary to give good primary care at the same time.

Any evaluation of the purported benefits of disease case management must take into account not only its impact on the disease and costs of its management but also the extent to which it affects (negatively or positively) all other aspects of the care of patients. The future of these "carve out" arrangements is not clear, and there are many who believe that they will disappear as managed care organizations become more integrated with specialty physicians in academic medical centers or in the community.

A related issue is the potential justification for having two "regular sources of care" when the two sources differ in their focus. In the United States, one-third of adult women indicate that both a family physician (or general internist) and an obstetrician/gynecologist are regular sources of care, with care for reproductive system concerns sought from the latter. Such women have higher numbers of visits overall and a higher likelihood of having received more recent Pap tests, mammograms, and cholesterol tests than women receiving care only from a family physician or internist (Weisman et al., 1995). Although it is possible that women who deliberately seek care from a primary care physician and a gynecologist also deliberately seek preventive care, it is likely that receipt of care from a gynecologist enhances receipt of preventive services in the realm of or related to that physician's area of interest and training. The extent to which these women receive other aspects of primary care (first-contact, interpersonal relationships, comprehensiveness overall, and coordination) is unknown. Because many integrated health systems, at least in the United States, are now permitting women to chose both a family physician or general internist and an obstetrician/gynecologist as their primary care practitioners, the need for assessment of the impact of these arrangements on receipt of high-level primary care (not only preventive care) is pressing.

Measurement of Longitudinality

As is the case for all of the four key features of primary care, the approach to measurement depends heavily on the definition of the characteristic. The definition posed by the Institute of Medicine, that is, "A sustained partnership refers to the relationship between the patient and clinician with the mutual expectation of continuation over time and predicated on the development of mutual trust, respect, and responsibility," may be equally pertinent in subspecialty care as in primary care if it is not clearly person focused rather than centered on the long-term management of some health problem.

Central to the measurement of longitudinality is the idea that individuals should be able to identify their source of primary care, and this source should be able to identify its eligible population (the "capacity" feature). Furthermore, individuals should use that regular source for all problems except those for which there is a referral elsewhere by the primary care physician (the "performance" feature). Measurement of this consistency of use over time requires a good system of information that documents where people go for unreferred care for different types of reasons. Therefore, it is not always possible to assess this performance feature of primary care. Furthermore, it may not even be the best approach. Freeman and Hjortdahl (1997) make a compelling case for the replacement of "temporal" longitudinality by "personal" longitudinality (which they designate as "continuity").

Temporal longitudinality connotes a relationship over a long period of time, whereas personal longitudinality focuses more on the strength of the relationship between patients and practitioners. It is possible, in their view, to have a long-term relationship that is based on a poor relationship and that a good relationship might develop even over a short period. Thus, it seems more reasonable and appropriate to assess the strength of the interpersonal linkage between the people and their source of care, which can be determined by observation, audiotape, or videotape or by interview. Studies have shown that ''trust,'' or confidence that the practitioner will do what is best for the patient, is highly correlated with satisfaction with care (Thom and Campbell, 1997) and therefore highly predictive of the seeking of services from that place or person. Thus, an appropriate measure of the likelihood of use of the regular source of care is the adequacy of the provider–patient interpersonal relationship. Because the need for ''trust'' in the physician is presumably important for all levels of care and not limited to primary care, assessment of its adequacy in primary care requires identification of those aspects of the interface that are particularly relevant to the establishment of person-focused (not disease-focused) care over periods of time.

Figure 8.1 shows these characteristics of the capacity and performance of health systems that are involved in the attainment of longitudinality.

The rest of this section discusses ways of measuring the regular source of care and the eligible population and then discusses the two approaches to measuring

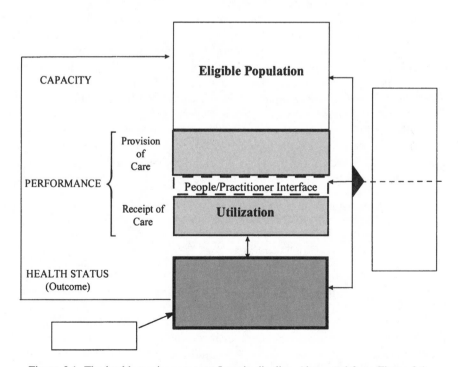

Figure 8.1. The health services system: Longitudinality. Abstracted from Figure 2.1.

appropriate use of the regular source of care: use over time for a variety of types of problems and, alternatively, the strength of the relationship between the primary care practitioner and patients.

Identification of a regular source of care and defining an eligible population

At the *population level*, the extent to which individuals have a regular source of care is often ascertained by means of a household survey, such as the U.S. National Health Interview Survey. This ongoing survey of a nationally representative sample of households periodically assesses whether people have a regular source of care and whether that source is a particular physician or a place. Data are available to determine time trends in the reporting of a regular source of care as well as changes in the type of source.

Over the years, there have been many ad hoc surveys conducted by researchers and pollsters, some of them periodic in nature. Among the most extensive are those conducted at the University of Chicago (Andersen et al., 1976; Aday et al., 1980, 1984). Later, the Robert Wood Johnson Foundation (through a professional polling organization) conducted several waves of interview by telephone (Freeman et al., 1987).

At the *facilities level*, identification with a regular source of care is reflected in the existence of patient rosters that indicate that the practitioner or group identifies an eligible population for which it is responsible. In the United States, the existence of such rosters is uncommon, although managed care organizations depend on the existence of such a roster to identify patients for whom they are responsible.

In many other countries, patient rosters ("lists") are an integral part of primary care and often serve as the basis for payment of practitioners. These lists are an integral part of primary care in countries such as the United Kingdom, Italy, the Netherlands, Portugal, and Denmark. In New Zealand and Ireland, the list is used for only part of the population. In Sweden, Finland, and Norway, the use of a list is experimental (Organization for Economic Cooperation and Development, 1995; BMJ, 1997). Patient lists are the basis for establishing a sense of responsibility for a group of people, and are the means by which practitioners can keep track of their patients' needs and the extent to which they are being met.

> Dr. G. is a general practitioner in Spain. Once a year, he and the nurse with whom he works review his lists to determine which individuals over age 75 have not had a visit within the past year. All of these patients are contacted to assess how well they are doing and to determine whether any services are indicated.

To study the validity of the roster of a health center in the province of Ontario Canada, where there is no required list, a mail and a telephone survey ascertained the extent to which patients and the facilities agreed that the facility was their regular source of care. The roster was made up of all individuals who indicated that they intended to use the practice as their regular source of care. In the case of patients already known to the practice at the time the register was developed, those whose records indicated a utilization pattern compatible with regular use were included. The roster was augmented with names of family members identified by new patients. The facility was considered the regular source of care if survey respondents indicated that it was their "usual" source. The accuracy of the roster as compared with the mail survey, in this one health center, was over 90% (Anderson et al., 1985).

The appropriate use of the regular source of care: Method based on utilization history

Research on *use* of the regular source of care has confused the concepts of longitudinal care, majority of care, and sequential care (Dietrich and Marton, 1982; Wall, 1981; Starfield, 1980). As a result, some of the methods described in this section have been referred to as "continuity" measures, whereas they really address the phenomenon of longitudinal care.

No standards for longitudinality have been proposed. Therefore, all of the measures described in this chapter are relative measures in that the results of one assessment are compared with another; better longitudinality is inferred from a higher score.

At the population level and in some facilities, it is possible to document where people have gone for care and whether it was a referral visit from existing data systems. Four measures have been used at the *population* level. It should be noted that methods mentioned below were neither developed for nor applied to primary care itself. To use them in the context of longitudinality, they would have to be modified to include in the numerator only those services sought from the primary care source. Some address temporal longitudinality (consistency of use one time). Others are intermediate in character between temporal and personal longitudinality.

1. The UPC (usual provider continuity). In this measure, the number of visits to the regular source of care is divided by the total number of visits in the same time period. The resulting ratio is known as the UPC (Breslau and Reeb, 1975). The closer the ratio is to 1, the higher the longitudinality.
2. COC (continuity of care). The score on the UPC is very sensitive to the total number of visits, for example, if an individual makes only one visit in a year and it is to the regular source of care, the UPC will be 1. The fewer the number of visits, the easier it is to achieve a high UPC. The COC corrects for this statistical problem by requiring detailed visit data and using it to correct for the effect of number of visits in its calculation. It also corrects for the total number of different providers that are seen and considers visits to specialists that are made *on a referral* from primary care as a visit to the primary care physician (Bice and Boxerman, 1977).
3. LICON (likelihood of continuity). This measure corrects for the effect of number of sources available as well as the total number of visits. The greater the number of sources available, the greater the likelihood that practitioners other than the regular source of care will be seen (Steinwachs, 1979).

Each of the three measures, when applied to all visits within a defined period of time (usually a year) indicates the extent to which a regular source of care is used over time. The measures do not determine the extent to which visits are for particular problems or are for a full range of services. They also do not determine whether any of the visits were made upon referral. Therefore, in applying any of these measures to an ascertainment of longitudinality, it is important to eliminate visits resulting from a referral by the primary care provider to another provider.

The UPC, COC, LICON, and place of visit for a variety of types of reasons are facility-based measures of longitudinality when the source of information is obtained either from records or patients in the facility. The "k" index (Ejlertsson and Berg, 1984) is a measure of longitudinality at the facility level. This measure is similar to the UPC (proportion of total visits that are to the regular source of care) except that the regular source of care is considered the individual seen by the patient at a particular visit rather than a physician identified by the patient as the regular source of care. The "f" index (Smedby et al., 1986) is similar to the "k" index in that it is the fraction of visits during a defined time that were made to a physician seen at a specified visit. A comparison of UPC, COC and the "k" index, with examples of different numbers and patterns of use of care, is provided by Ejlertsson and Berg (1984).

4. The modified continuity index (MMCI) was devised to take into account the number of providers seen and the number of patient encounters. The numerator of the rate is expressed as $1 - $ (number of providers $\div$ [the number of visits $+ 0.1$]) and the denominator $1 - (1 \div$ by [number of visits $+ 0.1$]). It was applied in a family medicine residency program to assess the attainment of longitudinality in the training context (Magill and Senf, 1987).

5. Another measure of longitudinality explicitly takes into consideration the nature of the problem for which care was sought. Individuals are contacted by survey to determine their regular source of care. Claims, medical records, or patient interviews are used to determine the nature of the care provided (optimally the reason for care but usually the diagnosis given) and the place it was provided. The extent to which nonreferred care was sought from the source of primary care (rather than from another source) for a variety of reasons is the measure of longitudinality. Although this measure has not been widely used, it was modified and applied in the Rand Health Insurance Experiment (Spiegel et al., 1983), a national demonstration of the effect of co-payments on utilization and health status. In this application, individuals were asked to indicate the name of their "personal" physician, that is, the individual to whom test results from a scheduled multiphasic screening examination should be sent. Records were reviewed to determine the physician providing the plurality of visits as well as to determine the type of physicians that patients consulted for upper respiratory infections, hypertension, and general examinations. Only 12% of patients said that a specialist was their personal physician, and only 6% named physicians who were listed as non-primary care specialists in the American Medical Association Masterfile and the American Medical Directory. When the primary care physician was defined as the one who provided the plurality of care, one in three patients was categorized as having a non-primary care specialist as the primary care physician. When the primary care physician was defined as the place where care

was sought for common problems, approximately 1 in 10 patients had a non-primary care specialist as their source of primary care.

An appropriate modification of this method would be useful in determining the extent of longitudinality of care. In this method, patients are queried as to their regular source of care, which can be defined as either the physician to whom they go for care when they have a new problem or the physician to whom they would want results of medical tests sent. Records of all visits over a period of time are reviewed to determine where the individual went for care for preventive or administrative reasons, for symptoms or signs of potential new illness, for care of existing problems, and for diagnostic or therapeutic reasons. Only visits that occurred on the patient's initiative are considered (i.e., visits that occurred as the result of a referral by the regular source of care are excluded from consideration). When medical records or claims forms do not contain information as to whether the visit was patient initiated, patients may be queried to determine where they went the last time they required a visit for these reasons and whether they went on referral from their regular source of care or on their own initiative. The extent to which unreferred visits for the variety of purposes were to the regular source of care indicates the extent of longitudinality of care that has been achieved.

An interesting approach to assessing longitudinality is found in the work of Sweeney and Gray (1995) in England. Defining absence of longitudinality as four consecutive consultations that did *not* take place with the doctor with whom the patients were registered, they found that patients without longitudinality were more likely to be in the lower social classes and with multiple types of problems.

Information about the attainment of longitudinality at the population level requires that information about the regular source of care be obtained by a population-based method, that is, by a method that contacts individuals independently of their visits at the facility. However, any of the above methods could be calculated using information provided by patients when they appear at the facility. In this case, the measure would be considered facilities based rather than population based. At the *facilities level,* methods of assessing longitudinality use information obtained from records within the facility. Therefore, the extent of longitudinality can be inferred only for those individuals who actually used the facility during the time period of interest.

One important aspect of longitudinality—the care of hospitalized patients by the primary care provider—has received little attention. In most health systems, hospitalized patients are cared for by hospital staff physicians rather than by primary care physicians (with appropriate consultation from hospital staff physicians). In many places in the United States, it is common for community-based physicians to care for their patients when hospitalized, as the "attending of record." Perrin and colleagues (1996) found that this practice varies widely from place to place and even within specific areas depending on the type of primary care facility. In general, salaried physicians in organized groups ("staff-model HMOs") are more likely to be in charge of their hospitalized patients, followed by community-based physicians in private offices; physicians working in neighborhood health centers (public aegis) and hospital clinics are least likely to do so (Perrin et al., 1996).

Other new methods of assessing the existence of a longitudinal source of care are presented in Chapter 13 in the context of overall evaluation of primary care.

Appropriate use of the regular source of care: Method based on characteristics of the clinician–patient interrelationship ("personal longitudinality")

As noted above, use of the primary care source for the wide variety of types of needs that constitute the content of primary care is difficult to assess because of an absence of data systems that document where people have gone for the variety of types of care they receive. An alternative method, employing surveys either among patients in facilities or in general populations, can assess the strength of the interpersonal relationship between the provider and patient that would be expected to be associated with consistent use over time.

"Trust" ("reliance on the character, ability, strength, or truth of someone or something"—*Websters New Collegiate Dictionary*, 1981) is sometimes considered to characterize this relationship; but it is not necessarily unique to primary care relationships. One small study (Thom and Campbell, 1997) in a primary care facility indicated that patients considered "trust" to be relationship specific and developing over time, but this might characterize long-term specialty care for the purpose of managing a particular disease as well as the person-focused relationship characteristic of primary care. Thus, the challenge to the assessment of the person-focused characteristic of the relationship is to distinguish those aspects of the relationship that are person specific from those that might be associated with the care of particular diseases or conditions. The importance of this is highlighted by the observation that about half of all consultations with primary care physicians are for problems that do not fit the conventional biomedical model (Leopold et al., 1996).

Leopold et al. (1996) specified six features of care that would facilitate the achievement of sustained, person-focused partnerships: whole-person focus; physician's knowledge of the patient; caring and empathy; patient trust in the physician; appropriately adapted care; and patient participation and shared decision-making. Because only the first two of these are specific to primary care, the approach to measurement of personal longitudinality should emphasize their assessment. (The others are more appropriately considered important aspects of doctor–patient relationships in general and are considered in Chapter 9.)

Many of the available instruments elicit people's satisfaction with the relationship with their provider rather than the actual characteristics of this relationship. Moreover, most instruments fail to distinguish between the nature of the relationship with the primary care provider and the provider seen at a visit or series of visits, which might be a disease-oriented specialist. Characteristics of primary care–patient relationships include the extent of understanding between provider and patient, the comfort of patients in telling providers about their concerns or worries, and the extent to which patients feels that their provider is interested in them as a person rather than as someone with a medical problem and understands which problems are most important to them.

Other methods of assessing both temporal and interpersonal aspects of longitudinality are presented in Chapter 13 in the context of overall evaluation of primary care.

What Is Known About the Attainment of Longitudinality

Various surveys indicate that generalists (family physicians, general practitioners, pediatricians, or general internists) are indicated as the regular source of care for the majority of the population. In the United States, where general internists and pediatricians as well as family physicians are considered to be primary care practitioners, family physicians and general practitioners account for about half of all physicians identified as the regular source of care; internists and pediatricians each account for about 14%, at least as of the 1980s. The remaining 20% of physicians identified as the regular source of care are other specialists. For the population of children, pediatricians are identified as the regular source of care for 56% of 1–5 year olds and 33% of 6–17 year olds. Income of the family is related to the type of physician who is indicated: Lower income families are more likely to identify a family physician or general practitioner and less likely to identify an internist or pediatrician than high-income families (Aday et al., 1980, p. 53). Moreover, even when a primary care specialist (such as an internist or pediatrician) is identified by low-income families, the physician is less likely to be board certified (Starfield et al., 1973).

In the Rand Health Insurance Experiment (which excluded people over age 62 and the 7% of the population in the highest income groups), 88% of the population in three areas of the country named a primary care physician as their personal physician. Almost half (49%) named general practitioners or family physicians, 16% named internists, and 22% named pediatricians. About one in eight people (12%) named a specialist: 5% named obstetricians/gynecologists, 4% surgeons, 2% internists/subspecialists, and the remainder named other types of physicians or physicians with unknown specialty (Spiegel et al., 1983).

Weiner (1981), in a study of the distribution and achievement of primary care within an entire metropolitan area (Baltimore) asked patients visiting a random sample of all types of physicians to indicate the year they first visited the physician. The duration of the physician patient relationship was calculated from this information and from the current year. The assumption was made that a longer duration would more likely be reflective of an ongoing relationship not associated with care of a particular problem or type of problem. Patients of both internists and family physicians reported durations of relationship approximately 7–8 years on average, about double that reported by patients of other types of physicians (about 3–4 years on average), suggesting that generalist physicians provide more longitudinality than specialists.

The National Ambulatory Medical Care Survey, a periodic survey of a representative sample of office-based physicians in the United States, provides a means of assessing longitudinality in its assessment of whether visits are first visits, follow-up visits (i.e., was a previous visit for the same problem), or first visits for a particular problem when the patient was previously seen for other problems. Puskin (1977) analyzed visits made by adults and calculated a longitudinality ratio for each type of physician. This ratio consisted of the number of patients seen before for other problems divided by the number of patients never seen before. General practitioners and family physicians had the highest ratios (2.36); general internists followed, with 1.65. Several types of other specialists had ratios slightly lower than that of internists (cardiovascular specialists at 1.54, general surgeons at 1.40, and obstetrician/gynecologists at 1.14), but the ratio of other specialists was much lower (0.23–0.42).

A similar analysis was done for visits by children except that only pediatricians and general practitioners/family physicians were compared (Fishbane and Starfield, 1981). The longitudinality ratio for pediatricians (4.65) was much higher than that for general physicians (2.27), although the ratio of 2.27 for generalists was similar to that found for adult patients and much higher than the ratio for other types of physicians in the adult study.

These findings indicate that generalists, pediatricians, and internists are more likely to provide longitudinal care than are other specialist physicians.

Studies that examine the extent to which physicians of different types provide care for a variety of types of problems also indicate that generalist physicians are more likely than other specialists to provide longitudinal care. For example, the study of Baltimore physicians, in which patients were asked where they last received a regular "check-up" and where they last received care for a cold or the flu, indicated that pediatricians, internists, and family physicians were two to three times more likely to be named as the source of care for both types of problems than were specialist physicians (Weiner, 1981).

Investigators in the Rand Health Insurance Study (Speigel et al., 1983) came the closest to assessing the achievement of longitudinality by determining the percentage of people who saw the same physician for all visits, for the majority of visits, and for less than a majority of visits over a year, according to the type of physician who was the "majority" source of care (defined as the physician seen for the most visits as derived from claims forms). Patients with a generalist as the majority source were over twice as likely to have seen the same physician for all visits as were patients with another specialist as the majority source (36% vs. 16%). Other analyses indicated that patients for whom a non-primary care specialist was the majority source were much *less* likely to see that physician for an upper respiratory infection (33%) than were patients for whom a generalist was the majority source; the latter saw that generalist 99% of the time. Even patients seen for a condition such as hypertension were more likely to be seen by their majority source if that source was a generalist than if it was another specialist. All patients whose source was a generalist saw that generalist for hypertension; only 53 percent of patients of other specialists saw that physician for hypertension, whereas 47% saw a generalist. These findings indicate that longitudinality is a much more frequent feature of the care of generalists than it is for other specialists.

All of these studies were conducted in the United States at a time when most people were free to visit any physician. Because this is not the case in many countries and is increasingly less the case in the United States, the particular findings may have little relevance to current practice. It is certainly the case that the extent to which people identify with a particular place or individual as their source of care varies from one health system to another and from place to place. In the United States in the early 1990s about 60% identified an individual and 40% identified a place as their regular source of care. In an entire city in Canada, where there is universal health insurance, fewer than one-third of children aged 1–5 years achieved longitudinality (defined as at least 80% of total care provided by the most frequently seen physician or physician practice or on referral from that practice) over a 5-year period (Mustard et al., 1996).

In countries without universal financial coverage for health services, individuals and families with low incomes are far less likely to report having a primary care physician or even a primary care facility. For example, in 1993, adults in the United States who were male, between ages 18 and 24 years, without having completed secondary school education, poor, black, Hispanic, or unemployed were more likely to be uninsured and, concomitantly, to lack a regular source of care (Centers for Disease Control and Prevention, 1995).

As noted above, the establishment of managed care in the United States should improve the extent to which its population reports an affiliation with a primary care physician and use that source consistently over time. In practice, however, yearly or more frequent and involuntary changes in insurance plans are interfering with the development of long-term relationships.

In health care systems in which the affiliation of a population or patients with a generalist is more part of the tradition of medical care, it is likely that the consistency of seeking of care from the chosen generalist is likely to be even greater than it has been in the United States.

Summary

Table 8.2 summarizes the nature of longitudinality. Longitudinality implies the existence of a regular physician or group of physicians and use of that source for care that is not limited to certain problems or types of problems. Its assessment involves the measurement of structural features of care (the identification of the regular source of care by people and the identification of the eligible population by the physician or group) and certain performance aspects (appropriate use of that regular source of care and the strength of interpersonal relationships).

There are several methods of assessing longitudinality of care. Most can be adapted for use for both population-based and facilities-based surveys and studies.

Longitudinality of care is less well achieved by certain segments of the population, especially individuals in the lower social classes and other relatively disenfranchised groups.

Longitudinality is associated with a variety of benefits, including less use of services, better preventive care, more timely and more appropriate care, less preventable illness, better recognition of patients' problems, less hospitalizations, and

Table 8.2. Summary of Longitudinality

	Capacity	Performance
Description: Person-focused care provided over time (at least 2 years)		
Involves	Linkage, through enrollment or informal contract (patient "list"), between providers and population	Proxy measure: Strength of person–practitioner relationship Unreferred use over time for the variety of problems experienced
Problem related	No	No
Personal relationship required	Yes	Yes
Time dependent	Yes, long periods of time	Yes, long periods of time
Specific measures	Population/patient survey Enrollment records	Population/patient survey Provider survey Audiotape or videotape Visit records UPC COC LICON k index

lower total costs. Longitudinality involving a relationship with a particular practitioner confers benefits that are more extensive than those involving only a relationship with a particular place.

Case management is a relatively new concept in health services. As a function that is focused on the patient over time, it is most closely related to the longitudinality feature of primary care. Its functions are both clinical and managerial and involve priorities that are focused on patients' needs as well as on professional imperatives. The functions that require clinical skills (such as first-contact care, comprehensiveness, and coordination of care) are logical components of case management, but further research and evaluation will be required to determine the feasibility and impact of assumption of more managerial functions by physicians. In a climate of managed care and disease case management, there should be ample opportunity for study of the way in which longitudinality is achieved and the success of the efforts at attaining it.

References

Aday L, Andersen R, Fleming G. Health Care in the U.S. Equitable for Whom? Beverly Hills: Sage Publications, 1980.

Aday L, Fleming G, Andersen R. Access to Medical Care in the U.S.: Who Has It, Who Doesn't. Chicago: Pluribus Press, 1984.

Alpert J, Charney E. The Education of Physicians for Primary Care. Pub. No. (HRA) 74-3113. Rockville, MD: U.S. Department of Health, Education, and Welfare, Public Health Service, Health Resources Administration, 1974.

Alpert J, Robertson L, Kosa J, Heagart M, Haggerty R. Delivery of health care for children: Report of an experiment. Pediatrics 1976; 57:917–30.

Andersen R, Aday LA. Access to medical care in the U.S.: Realized and potential. Med Care 1978; 16:533–46.

Andersen R, Kravits J, Anderson O. Two Decades of Health Services: Social Survey Trends in Use and Expenditure. Cambridge, MA: Ballinger Publishing Co., 1976.

Anderson J, Gancher W, Bell P. Validation of the patient roster in a primary care practice. Health Serv Res 1985; 20:301–14.

Angell M, Kassirer J. Quality and the medical marketplace—Following elephants. N Engl J Med 1996; 335(12):883–5.

Baker R. Characteristics of practices, general practitioners and patients related to levels of patients' satisfaction with consultations. Br J Gen Pract 1996; 46:601–5.

Baker R, Streatfield J. What type of general practice do patients prefer? Exploration of practice characteristics influencing patient satisfaction. Br J Gen Pract 1995; 45:654–9.

Becker M, Drachman R, Kirscht J. Predicting mothers' compliance with pediatric medical regimens. J Pediatr 1972; 81:843–54.

Becker M, Drachman R, Kirscht J. Continuity of pediatrician: New support for an old shibboleth. J Pediatr 1974; 84:599–605.

Benson P, Gabriel A, Katz H, Steinwachs D, Hankin J, Starfield B. Preventive care and overall use of services: Are they related? Am J Dis Child 1984; 138:74–8.

Bice T, Boxerman S. A quantitative measure of continuity of care. Med Care 1977; 15:347–9.

Bindman A, Grumbach K, Osmond D, Vranizan K, Stewart A. Primary care and receipt of services. J Gen Intern Med 1996; 11:269–76.

Breslau N, Reeb K. Continuity of care in a university based practice. J Med Educ 1975; 50: 965–9.

British Medical Journal. Norwegian GPs move to list based system. BMJ 1997; 7098:1852

Brown RS, Clement DG, Hill JW, Retchin SM, Bergeron JW. Do health maintenance organizations work for Medicare? Health Care Financ Rev 1993; 15(1): 7–23.

Butler J, Winter W, Singer, J, Wenger M. Medical care use and expenditure among U.S. children and youth: Analysis of a natural probability sample. Pediatrics 1985; 76:495–507.

Centers for Disease Control and Prevention. Health Insurance Coverage and Receipt of Preventive Health Services—United States, 1993. MMWR 1995; 44:219–25.

Chambers C, Balaban D, Carlson B, Ungemack J, Grasberger D. Microcomputer-generated reminders, improving the compliance of primary care physicians with mammography screening guidelines. J Fam Pract 1989; 29:273–80.

Charney E, Bynum R, Eldredge D, Frank D, MacWhinney J, McNabb N, Scheiner A, Sumpter E, Ikor H. How well do patients take oral penicillin? A collaborative study in private practice. Pediatrics 1967; 40:188–95.

Child Health Financing Report. New York Hikes Medicaid Fees. American Academy of Pediatrics 1990; VII:1.

Commonwealth Fund. Survey of Women's Health. New York: Louis Harris and Associates, 1993.

Commonwealth Fund Quarterly. Physicians experiencing turbulent times. Commonwealth Fund Quarterly 1996; 2:1.

Davis K, Collins K, Schoen C, Morris C. Choice: Enrollees' views of their health plan. Health Aff 1995; 14(2):99–112.

Dietrich A, Marton K. Does continuous care from a physician make a difference? J Fam Pract 1982; 15(5):929–37.

Duggar B, Balicki B, Keel K, Yates T. Health Services Utilization and Costs to Medicaid of Afdc recipients in New York and California Served and Not Served by Selected

Community Health Centers. Final Report. Columbia, MD: Center for Health Policy Studies, 1994.

Ejlertsson G, Berg S. Continuity-of-care measures. An analytic and empirical comparison. Med Care 1984; 22:231–9.

Ettner SL. The timing of preventive services for women and children: the effects of having a usual source of care. Am J Public Health 1996; 86(12):1748–54.

Evang K. Health Service, Society, and Medicine. London: Oxford University Press, 1960. pp 87–8.

Fishbane M, Starfield B. Child health care in the United States: A comparison of pediatricians and general practitioners. N Engl J Med 1981; 305:552–6.

Flint S. The Impact of Continuity of Care on the Utilization and Cost of Pediatric Care in a Medicaid Population. Dissertation. Chicago: University of Chicago, 1987.

Flocke S, Stange K, Zyzanski S. The impact of insurance type and forced discontinuity on the delivery of primary care. J Fam Pract 1997; 45:129–35.

Freeman G, Hjortdahl P. What future for continuity of care in general practice? BMJ 1997; 314:1870–3.

Freeman G, Richards S. How much personal care in four group practices? BMJ 1990; 301: 1028–30.

Freeman GK, Richards SC. Personal continuity and the care of patients with epilepsy in general practice. Br J Gen Pract 1994;44;395–9.

Freeman H, Blendon R, Aiken L, Sudman S, Mullinix C, Corey C. American report on their access to health care. Health Aff 1987; 6:6–18.

German P, Skinner A, Shapiro S, Salkever D. Preventive and episodic health care of inner-city children. J Community Health 1976; 2:92–106.

Gill J, Mainous A. The role of provider continuity in preventing hospitalizations. Arch Fam Med 1998 7(4):352–7.

Gordis L. Effectiveness of comprehensive care programs in preventing rheumatic fever. N Engl J Med 1973; 289:331–5.

Gulbrandsen P, Hjortdahl P, Fugelli P. General practitioners' knowledge of their patients' psychosocial problems: Multi-practice questionnaire survey. BMJ 1997; 314:1014–8.

Hjortdahl P. Continuity of care: General practitioner's knowledge about, and sense of responsibility toward, their patients. Fam Pract 1992; 9:3–8.

Hjortdahl P, Borchgrevink C. Continuity of care: Influence of general practitioners' knowledge about their patients on use of resources in consultations. BMJ 1991; 303:1181–4.

Hjortdahl P, Laerum E. Continuity of care in general practice: Effect on patient satisfaction. BMJ 1992; 304:1287–90.

Hurley R. Toward a behavioral model of the physician as case manger. Soc Sci Med 1986; 23:75–92.

Institute of Medicine. Primary Care: America's Health in a New Era. Washington, DC: National Academy Press, 1997.

Kelleher K, Childs G, Wasserman R, McInerny T, Nutting P, Gardner W. Insurance status and recognition of psychosocial problems. A report from PROS and ASPN. Arch Pediatr Adolesc Med 1997; 151:1109–15.

Lambrew J, DeFriese G, Carey T, Ricketts T, Biddle A. The effects of having a regular doctor or access to primary care. Med Care 1996; 34:138–51.

Lawrence R, Dorsey J. The Generalist–Specialist Relationship and the Art of Consultation. In Noble J (ed): Primary Care and the Practice of Medicine. Boston: Little Brown, 1976. Pp 229–45.

Leopold N, Cooper J, Clancy C. Sustained partnership in primary care. J Fam Pract 1996; 42:129–37.

Liptak G, Revell G. Community physician's role in case management of children with chronic illnesses. Pediatrics 1989; 34(3):465–71.

Lieu T, Black S, Ray P, Chellino M, Shinefeld H, Adler N. Risk factors for delayed immunization among children in an HMO. Am J Public Health 1994; 84:1621–5.

Magill M, Senf J. A new method for measuring continuity of care in family practice residencies. J Fam Pract 1987; 24:165–8.

Marcus A, Stone J. Mode of payment and identification with a regular doctor. Med Care 1984; 22:647–60.

McDaniel D, Patton E, Mather J. Immunization activities of private practice physicians: A record audit. Pediatrics 1975; 56:504–7.

Miller M. Who receives optimal medical care? J Health Soc Behav 1973; 14:176–82.

Mustard CA, Mayer T, Black, C, Postl, B. Continuity of pediatric ambulatory care in a universally insured population. Pediatrics 1996; 98:1028–34.

Nazareth I, King M. Decision making by general practitioners in diagnosis and management of lower urinary tract symptoms in women. BMJ 1993; 306:1103–6.

O'Malley AS, Forrest CB. Continuity of care and delivery of ambulatory services to children in community health clinics. J Community Health 1996; 21(3):159–73.

Organization for Economic Cooperation and Development. New Directions in Health Care Policy. Health Policy Studies No. 7. Paris: Organization for Economic Cooperation and Development, 1995.

Perrin JM, Greenspan P, Bloom SR, Findelstein D, Yazdgerdi S, Leventhal JM, Rodewald L, Szilagyi P, Homer CJ. Primary care involvement among hospitalized children. Arch Pediatr Adolesc Med 1996; 150:479–86.

Puskin D. Patterns of Ambulatory Medical Care in the United States: An Analysis of the National Ambulatory Medical Care Survey. Dissertation. Baltimore: Johns Hopkins University, 1977.

Salkever D, German P, Shapiro S, Horky R, Skinner E. Episodes of illness and access to care in the inner city: A comparison of HMO and non-HMO populations. Health Serv Res 1976; 11:252–70.

Schmittdiel J, Selby J, Grumbach K, Quesenberry C. Choice of a personal physician and patient satisfaction in an HMO. JAMA 1997; 278:1596–99.

Scitovsky A, Benham L, McCall N. Use of physician services under two prepaid plans. Med Care 1979; 17:441–60.

Smedby O, Eklund G, Eriksson E, Smedby B. Measures of continuity of care: A register-based correlation study. Med Care 1986; 24:511–8.

Spiegel J, Rubenstein L, Scott B, Brook R. Who is the primary physician? N Engl J Med 1983; 308:1208–12.

Spivak H, Levy J, Bonanno R, Cracknell M. Patient and provider factors associated with selected measures of quality of care. Pediatrics 1980; 65:307–13.

Starfield B. Continuous confusion. Am J Public Health 1980;70:117–9.

Starfield B. Effectiveness of Medical Care: Validating Clinical Wisdom. Baltimore: Johns Hopkins University Press, 1985.

Starfield B, Bice T, Schach E, Rabin D, White KL. How "regular" is the "regular source of medical care?" Pediatrics 1973; 51:822–32.

Steinwachs D. Measuring provider continuity in ambulatory care. An assessment of alternative approaches. Med Care 1979; 17:551–65.

Steinwachs D, Yaffe R. Assessing the timeliness of ambulatory medical care. Am J Public Health 1978; 68:547–56.

Stewart A, Grumbach K, Osmond D, Vranizan K, Komaromy M, Bindman A. Primary care and patient perceptions of access to care. J Fam Pract 1997; 44:177–85.

Sturm R, Meredith LS, Wells KB. Provider choice and continuity of the treatment of depression. Med Care 1996; 34(7): 723–34.

Sweeney KG, Gray DP. Patients who do not receive continuity of care from their general practitioner—are they a vulnerable group? Br J Gen Pract 1995; 45(392):133–5.

Thom D, Campbell B. Patient–physician trust: An exploratory study. J Fam Pract 1997; 44: 169–76.

Wall EM. Continuity of care and family medicine: Definition, determinants, and relationship to outcome. J Fam Pract 1981; 13(5):655–64.

Wasson J, Sauvigne A, Mogielnicki R, Frey W, Sox C, Gaudette C, Rockwell A. Continuity of outpatient medical care in elderly men. A randomized trial. JAMA 1984; 252:2413–7.

Weiner J. An Analysis of Office-Based Primary Care in Baltimore City. Dissertation. Baltimore: Johns Hopkins University, 1981.

Weisman C, Cassard S, Plichta S. Types of physicians used by women for regular health care: Implications for services received. J Womens Health 1995; 4:407–16.

Weiss LJ, Blustein J. Faithful patients: The effects of long-term physician-patient relationships on the costs and use of health care by older Americans. Am J Public Health 1996; 86(12):1742–7.

Woolhandler S, Himmelstein D. Patients on the auction block. Am J Public Health 1996; 86:1699–700.

— 9 —

Practitioner–Patient
Interactions

Dr. K. practices medicine on the lower east side of Manhattan. He says, "Many times patients will come in and give all sorts of exotic stories until they are brave enough to tell you the real reason they are here. Yesterday a patient came in and told me about aches and pains and headaches and problems in all parts of her body and she was sure it wasn't the flu and that there was something wrong with her and she didn't know what it was. I examined her but I couldn't find anything abnormal. So I kept encouraging her to just talk to me about what she was feeling. I noted an anxious look on her face and I watched her. Finally she broke down and said "Listen, I've been taking drugs." Then it became clear that the problems she was having were withdrawal symptoms. I don't think that if I had asked her a lot of questions, or even asked her about whether she was taking drugs, she would have told me. She had to work up the courage to do it and that took a little time and my encouragement. The thing is, if you can break the barriers down, you can find out why they really came to see you and solve the problem without a lot of visits, tests, and drugs. I could have said "You've got a lot of aches and pains, so I'll take a few tests and give you some aspirin to take home and come back in two days and let's see what happens." If you just listen and watch patients, you learn from them. When you see an anxious look, you know that the patient wants to tell you something, and you just have to let it come out when it's ready to come out. A doctor treats patients, not toilets, electrical appliances or air conditioners. A human being is complex, not a machine, so you really have to try to understand things. Anybody can order a test or write a prescription. The whole thing about practicing medicine is to find out why.

Interactions between practitioners and patients contribute to the establishment of long-term relationships, which facilitates effectiveness in primary care. They are the means by which physicians learn about many if not most patients' problems and how patients learn about most aspects of their care. Although interactions between patients and practitioners take place in the course of consultation and referral practice, it is the breadth and depth of the context that distinguishes interactions in primary care from those in other care.

169

People are often frightened to tell the doctors things. They might get angry, or say you are imagining it, or think it is trivial. A lot of people are afraid of doctors. Maybe the doctor will classify them as a "mental patient." Because they are afraid, they learn to hide things from doctors, assuming that the doctors will find out anyway because of their training. I think doctors should act as human beings, not as doctors. Doctors should know that each patient is a living person, with feelings. Even if the doctor has treated the same medical problem over and over again, each patient is different.   Mr. M., a 50-year-old contractor

Both practitioners and patients contribute to the process of medical care. When patients seek care, they present themselves and their problems, concerns, and needs by using the system (utilization); the practitioner bears responsibility for recognizing the patient's problems, needs, or concerns (problem recognition) and for formulating those needs into a diagnosis for which appropriate management can be suggested. Patients participate through their understanding of the suggestions and recommendations and for accepting them as appropriate. They also participate in the suggested regimen either by carrying it out and by returning at the recommended time or by seeking alternatives when the recommendations do not appear appropriate or are inadequate. Practitioners then reassess the situation by determining whether the problem is resolved, the concerns ameliorated, or the needs adequately met.

The long-term relationship that characterizes primary care will be difficult to sustain if either party is uncomfortable with their encounters. Because many problems that patients bring to primary care physicians are of uncertain cause or prognosis, the relationship must be strong enough to tolerate ambiguity, at least at some stages in the development of problems. This strength is built in part on a free flow of relevant information between both parties and on the rapport that provides the context for the relationship. Much communication serves to convey specific items needed to deal directly with the problem, concern, or need. Verbal conversation is the most common mode of communication. The practitioner asks questions to elucidate the problem, and informs the patient about the diagnosis, the plan of intervention directed at resolving or ameliorating the problem, and the plan for reassessment. Patients provide information about their problems, concerns, and needs and later query the physician if they are unclear about aspects of the diagnosis, therapy, or follow-up plan.

This is the ideal situation. In practice, short-cuts may occur, or patients may not be permitted to say as much about their problem as they would like to either because the practitioner directs the flow of information by asking only certain questions or because the patient is not allowed enough time. Sometimes the practitioner may provide too little information so that the patient is unable to understand the diagnosis, the plan of intervention, or the plan for reassessment.

My mother was found to have a positive stool guaiac on routine screening. She has a prior history of ulcers and we suspected a recurrence, but she was sent to a gastroenterologist for a colonoscopy. During the procedure, the physician verbalized his observations, at one point audibly exclaiming to himself and the attending nurse, "There it is; there's the cancer." At the conclusion of the examination, I asked the doctor if my mother and I could sit down and talk with the doctor, who replied effusively, "Of course." In the consultation room, the physician fielded questions from me while simultaneously dictating notes from his examination.

Dr. C.D., an eminent pediatrician

The importance of the limitations in physician–patient communication is indicated by their relationships with malpractice suits. Primary care physicians with a history of malpractice claims are much more likely to have poor communication skills (based on audiotapes of their visits with patients) than other physicians. The most important characteristics of the interaction are educating patients about what to expect and about the flow of the visit; physicians without malpractice claims had spent longer times with their patients (Levinson et al., 1997).

In traditional theories of physician–patient interaction, the role of the practitioner received a disproportionately large share of attention. Social theorists assumed that the physician had a commanding role because of the functions ascribed to the physician–patient interaction. Some theorists considered the physician to be an agent of social control who legitimized a "social deviance," such as absence from work because of illness. According to these traditional theories, the role of the patient is relatively passive and that of the professional is dominant. Others believed that economic interests of the physician dictate that they keep patients satisfied so that they will not seek care from other sources. This requires the maintenance of a "professional" demeanor involving specialized knowledge and an arcane language. In these theories, the patient might not be passive, but any conflict between the patient and physician would be minimized so as to enhance the physician's stature (Freidson, 1972).

The assumption by the physician of a dominating role interferes with the appreciation of the role of the myriad determinants of health and influences acting on patients and with the fact that patients do not necessarily regard their medical care as the most salient determinant or influence. Moreover, physicians and patients often disagree on the nature of the patient's problem; in general, physicians and patients are in agreement only about half of the time (Starfield et al., 1979, 1981; Connelly et al., 1989). Only about half of all patients report playing an active role in the interaction with their physician; the other half believe their role to be passive (Brody et al., 1989a).

> Mr. R. is a 42-year-old engineer who experienced a sharp pain in his chest when lifting a 20-pound load. Because he has a family history of heart disease, he sought care from a cardiologist. The following dialogue ensued:
>
> Physician: "One of the advantages of being a cardiologist is that I can allay your fears. I've looked at your tests and I do not believe that you have had a significant coronary event."
>
> Mr. R.: "Thank you doctor. But you have not allayed my fears. I am an educated man and when I hear you use the words "believe," "significant," and "event" in one sentence, I worry about what you are telling me. I am not at all reassured."
>
> Charge for consultation: $400.
>
> Charge for laboratory tests: $375.

Some conceptualizations of the physician-patient interaction assign a larger role to the patient. Szasz and Hollander (1956), for example, describe three models for physician–patient interaction. In the first, the activity–passivity model, the physician makes the decisions. This occurs in situations where the patient is anesthetized or unconscious. In the second, the guidance–cooperation model, the physician provides the instructions and the patient carries them out (cooperates). In the third, the mutual participation model, the physician assists patients in helping themselves; patients participate in decision-making. In this third model, the physician does not presume to know what is best for the patient; patients are aware of constraints in their own life circumstances that make certain methods of intervention more or less feasible. What is best for the patient emerges from the interaction between patient and physician in which both contribute their own unique information and then negotiate the most appropriate approach to management (Szasz and Hollander, 1956).

The rise of the consumer movement and the increasing sophistication of the population inevitably narrowed the gap between professional competence and consumer knowledge (Haug and Levin, 1981), leading to different types of exploration of the dynamics of the interaction.

Depending on the degree of practitioner control over the interaction versus that of the patient, four types of interaction are now recognized. When both the patient and the physician have high control, the interaction is characterized as "mutuality." When the patient has high control but the physician has low control, the interaction is "consumerist." Low patient and high practitioner control produces a "paternalistic" interaction, whereas low control by both participants produces a "default" interaction (Stewart and Roter, 1989).

This categorization is similar to one designed to be a framework for describing physician–patient communication. This framework has four "models": paternalistic (physician articulates the problem and treatment); informative (physician provides information for patient to choose among alternatives); interpretive (physician clarifies patient's values and helps patients to select an intervention); and deliberative (physician helps patient determine and choose among their own values) (Emanuel and Emanuel, 1992).

Green (1988), a defense attorney in malpractice suits, observed that almost all medical malpractice litigation stemmed from misunderstandings about the decision-making process and argued that the doctrine of "informed consent" should be replaced by some tangible manifestation of shared decision-making, perhaps in the form of "contracts" that reflect agreement on decisions by patients and physicians. His suggested approach involves a short form that explains the four decision-making models (traditional, informed consent, collaboration, and patient choice) and requests both patients and physicians to indicate which they prefer.

Despite its importance, the verbal content of the interaction cannot alone sustain the practitioner–patient relationship. Both practitioners and patients respond to the context of the interaction, how each feels about the other, and how those feelings are conveyed. This context can be assessed by analyzing the voice tones rather than the content of the interaction or by observing physical postures and mannerisms. Voice tone and affect have more influence on what patients carry away from their encounter than does the content of the interaction, even when specific items of information are concerned.

The literature on the dynamics of the medical encounter focuses on both parties in the encounter by examining the nature of both the verbal communication and nonverbal behaviors. Although communication between professional and patient is not limited to primary care, most knowledge about the subject derives from studies in primary care facilities. It is possible to code the content of the interaction as well as the tone of the vocal communication. Several methods to code the components of the interaction are available (Roter and Hall, 1989), the two main categories of components being verbal information transfer between patients and physicians and socioemotional behaviors. Information transfer involves question-asking, giving information relevant to the illness or health problem and its management, and concordance on problem identification and treatment. Techniques for ascertaining and evaluating information transfer usually involve audiotaping the encounter, although direct observation and listening by a neutral observer has also been effective. The content of the verbal interaction is then analyzed. Socioemotional components involve explicit communication of feelings; feelings conveyed as nervousness or anxiety; warmth or empathy; or expressions of satisfaction and confidence. The socioemotional content of the interaction is also assessed from audiotapes, but here the voices are passed through an electronic filter that eliminates the highest voice frequencies and makes the verbal content unintelligible while preserving rhythm, tempo, and other nonverbal qualities (Hall et al., 1987).

The characteristics of the physician–patient interaction contribute substantially to what patients think and do as reflected in their satisfaction, their recall of information pertinent to their problem, their understanding of that information, and their compliance with advice.

Patients' satisfaction with their care is most related to the amount of information given by practitioners, especially of general rather than technical information (Roter and Hall, 1989). Examples of general information include explanation about the health problem and its treatment, stress counseling, and discussion of patient's ideas about the problem and its management. Technical information includes such items as the results of examinations or tests (Brody et al., 1989b). Patient satisfaction is also improved by greater communication overall, especially by social conversation, partnership-building conversation, positive feelings, and positive talk, but is reduced by conveying negative feelings or information.

While physicians are taught to ask questions, most patients do not ask many questions even though they may want information. The challenge for the physician is to establish a dialogue in which patients' concerns emerge in a context other than by direct questioning. Patients are more satisfied, both with the technical and with the interpersonal aspects of care, when physicians involve them in decision-making by asking whether the patient agrees with the decision about the problem, its causes, and its management. Physician-initiated interest in the patient's views has a greater impact on satisfaction than does the patient's perceived ability to ask questions or the patient's report of self-initiated comments. In fact, the patient's ability to ask questions or to initiate comments improves satisfaction only with the technical aspects of care and has no effect on the interpersonal aspects (Lerman et al., 1990). Thus, when physicians solicit the involvement of patients, the latter are more satisfied with the care, a phenomenon that supports the newer "sharing" theories of the physician–patient interaction rather than the older authoritarian models.

> I went to see the dermatologist and the nurse showed me inside the examining room and told me to take off my clothes and lie down on the table. The doctor came in and examined me. It was like being in a pathology lab. He was dictating a very beautiful description of my rash into a microphone in the ceiling. After he looked me all over, the first thing he said was "Well, I'm 99 percent sure that it's not a fungus but I'm going to take a test to be 100 percent sure. What he didn't tell me at the time was that the test would cost $20. He might have said "Would you like me to take the test now or if it doesn't go away in a few days to take it then?" but his nurse came in and scraped me with a little knife, and then the doctor told me to turn over. There I was naked on my stomach and he said "I'm going to give you a cortisone shot. I think that will probably take care of it or at least I hope it will take care of it." And then the nurse stuck me with a needle. Now I don't like to take a lot of medication but I didn't have much time to think about anything and when you are lying there with your behind sticking up, you're sort of vulnerable, and so, before I had chance to decide anything, I had the shot. Then he handed me a bottle of pills and when I asked what they were he said that they were cortisone pills and he wrote out a prescription and told me these were for more pills. I then said "Do I have to take these pills? Maybe the shot will do it?" "Well," he said, "You don't have to take the pills," and he took then from me and threw them in the basket. So I said, "I'll just take the prescription and if the rash doesn't go away I'll get the prescription filled." "No," he said, "you know best," and he tore up the prescription.   Mr C., a 30-year-old accountant

Patients are more likely to accept advice and instructions when the practitioner provides more information, asks fewer questions overall (but more questions about compliance), and provides more positive and less negative feedback. In addition, patients have a better understanding of advice particularly when the practitioner makes efforts to build a partnership. Useful strategies for improving patient's understanding of advice (Roter and Hall, 1989) include

• Presenting information early in the visit
• Taking care to be specific rather than general with instructions
• Organizing information into clear blocks
• Repeating the most important information
• Asking patients for feedback as to their understanding
• Summarizing information at the close of the visit

The characteristics of the interaction between physicians and patients also influence the outcomes of medical care. When both agree on the nature of the problem, the outcome is more likely to be reported as improved when judged by both patient and physician at the time of a follow-up visit (Starfield et al., 1979, 1981; Bass et al., 1986; Headache Study Group, 1986). In addition, when patients believe that they were active participants in the medical encounter, they report less discomfort, greater alleviation of their symptoms, and more improvement in their general condition on follow-up a week after their visit. They also report less concern with their illness and a greater sense of control over it (Brody et al., 1989a;

Wasserman et al., 1984). Objective signs of better disease control are also evident when patients actively participate in the physician–patient interaction. For example, greater patient involvement results in better diabetes control, better blood pressure control, and improved quality of life (Greenfield et al., 1985, 1988; Roter, 1977; Kaplan et al., 1989; Orth et al., 1987; Stewart, 1995).

A large study conducted in three U.S. cities and involving adults with chronic illness under care of primary care physicians, endocrinologists, or cardiologists showed that mutual decision-making ("participatory style") in visits increased linearly as the duration of relationship increased from the first visit to 5 years or longer (Kaplan et al., 1995). A scale for participation in decision-making was derived from answers to three questions asking if the doctor would ask the patient to help make a decision about treatment choice, would make an effort to give patients some control over the treatment, and would ask the patient to take some responsibility for the treatment. Even more significant, however, was the importance of participatory style on the subsequent duration of the relationship. Patients of physicians with higher participatory decision-making styles were less likely to change physicians during the subsequent 1-year follow-up. Family physicians and endocrinologists were more likely to be rated as having good skills than were cardiologists, particularly if they were in low-volume practices (Kaplan et al., 1996).

Despite the many studies and the extensive literature on physician–patient communication, much remains to be learned. Although most of the studies have been conducted in primary care settings, there has been no attempt to ascertain the relationship between communication styles and extent of attainment of primary care characteristics. As a result, we do not know whether physicians who provide better primary care in general also have better communication skills. Apart from the study mentioned above (Kaplan et al., 1996), which examined the influence of communication style on duration of the physician–patient relationship, studies have not explored the extent of its association with first-contact care, comprehensiveness, or coordination of care. Moreover, there has been considerable confusion in the concepts that have been studied, particularly with regard to the apparently overlapping phenomena of trust, communication, and satisfaction (Thom and Campbell, 1997). All three may be important in the context of longitudinality, which involves a person-focused, sustained relationship over time (Leopold et al., 1996). Yet, trust is not something that is unique to primary physician–patient relationships in primary care, and it is equally important for patients to be satisfied with care received from subspecialists as from primary care physicians. Little is known, however, about the importance of the various aspects of physician–patient communication in different types of practices. Evidence that malpractice suits in specialty care, particularly concerning surgeons, are unrelated to communication styles suggests either that communication patterns are relatively much less important or that the nature of the basis for the suit differs. For example, if malpractice suits filed against surgeons are primarily prompted by errors of commission whereas those filed against primary care physicians are for errors of omission, the implications for the nature of physician–patient communication will differ.

Although "trust" has been defined as "a person's belief that the physician's words and actions are credible and can be relied on" (i.e., confidence), the instruments that have been used to measure it do not precisely address "confidence." The most often used tool (Anderson and Dedrick, 1990) contains questions such as "I doubt that my doctor really cares about me as a person" and "my doctor is usually considerate of my needs and puts them first"; these reflect the nature of patient–physician interactions rather than states of belief. Moreover, 5 of the 11 questions in the scale use the word "trust" without defining it. Studies have failed to clarify the nature of the overlap and interactions among "trust," satisfaction, and communiction, and it is unclear as to the underlying cause of the benefits accruing from their relative influences. "Satisfaction" with a physician and styles of communication are related, but not highly. That is, high satisfaction is not always associated with good communication, and good communication is not always related to high satisfaction; at least part of the association may be that the same questions are used to measure both. Both have been associated with better concordance, but participatory communication styles (and, therefore, agreement between physician and patient on the nature of the patient's problem) are more highly associated with better outcomes, thereby suggesting the greater salience of the nature of the communication. That is, it seems likely that the chain of effect is from type of communication to practitioner–patient agreement on problems and strategies for intervention, to better concordance and patient understanding, and hence to better outcomes. "Trust" and "satisfaction," in this conceptualization, are by-products of these relationships.

Unfortunately, no studies have been designed to test the pathways that result in better outcomes of care and the applicability of the results to different types of patient's needs in different settings. From the viewpoint of primary care, the need for clarity is particularly acute because of the greater diversity of types of needs that must be addressed. Subspecialists deal primarily with one type of need: management of a presenting problem that has already reached some definition. Primary care physicians not only have to deal with presenting problems, at least half of which are sufficiently vague that they cannot be explained by conventional medical diagnoses (Weston and Brown, 1989; Pollack et al., 1993), but they also have to deal with the impact of what they do on the individual's future patterns of utilization and help-seeking, with the management of ongoing problems, and with opportunistic health promotion (Stott and Davis, 1979). The nature of the challenges to practitioner–patient communication may not be the same for all, and no studies have considered possible differences in impact of different communication styles in each of these situations.

Although the medical encounter has long been considered an art rather than a science, new avenues of research demonstrate how old techniques are amenable to study and change. There is a "technology" that can be taught. Talking with patients may be an ancient art, but there is also a modern science based on empirical evidence. Training in communication skills does improve the performance of physicians, at least as judged by their patients (Kaplan et al., 1995). Physicians trained in skills that result in patients becoming more active participants in the medical encounter obtain better diagnostic information from them (Maguire et al., 1986). This training also improves the quality of the explanation that the physician gives to patients and enhances the usefulness of what the patient tells the physician (Putnam et al., 1988). Checklists to evaluate medical interviewing skills at the undergraduate level are available (Kraan et al., 1989). There are models for teach-ing doctor–patient communication skills during residency (Schofield and Arntson, 1989). Given such training, primary care residents are better able to detect psy-chiatric illness among their patients (Goldberg et al., 1980). If skills in communi-cation are not part of medical training, they can be learned afterwards (Kurtz, 1989).

> In an era in which patients are encouraged to be more active participants in medical encounters and doctors are exhorted to devote more attention to the socioeconomic causes of illness and disease, it is telling that in medical advertisements the ways in which patients are represented are increasingly as dismembered specimens, me-chanical beings, gendered, physically active. These all are biomedical representa-tions of people. They support the tendency of biomedical medicine to place impor-tance on technology and drug treatment to treat localized conditions, to encourage the anonymity of the patient, to promote the vision of the "divided self," and devalue the affective aspects of the doctor–patient relationship.
>
> D.L., *International Journal of Health Services* (Lupton, 1993)

The adequacy of the patient–physician interaction includes more than the mere transfer of information. What patients know about their problems and their treat-ments is determined by more than what practitioners tell them. Illness has meaning to patients far beyond its physical manifestations because every illness produces some disturbance in the life of a person. Cure of an illness removes the physical abnormality, but healing requires restoration of the relationships disturbed by the illness. If a practitioner does not attend to the nonphysical correlates of the illness by failing to explore their meaning to the patient, the outcome may turn out to be unsatisfactory (McWhinney, 1989). Patients come with preconceptions that influ-ence the way they interpret both their illness and the physician's advice. When practitioners explore with patients as to what they know and what they think about their illness, its effects, and its management, these preconceptions can be revealed. Then the physician can furnish information in a context meaningful to the patient. For this reason, straightforwardness in providing factual advice is not generally the best approach, although it may seem efficient (Maynard, 1990). The way in which information is conveyed to patients and their involvement as active participants in the dialogue has a powerful impact on what they think, how they feel, and how they respond to medical advice.

Because health is heavily influenced by the social context in which people live and work, it might be expected that social factors should be an important com-ponent of physician–patient interactions. Many studies have shown that this is not the case. The training of physicians generally focuses on biological determinants of illness rather than on social determinants, and there is no accepted method of categorizing social factors as there is for biological factors. Waitzkin's philosoph-ical and empirical analysis (1991) of the nature of the interaction between physi-cians and patients shows how ideology determines the content of the discourse and how it leads physicians to avoid the social issues that cause illnesses and influence their course and response to treatment. For example, a well-accepted goal of medical care is to return individuals to their jobs. Because patients have different value systems and may not share these goals, open discussion of strategies to reduce illness, disability, and discomfort can produce disagreement and conflict. Many of the determinants of disease and health status are beyond the control of individuals. Even those individual behaviors that are commonly believed to be initiated and maintained by individual choice are heavily influenced by the social and environmental context (see Fig. 1.2). Thus, solving many health problems requires much more than dealing with individuals alone; practitioner–patient interactions often must take the population context into account. As a result, the solution to many health problems lies in collective action leading to environmental and social alteration of the conditions that predispose to and maintain illness.

Medical teaching conventionally fails to recognize that individuals themselves cannot alter many of the circumstances in which they find themselves. The result of this failure leads to medical interventions that palliate rather than cure because they are addressed at increasing the individual's ability to accommodate to situations that are adversely affecting health rather than to change them. For example, stress and its influences on predisposing to illness are often treated with medications that help people to adapt to environmental conditions even though they continue to cause harm both to the individual and to others exposed to the same adversity.

Appropriate recognition of the nature of these determinants of ill health that comes from interactions with individual patients can become an important tool for practitioners in their role as protectors of the health of populations. Without such recognition, the underlying tensions in the practitioner–patient interaction remain unresolved, as individuals come to recognize that their practitioners have little to offer in the way of definitive solutions to their health problems. The short-term approach to changing this underlying tension in medical discourse lies in a conscious attempt by physicians to recognize the existence of this underlying tension, to understand the basis for it, and to avoid technical solutions such as medications to reduce work-related and environmentally induced stress and its physiological effects. Rather than "over-medicalizing" health problems, physicians could help patients to understand the genesis of their problems and to encourage their involvement in collective rather than individual activities to dealing with the underlying determinants of problems. In the long run, more fundamental restructuring of health systems and practitioner–patient interactions to bring them into closer relationship to other social systems, in the context of health care of populations, will be needed to make medical care more effective and equitable in preventing, caring for, and healing illness, and in promoting health.

References

Anderson L, Dedrick R. Development of the trust in physician scale: A measure to assess interpersonal trust in patient–physician relationships. Psychol Rep 1990; 67:1091–100.

Bass M, Buck C, Turner L, Dickie G, Pratt G, Robinson H. The physician's actions and the outcomes of illness in family practice. J Fam Pract 1986; 23:43–7.

Brody DS, Miller SM, Lerman CE, Smith DG, Caputo GC. Patient perception of involvement in medical care: relationship to illness attitudes and outcomes J Gen Intern Med 1989a; 4:506–11.

Brody DS, Miller SM, Lerman CE, Smith DG, Lazaro CG, Blum MJ. The relationship between patients' satisfaction with their physicians and perceptions about interventions they desired and received. Med Care 1989b; 27(11):1027–35.

Connelly J, Philbrick J, Smith Gr, Kaiser D, Wymer A. Health perceptions of primary care patients and the influence on health care utilization. Med Care 1989; 27:S99–S109.

Emanuel E, Emanuel L. Four models of the physician–patient relationship. JAMA 1992; 267; 2221–6.

Freidson E. Client control and medical practice. In Jaco EG (ed): Patients, Physicians and Illness. A Source book in Behavioral Science & Health. 2nd Ed. London: Collier Mac-Millan, 1972. pp 214–221.

Goldberg D, Steele J, Smith C, Spivey L. Training family doctors to recognize psychiatric illness with increased accuracy. Lancet 1980; 2:521–3.

Green J. Minimizing malpractice risk by role clarification: The confusing transition from tort to contract. Ann Intern Med 1988; 109:234–41

Greenfield S, Kaplan S, Ware JE. Expanding patient involvement in care. Ann Intern Med 1985; 102:520–8.

Greenfield S, Kaplan SH, Ware JE Jr, Yano EM, Frank HJL. Patients' participation in medical care. J Gen Intern Med 1988;3:448–57 .

Hall J, Roter D, Katz N. Task versus socioemotional behaviors in physicians. Med Care 1987; 25:399–412.

Haug M, Levin B. Practitioner or patient—Who's in charge? J Health Soc Behav 1981; 22: 212–29.

Headache Study Group of the University of Western Ontario. Predictors of outcome in headache patients presenting to family physicians—A one year prospective study. Health J 1986; 26:285–94.

Kaplan S, Gandek B, Greenfield S, Rogers W, Ware J. Patient and visit characteristics related to physicians' participatory decision-making style. Med Care 1995; 33:1176–87.

Kaplan S, Greenfield S, Gandek B, Rogers W, Ware J. Characteristics of physicians with participatory decision making styles. Ann Intern Med 1996; 124:497–504.

Kaplan S, Greenfield S, Ware JE Jr. Impact of the doctor–patient relationship on the outcomes of chronic disease. In Stewart M, Roter D (eds): Communicating With Medical Patients. Newbury Park, CA: Sage Publications, 1989. pp 228–245.

Kraan HF, Crijnen A, Zuidwed J, der Vleuten C, Imbos T. Evaluating undergraduate training—A checklist for medical interviewing skills. In Stewart M, Roter D (eds): Communicating With Medical Patients. Newbury Park, CA: Sage Publications, 1989. pp 167–77.

Kurtz SM. Curriculum structuring to enhance communication skills development. In Stewart M, Roter D (eds): Communicating With Medical Patients. Newbury Park, CA: Sage Publications, 1989. pp 153–66.

Leopold N, Cooper J, Clancy C. Sustained partnership in primary care. J Fam Pract 1996; 42:129–37.

Lerman C, Brody D, Caputo C, Smith D, Lazaro C, Wolfson H. Patients' perceived involvement in care scale: Relationship to attitudes about illness and medical care. J Gen Intern Med 1990; 5:29–33.

Levinson W, Roter D, Mullooly J, Dull V, Frankel R. Physician–patient communication: The relationship with malpractice claims among primary care physicians and surgeons. JAMA 1997; 277:553–9.

Lupton D. The construction of patienthood in medical advertising. Int J Health Serv 1993; 23(4):805–819.

Maguire P, Fairbairn S, Fletcher C. Consultation skills of young doctors: I—Benefits of feedback training in interviewing as students persist [published erratum appears in BMJ 1986; 293(6538):26]. BMJ 1986; 292:1573–6.

Maynard D. Bearing bad news. Medical Encounter Newsletter on the Medical Interview and Related Skills. Summary. 1990; 7:2–3.

McWhinney I. The Need for a Transformed Clinical Method. In Stewart M, Roter D (eds). Communicating With Medical Patients. Newbury Park, CA: Sage Publications, 1989. pp 25–40.

Orth J, Stiles W, Scherwitz L, Hennrikus D, Valbona C. Patient exposition and provider explanation in routine interviews and hypertensive patients' blood pressure control. Health Psychol 1987; 6:29–42.

Pollack M, Cummings N, Dorken H, Henke C. Managed mental health, Medicaid, and medical cost offset. New Directions Ment Health Serv 1993:27–40.

Putnam S, Stiles W, Jacob C, James S. Teaching the medical interview: An intervention study. J Gen Intern Med 1988; 3:38–47.

Roter DL. Patient participation in the patient provider interaction: The effects of patient question asking on the quality of interaction, satisfaction and compliance. Health Educ Monogr 1977; Winter:281–315.

Roter DL, Hall JA. Studies of doctor–patient interaction. Annu Rev Public Health 1989; 10: 163–80.

Schofield T, Arntson P. A model for teaching doctor–patient communication during residency. In Stewart M, Roter D (eds): Communicating With Medical Patients. Newbury Park, CA: Sage Publications, 1989. pp 138–52.

Starfield B, Steinwachs D, Morris I, Bause G, Siebert S, Westin C. Patient–provider agreement about problems. Influence on outcome of care. JAMA 1979; 242:344–6.

Starfield B, Wray C, Hess K, Gross R, Birk P, D'Lugoff B. The influence of patient–practitioner agreement on outcome of care. Am J Public Health 1981; 71:127–32.

Stewart M. Effective physician–patient communication and health outcomes: A review. Can Med Assoc J 1995; 152:1423–33.

Stewart M, Roter D (eds). Communicating with Medical Patients. Interpersonal Communications, vol 9. Newbury Park, CA: Sage Publications, 1989.

Stott NC, Davis RH. The exceptional potential in each primary care consultation. J R Coll GP 1979; 29(201):201–5.

Szasz T, Hollander M. A contribution to the philosophy of medicine. Arch Intern Med 1956; 97:585–92.

Thom D, Campbell C. Patient–physician trust: An exploratory study. J Fam Pract 1997; 44: 169–76.

Waitzkin H. The Politics of Medical Encounters: How Doctors and Patients Deal With Social Problems. New Haven:Yale University Press, 1991

Wasserman R, Inui T, Barriatua B, Carter W, Lippincott P. Pediatric clinicians' support for parents makes a difference: An outcome-based analysis of clinician–parent interaction. Pediatrics 1984; 74:1047–53.

Weston W, Brown J. The importance of patients' beliefs. In Stewart M, Roter D (eds): Communicating With Medical Patients. Newbury Park, CA: Sage Publications, 1989. pp 77–85

— 10 —

Comprehensiveness of Care: Who Should Provide What

Alisa is a 4-year-old child whose growth and development have been normal. For the past year, however, she has had acute otitis media that never seems to clear despite apparently adequate antibiotic therapy. Several doctor's appointments have not been kept, and her mother does not call to cancel or re-schedule them. At a monthly case conference, the situation was discussed and a decision was made to have Dr. S. make a home visit.

The family lives in an apartment house in a low-income neighborhood. The building has an elevator but the corridors are dark. The family's apartment is, however, light and well kept. When Dr. S. rang the bell, she was greeted warmly by Mrs. M. and her three children, who were not in school that day. In the course of discussing the family and their health problems, Dr. S. asked where the children slept and Mrs. M. volunteered to show her the apartment. As they sat talking in the living room over coffee that Mrs. M. had prepared, Dr. S. noticed a closed door leading off the room and inquired about what it was. Mrs. M. offered to show her and opened the door. Sitting in the corner was an elderly-appearing white-haired woman, rocking back and forth and talking to herself. A few minutes of observation convinced Dr. S. that the woman, the maternal grandmother, was actively hallucinating.

Subsequent social work intervention resulted in appropriate placement of the grandmother. Alisa's ear problem, which persisted because of Mrs. M.'s distraction with her own mother's schizophrenia and her consequent inability to focus on the prescribed therapy, resolved.

Comprehensiveness requires that primary care adequately recognize the full range of patients' health-related needs and arrange for the resources to deal with them. Decisions as to whether primary care rather than some other level of care maintains the capacity to provide specific services will vary from place to place and from time to time, depending on the nature of the health problems of different populations.

Individual practitioner–patient interactions not only provide insight as to the likely determinants of ill health and possible interactions for them in individual patients. They also provide clues as to the likelihood of ill health among other

181

people who may be seen by the practitioner or by the health facility or plan. That is, the same predispositions to illness that occur in the particular patient may also exist in others who live in the same community or are exposed to the same social, environmental, or occupational conditions. Adequate recognition of the genesis of a patient's problem thus provides a powerful tool for the practitioner to influence the nature of the services that should be provided to the population under care in the practice, facility, health plan, or integrated health system.

Primary care is the entry point for individual health care, the locus of continuing responsibility for patients in populations, and the level of care in the best position to interpret presenting problems in the context of the patient's history and social milieu. Thus, the way in which it is designed to provide appropriate services and the adequacy of doing so are key components of a strategy for improving effectiveness and equity of health services.

Primary care is, however, but one component (albeit the cornerstone component) of health systems. Its role is to directly provide all services for common needs and act as an agent for the provision of services for needs that must be met elsewhere.

Continuing experience is required to maintain competence in dealing with problems; no type of practitioner should be expected to deal alone with all needs in the population. Rather, comprehensiveness requires that services be available and provided when needed for problems occurring with a frequency sufficient for practitioners to maintain their competence. The range of services available and provided in primary care may thus vary from community to community as the incidence or prevalence of problems differs.

Because primary care focuses on meeting peoples' needs, it must have available a range of services targeted to those needs and achieve a high level of performance in recognizing existing needs in its population. "Needs" may be symptoms, dysfunctions, discomforts, or diseases; they also might be indicated preventive interventions or even health-promoting interventions. The challenge is to recognize situations in which an intervention is both needed and justified. The range of types of health problems in primary care is much greater than in any other type of care, and therefore the range of all types of interventions is wider. Recognizing when services are required is a challenge not only for those who are ill and appear for care. Because primary care is ongoing, the caring and healing functions are likely to be more prolonged, extensive, and far-ranging. More extensive types of resources must often be brought to bear. Services not normally provided in subspecialty care, such as home visits and other efforts at outreach, are often required as part of comprehensive care. Because primary care deals with a broader array of health concerns and does so within a broader social context, it must have a wide array of types of resources at its disposal.

Although it may appear that the greater the range and application of available services the better the care, this is not necessarily true. Some types of services may not be effective, some may be effective but not worth their cost, and some may be harmful. As is noted later in this chapter, deciding on an appropriate range of services is an important policy issue and a key component of the role of primary care services.

In small facilities, such as the office of an individual practitioner, the range of available services will be necessarily narrower than in larger facilities because efficiency dictates that equipment and facilities be available only if use is sufficiently high. In the small facilities, where the range of services is narrow, the provider must ensure that an appropriate referral is made and that the needed services will be received. Health care reform for the 21st century will increasingly involve larger organizations and target populations; policy decisions concerning an appropriate range of services will, at the same time, become easier and more complex. Greater ease will accrue because there will be increased capacity to use information to learn about the nature and distribution of health problems. On the other hand, greater complexity will result because of increasing recognition that different populations have different needs and therefore require a different mix of services.

Comprehensiveness of care is an important mechanism because it ensures that services are tailored to health needs. When services are too narrow in scope or depth, preventable illnesses may not be prevented, illnesses may be allowed to progress longer than is justifiable, quality of life may be jeopardized, and people may die sooner than they should. Patients themselves recognize the importance of comprehensiveness and express dissatisfaction in its absence. For example, Fletcher and colleagues (1983) found comprehensiveness to be the second most important characteristic of care (after continuity) for patients attending a primary care clinic for adults. Hickson and colleagues (1988) found that the third most common reason for parents' dissatisfaction, after lack of response to treatment and inconvenient location of office, was the failure of physicians to be interested in the behavior problems of their children.

Comprehensiveness is thus judged by the extent to which the available range of services meets needs that are common in all populations and the needs that are common in the population served, as well as the extent to which there is evidence that the services are being applied adequately to meet those needs.

> I went to see an ENT doctor because of pain in my ear. He poked in my ear, poked it this way and that way and he said that he didn't see anything wrong. I said "But doctor, it hurts me so bad that it even hurts me in my eye." He looked in my ear again with that light and he poked around and then he said that it's all in my imagination. When he said that it's all in my imagination I started to get angry, and when he said that, I stood up and said "Thank you very much for not finding anything wrong with my ear, Doctor. How much is your fee?" He told me and I said "Why don't you imagine that I just paid you?" And I walked out.
>
> They get angry with you and it makes you want to start screaming "Hey , I'm having the pain. Why don't you listen to me for five minutes? I come to you for help and you tell me I'm not having those pains and its all in my mind." I don't feel they should tell me anything until they listen to me first and then come to a conclusion of what's wrong. If there isn't anything wrong with my ear, then the doctor should find out what is giving me the pains and not assume that, just because I don't have a problem in the part of the body they take care of, that there's nothing wrong. I like doctors, but they have to listen and have a little compassion for the patient and not just think about their little piece of my body.
>
> Mrs. R., a 60-year-old secretary

The Benefits of Comprehensiveness: Prevention as One Example

The benefits of comprehensive care can be inferred from the known benefits of preventive care (Russell, 1986) and from the benefits of providing services known to be effective for populations with particular health needs. One cross-national study, however, takes issue with the assumption that all needed services should be provided or arranged for by the source of primary care. After comparing the health systems in the United States with those in several western European nations, Silver (1978) concluded that children were more likely to have received indicated preventive care such as immunizations in those systems where responsibility for these preventive procedures was divorced from the primary care practice and was assumed by a public authority. Whether this is generally the case or just the case when primary care services are not adequate remains to be determined. The critical factor may be the extent to which the public authority is sufficiently well organized to provide the service in a systematic and integrated way. In the United States, where local public health involvement in delivering services has been greatly weakened over the most recent several decades, it may not have adequate resources to mount such efforts. For example, when access to primary care providers is improved as a result of better insurance coverage for preventive care (including immunizations and prenatal care), previously underinsured and uninsured families are more likely to receive these services from their primary care provider than from separate public health facilities (Rodewald et al., 1997; Simpson et al., 1997).

Prevention is a special need in primary care. Historically, prevention has been a public health function; most preventive activities were directed at populations, largely to protect the public welfare rather than individual health. Often governed by laws and regulations, they treated everyone equally: Everyone needed immunizations. Everyone needed protection against environmentally induced disease. However, prevention has expanded from the simple concept of protection of populations against disease by intervening at its environmental source. Prevention now considers risks that only some individuals face because of particular biological or social susceptibilities. When everyone is at risk, or when the likelihood of being at risk is unknown, there is often a good case for a public health rather than a clinical strategy toward prevention. Population-based strategies may not always be the most efficient or even the safest when not everyone is at risk, and they become less justifiable as the likelihood of risk decreases. Furthermore, not everyone wants to engage in prevention when it requires personal actions or when it is imposed by a perceived bureaucracy.

Providing preventive services to all individuals has the advantage of appearing to be equitable; a case in point was the U.S. recommendation to screen all infants for sickle cell anemia, even though it is 168 times more common among African-Americans than among white Americans, on the grounds that "screening should benefit all babies equally" (Sickle Cell Disease Guideline Panel, 1993). However, every intervention (including preventive interventions) has risks, and subjecting individuals at low risk of the condition to the risks of the intervention is likely to cause more harm than would be expected from the unlikely occurrence of the condition itself. Moreover, there is no assurance that even a strategy to reach everyone in the population will reach those who are hardest to reach and who may be in most need.

Many clinical prevention activities are related to specific diseases; others are more oriented toward generally improving resilience against a variety of threats to health. Examples in the first category are mammography to detect breast cancer, hypertension screening to detect susceptibility to cardiovascular disease, and newborn screening to detect congenital metabolic disease at an early presymptomatic stage. In the latter category are primary preventive activities such as seat belts and helmets, breast feeding, and smoking cessation. Because not everyone is at risk for adverse effects of either the specific diseases or the multiplicity of conditions that might be averted by the intervention, the likelihood of being at risk requires ascertainment. The challenge to health services is to determine when ascertainment is best carried out through a population-based approach and when a clinical medicine function is more appropriate.

Population-wide interventions, which generally are more appropriately carried out by public health activities, are most appropriate when individual risk assessment is impossible or difficult, when there is a low risk of adverse effect, and when the problem to be prevented is either common or has serious implications for the population. (Population-wide approaches are also more appropriate when everyone is known to be at risk, as is the case for environmentally induced conditions or injuries.)

The choice between generalized (whole population) and selective (selected populations) approaches to ascertaining risks, and therefore the relative merits of a public health or clinical medicine approach, often is not easy to make. Selection of the most appropriate approach requires pre-existing knowledge of the likelihood of risk (Rose, 1992). It requires a tool that is able to identify risks in a way that is of acceptable sensitivity and specificity, has reasonably precise cut-off points and little ambiguity in the border zone between abnormal and normal, is acceptable to patients and providers, does not cause adverse effects when people are falsely labeled, is feasible in practice, and is not unacceptably expensive to undertake. The matter of avoidance of unnecessary adverse effects from false labeling is more critical in general population approaches than in selective ones because more side effects may be tolerated in populations already at high risk. High cost is more easily tolerated in selective approaches for the same reason: High cost is more acceptable when risk is higher. Sometimes generalized approaches are better just because opportunities for reaching people are better; selective approaches usually require that there be a special mechanism for reaching those at risk. Generalized approaches are better for problems that are common in the population or pose a public health problem. This is why immunizations sometimes are carried out as a public health rather than as a clinical medicine function. Dedicated public health approaches are also often justified as more effective because clinical medicine has been slow to assume the challenge of prevention (Starfield and Vivier, 1995).

Table 10.1 indicates the different practice characteristics, as viewed from the perspective of health system components, that influence whether a population ap-

Table 10.1. Health System Requirements for Successful Prevention of Population Versus Selective Approaches

Health System Characteristics	Approach to Prevention	
	Population	Selective
	Structural	
Personnel	Dedicated public health/community medicine specialists *or* (in office-based practice) physicians trained in preventive medicine *or* (in practice teams involving personnel with public health/community medicine expertise	
Continuity mechanisms	Information/medical record systems containing, at a minimum, basic demographic characteristics (age, gender, race) and a recall system to identify individuals in a timely fashion	Information/medical record systems containing, at a minimum, data on relevant risk characteristics and a recall system to identify individuals when indicated
Financing	Financial coverage targeted to preventive services through public mechanisms	Universal and comprehensive third-party coverage for preventive services
Population eligible	Well defined	Well defined
	Process	
Problem (needs) identification	Little information required	Personnel trained in biopsychosocial approaches *or* adequate automated problem identification
Diagnosis, management	Mechanisms for assessing the adequacy of the trajectory of care (i.e., quality management)	
Utilization, acceptance, understanding, participation	Population unable to assume responsibility for initiating care and carrying through to adequate completion	Population able to assume responsibility for initiating care and carrying through to adequate completion *or* adequate outreach activities to defined populations

proach (everyone gets the preventive intervention, either in a health plan or center or through a public health effort) or a selective approach (intervention is targeted at high-risk populations only) is likely to be the best strategy when there is a choice to be made. The types, training, and motivation of personnel in the practice, the adequacy of available information and its transfer, financial incentives, and clear definition of the population covered by the practice are all relevant structural considerations.

A variety of past efforts, including conventional continuing medical education and the use of guidelines to improve the extent to which preventive activities are carried out in clinical practice, have had limited effectiveness. The complexity of primary care practice is associated with extraordinary variability in performance (Crabtree, 1997). The completeness with which practices are able to recognize problems and needs in the population, the adequacy of their diagnostic and treatment procedures, and the characteristics of the population that signify likelihood of acceptance of the preventive activities all will influence the choice between primary care and public health approaches.

Policy and Research Implications of Comprehensiveness of Care: Services To Be Provided by Primary Care

In some countries, specification of services that should be provided in clinical practice rather than by public health activities are set by national policy. Often, decisions as to what should be covered are made by limiting the availability of resources for clinical care; where there are few or no resources to provide a defined service, no individual decisions about its utility for any specific individual are required because it is simply not available to anyone (Grogan, 1992). This clearly is the most equitable approach to specifying the range of services to be provided. In other countries, the only limit on the services that are available is demand of the providers and patients; because markets can generate their own demand, there is generally a high degree of inequity in the range of services available to their populations. The effect of this difference is demonstrated by consideration of the frequency with which certain technologies are used in different countries (Fig. 10.1). Although none of these are primary care interventions, the same types of differences are found for technology available in primary care as well, as is particularly notable in France and Germany. Even in countries in which demand drives

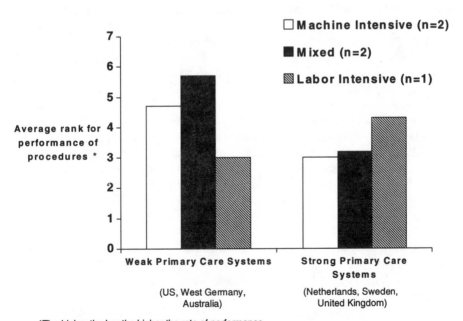

*The higher the bar the higher the rate of performance

Figure 10.1. Ranks for rates of technology use. Source: based on Battista et al. (1994).

the range of services that are provided, increasing mandates for accountability resulting from increased public expenditures of funds are likely to produce greater homogeneity of the range of services available to different population groups. However, where privatization of funding is increasingly the case, greater heterogeneity and inequity is likely to result.

Policy decisions concerning the appropriate locus of responsibility are not limited to preventive services. The relevant policy issue for comprehensiveness in general lies in deciding which services appropriately belong in primary care and which should be arranged for elsewhere.

In the best of all possible worlds, the range of services provided would be determined only by need and delivered at levels of care where clinicians encounter them frequently enough to maintain competence in dealing with them. In reality, compromises are necessary because resources are limited and there are competing needs for various types of health services and for social services other than health, such as housing and education.

In any health system, health care organization, or office practice, decisions must be made concerning the services to be directly provided or arranged for. Although not all services will be provided in the primary care sector, the primary care provider bears the responsibility for recognizing health care needs and for arranging and coordinating the provision of services to be provided elsewhere. Therefore, the nature of the benefit package has high salience in primary care, even if it does not provide all needed services.

In many (if not most) health systems, hospitalizations and the most expensive specialty services are covered by insurance plans or national health systems. In contrast, many primary care services are often not included, sometimes on the grounds that they are more "discretionary" and therefore will be used excessively if reimbursed, that they are predictable and therefore not requiring "insurance" against uncertainty, or that they do not need to be covered by insurance because they are relatively inexpensive and hence affordable.

Several considerations dictate the services that are to be available. These considerations are of several types: the availability of standards, the specification of needs to be addressed, evidence-based criteria, and the marketplace. The resulting policy depends on which approach is taken. A discussion of each of these four considerations follows. Although none of the four is helpful in determining exactly what should be provided in primary care, each might serve as a model for doing so.

Standards

The Health Policy Agenda was the product of several years of deliberation by representatives of the major professional associations in the United States. In general, its package of specified benefits includes "physician services both inpatient and outpatient, hospital services, laboratory and roentgenogram services, prescription drugs, institutional care for the elderly and physically or mentally disabled, dental services, early and periodic screening including diagnosis and treatment services, family planning services, home health and personal care services, and other medically necessary services" (Tallon, 1989).

More detailed is the policy on health benefits proposed by the American Academy of Pediatrics in 1989. "Health insurance plans should cover the following services for children from birth through 21 years old. These services should be ordered by a doctor and delivered in either a hospital or doctor's office . . . the following is an ideal list of benefits . . . by which each plan's covered services should be compared." The list includes the following:

- Medical care, including health supervision and treatment of acute conditions and diagnosis of severe and long-term illness
- Treatment of pre-existing conditions
- Surgical care, including steps to correct birth defects
- Mental health, alcohol, and other substance abuse services
- Emergency and trauma services
- Inpatient hospital services
- Consultations with pediatric subspecialists
- Family planning services
- Pregnancy services, including prenatal care, prenatal consultation with a pediatrician, and care for the pregnancy of a single dependent of the policy holder
- Care of all newborn infants, including a pediatric specialist to attend high-risk pregnancies
- Examinations and health checks from the time of birth and treatment of birth defects and other illnesses or injuries
- Laboratory and pathology services
- Diagnostic and therapeutic radiology services; anesthesia services
- Services ordered by the doctor to help a child recover from an illness or injury, including physical therapy
- Speech therapy and occupational therapy
- Home health care or the services of a licensed private duty nurse
- Hospice care for the terminally ill child
- Help for parents or guardians who need relief from the constant demand of caring for children with long-term illnesses
- Long-term care services delivered in an intermediate care or skilled nursing center instead of in hospitals
- Case management and supervision of the special medical and social services needed by chronically ill or disabled children
- Medical and social services to check for and treat suspected child abuse or neglect
- Transport to the hospital or health center
- Preventive and restorative dental care
- Nutrition counseling and check-ups
- Prescription drugs, medical and surgical supplies
- Corrective eyeglasses or lenses
- Hearing aids and special nutritional supplements
- Rental or purchase of durable medical equipment, such as special beds or crutches

The list of services, extensive as it is, still excludes certain services such as home visits by physicians and is vague about the extent of other services. Does surgical care include cosmetic surgery other than correction of birth defects? What is included under laboratory services? Nonetheless, it is obvious that the proposal of the American Academy of Pediatrics is far more comprehensive than are most existing insurance benefits packages and public programs.

Standards for preventive care may be derived from published guidelines for a wide variety of types of procedures, including screening, counseling, and immunizations or chemoprophylaxis. These guidelines (U.S. Preventive Services Task Force, 1996) provide a review of the effectiveness of more than 100 clinical interventions for the prevention of 60 diseases and conditions and make recommendations as to their indications and the timing and frequency of the services that were judged to be effective by a large panel of experts who reviewed the evidence.

Community health needs

Another approach to specifying the scope of benefits packages is based on the range of needs of a community. In one method for defining it, an organization providing health care documents the health needs of its population and uses the data to set priorities. In contrast to the setting of priorities according to goals and objectives, as described above, this method could lead to different priorities from one community to another and depends on what data each community decides to collect and the criteria used to interpret it. This approach is discussed in greater detail in Chapter 14.

Evidence of the effectiveness of services

The third element of the benefits package sets priorities according to the degree of benefit afforded. Instead of using data to determine community health needs, this approach establishes priorities according to the public's perception of value of an intervention, its impact on outcome of care, and its cost. It was attempted in Oregon where a governmental commission had the responsibility for obtaining the needed information and for developing the range of services that would be made available. The commission sought public input through town meetings and random surveys. People were asked how highly they value such conditions as mobility, mental capacity, freedom from pain, and ability to continue working. The data then become part of a cost–benefit calculation involving consideration of the extent to which a specific intervention achieves the desired outcomes, including such criteria as improving life expectancy, quality of life, and the number of people it would benefit. A prioritized list was developed such that the treatment of conditions below certain ranking would not be reimbursed. Although designed and implemented only for the Medicaid program (i.e., for uninsured people with very low incomes), it succeeded in increasing the amount of money available to raise the income levels for eligibility for Medicaid and hence reduce the number of individuals without health insurance (Bodenheimer, 1997).

Proposed coverage criteria for inclusion of interventions in health plans in general (not primary care in specific) are (1) intervention is used for a medical condition, (2) there is evidence for its effectiveness on health outcomes, (3) its application is expected to produce the desired effect on application, (4) its benefits outweigh its harmful effects, and (5) it is the most cost-effective for the purpose intended (Eddy, 1996). This approach is based on evidence of effectiveness of management for problems that are believed to be most important in the population rather than most common. Thus, it is an approach to providing services where resources are insufficient to meet the standards of comprehensiveness that might be set by methods based on population needs.

The marketplace

In a market-based health system, different facilities often use comprehensiveness of services to gain an edge over competitors. A baseline of comprehensiveness is often determined by governmental regulations that mandate services such as office-based medical care; hospitalization; heart, kidney, or cornea transplants; and infertility control. Most additions to these basic packages, which sometimes increase costs considerably, derive from negotiations with employers or insurance companies, who often put their requirements out for bids by different health providers. The final negotiated benefit package is often revised based on experience and subsequent annual negotiations.

In the United States, comprehensiveness of benefits is generally based on conditions in the marketplace. As a result, the benefits available to individuals, families, enrolled groups, or employees in various industries or firms are widely discrepant. A comparison of 15 insurance plans (Alpha Center, 1990), each developed to provide financing for the previously uninsured, found that some services were always covered, some were usually covered (in 10 to 12 plans), some were covered only sometimes (six to eight plans), and some were covered only rarely (one to three of the plans). The following were *always* covered:

- Visits to doctor's office
- Outpatient diagnostic x-ray and laboratory testing
- Outpatient surgery, including doctor and facility charge
- Well-baby care
- Ambulance services
- Emergency room services
- Hospital inpatient services, including semiprivate room and board, surgeon's fees, anesthesiologist's fees, doctor visits in the hospital, and prescriptions

However, not all plans covered these services to the same extent. Those services that were *almost always* covered included outpatient routine physicals; outpatient immunizations; outpatient physical therapy; and private duty nursing in the hospital. Again, however, the extent of the benefit varied.

Services that were *usually* covered included outpatient prescriptions; home health visits; and routine hearing and eye examinations.

Services that were covered only *some of the time* included convalescent care or care in a skilled nursing facility; outpatient mental health services; inpatient mental health services; and hospice care. Typically, these benefits had limitations on the number of such services or on the dollar amount provided.

Services that were provided only *rarely* included durable medical equipment; prosthetic and orthotic appliances; podiatry; and genetic testing and counseling.

In general, decisions about the content of the benefits package have largely been determined by professional opinion and by cost considerations. Where needed services are not included, they are either not received at all, purchased by those who need them, or provided directly by the public health sector. Providing services through the public health sector runs the risk of fragmenting services and reducing the likelihood of achieving longitudinality, first-contact care, and coordination of care. In developing nations, the focus on selective rather than integrated care may be justified, given the stage of underdevelopment of the health services sector and the type of population needs (Walsh and Warren, 1979). But even in this situation, a case can be made that integrated care is a more appropriate strategy in the long run (Rifkin and Walt, 1986).

An approach to defining what is appropriate for coverage by primary care is provided by deliberations within the British Medical Association (General Medical Services Committee, 1996). These deliberations resulted from changes in the way general practitioners (the primary care physicians in the United Kingdom) are paid for their services. New contract mechanisms are calling into question many of the services heretofore provided by many if not most general practitioners. Table 10.2 lists the services that are considered ''core'' and those that are considered to require additional payment if performed (non-core).

According to principle, what is considered to be in the purview of primary care rather than through referral elsewhere should depend on the frequency of the prob-

Table 10.2. Core and Non-Core Services: Proposals of The British Medical Association—1996

Core Services

Responding to patients' problems
Proactive services: Health promotion and preventive activities
Minor surgery and intrapartum care
After-hours care, child health surveillance, chronic disease management
Organizing the primary health care team

Non-Core Services

Participation in professional teaching, audit activities, commissioning, and purchasing
Care of patients in nursing home, residential facilities, and highly dependent patients at home
Care associated with or derived from hospitalization of patients, removal of sutures or care of dressings done in secondary care, treatment of minor injuries
Prescribing of complex medical regimens (e.g., cytotoxins, ritalin, hormone implants, intravenous nutrition)
Complex mental health care (e.g., not yet discharged from psychiatrist care)
Activities related to drug trials
Uncommon procedures (e.g., unblocking shunts)
Procedures requiring special training (e.g., acupuncture, endoscopy, colonoscopy, sigmoidoscopy, varicose vein ligation, vasectomy, colposcopy)
Shared care arrangement with other providers (e.g., anticoagulant therapy, dialysis, diabetic retinopathy screening)
Organization of services provided by other professionals (e.g., physiotherapists, dietitians, chiropractors)
Non-practice professional services (e.g., part-time prison duties)
Medicolegal reports, occupational health work, sports examinations, drivers' examinations

lem or need; primary care practitioners should be trained (initially or through continuing education) to provide for these common needs. If more time-consuming procedures or more risky procedures are indicated in the practice, panels of patients should be smaller or compensation for extra time required should be provided to allow the practitioner to include the service in the primary care practice. A recent report of the successful incorporation of colonoscopy (generally done by non-primary care specialists) in general practice is an example of the response of a group of U.S. family physicians to an increasingly common need for a preventive service (Pierzchajlo et al., 1997). In this practice, 100 colonoscopies were done per year by a family physician in a rural area who had been trained to do the procedure. Over a 7-year period, there was only one major procedural complication successfully managed by the practitioner.

Empirical support for the proposition that need for referral is related to frequency with which problems are encountered in the population comes from a large national study of office-based primary care pediatricians. The likelihood of referral for a wide variety of children's problems was highly and directly related to the infrequency with which the problem was encountered by the practitioners in their daily practice (CB Forrest et al., in preparation).

In the future, decisions concerning the appropriate range of services to be provided in primary care, as well as secondary and tertiary care, will be based increasingly on public accountability, taking into consideration community needs, equity of access, and the effectiveness of services. Although methods for setting priorities are still primitive and there is no consensus concerning the approach to be used, recognition of the limits on resources will focus attention on the challenge and compel careful consideration of the various alternatives.

> Dr. M. is a postgraduate research fellow studying the primary care experiences of patients who are being seen in three pediatric specialty clinics at a highly regarded hospital. Because he was interviewing physicians about their patients, he also asked them about the likely duration of their relationship with each patients. None of the physicians could answer the question, as they had not even thought about what role they were playing in the care of these children over time.

Measurement of Comprehensiveness

As is the case with the other attributes of primary care, the assessment of comprehensiveness can focus either at the system/population level or at the facilities/patient level. At the population level the needs of the community define the range of services that should be provided, and comprehensiveness is measured by the penetration of these services in the community. At the facilities level, the range of services is usually set according to professional guidelines such as immunization schedules or recommendations for procedures such as mammograms. Assessment at this level generally uses chart audits or other records such as claims forms.

Figure 10.2 depicts the components of comprehensiveness in the context of the health services system for populations and patients.

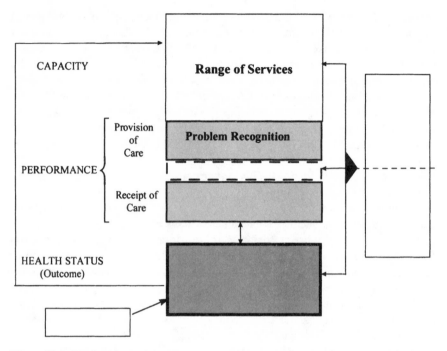

Figure 10.2. The health services system: Comprehensiveness. Abstracted from Figure 2.1.

Range of services

The range of services that are available should consist of a core that is relevant to every population as well as additional services for populations with special health needs that are common.

At the *population level*, standards for the range of services needed by communities are stated in such general terms that measurement of a range is generally not feasible. For example, the World Health Organization (WHO) recommends that

> for primary care to be comprehensive, all development-oriented activities should be interrelated and balanced so as to focus on problems of the highest priority as mutually perceived by the community and health system, and that culturally acceptable, technically appropriate, manageable, and appropriately selected interventions should be implemented in combinations that meet local needs. This implies that single-purpose programs should be integrated into primary health care activities as quickly and smoothly as possible.   WHO, 1978

This statement makes it clear that comprehensiveness does not consist of single-purpose programs, but it gives little guidance to determine which problems are of highest priority and how decisions are to be made concerning the measurement of cultural acceptability, technical appropriateness, and manageability.

The range of services appropriate to primary care consists of three components: the problems and needs of populations and patients, the tasks that are required to address these problems, and the place where they are carried out. That is, they consider *what* problems are dealt with, *how* they are most appropriately handled, and *where*. Rivo and colleagues (1994) used the findings of a national survey of practices in the United States to identify the frequency of problems encountered in primary care practices and compiled a list of competencies associated with them.

Table 10.3 lists a subset of types of problems that are appropriately considered primary care problems. (Problems that are unarguably in the purview of primary care because of their very high frequency, e.g., the common cold, are not included in this list.)

Table 10.4 lists the tasks and skills that are associated with recognition and management of problems encountered in primary care.

Primary care practitioners also have to be familiar with, and use, other ambulatory care services, hospital-based services, home care, and nursing homes and hospices when appropriate.

Rivo et al. (1994) used this list to establish the comprehensiveness of training programs for different specialties commonly thought to be providing primary care. Counts of the number of competencies addressed in the different programs clearly indicated the greater range of services provided in family practice, pediatric, and internal medicine compared with emergency medicine and obstetrics/gynecology.

Comparisons between various systems of care might provide information to establish relative (rather than absolute) adequacy of comprehensiveness of the services available. For example, a population-based approach to assessing "range of services" might entail comparing programs between countries to determine the extent to which various types of primary care services are included in primary care (e.g., mental health services, preventive health services and screening, or dental health services). Few studies of this type exist: A notable one is the International Collaboration Study of Medical Care Utilization (Kohn and White, 1976). One part of this study described selected aspects of health care provisions in the late 1960s in seven study countries: Canada, the United States, Argentina, the United Kingdom, Finland, Poland, and Yugoslavia (Kohn and White, 1976, pp. 420–37).

Table 10.3. Problem Types and Examples of Problems in the Purview of Primary Care

---

Musculoskeletal: Fibromyalgia, tendinitis, rheumatoid arthritis, osteoarthritis
Gynecologic: Vaginitis
Urologic: Urinary tract infection, urinary incontinence
Ear, nose, and throat: Otitis media, sinusitis
Ophthalmologic: Corneal abrasion, conjunctivitis
Dermatologic: Acne, scabies, pediculosis
Infectious: Cellulitis, pneumonia
Cardiovascular: Angina, hypertension, stroke
Endocrine: Diabetes, thyroid disease
Pulmonary: Asthma, bronchitis, emphysema
Gastrointestinal: Ulcer, irritable bowel
Psychosocial: Depression, anxiety disorders, stress and grief reactions, substance abuse

---

Adapted from Rivo et al. (1994).

Table 10.4. Tasks and Skills Needed in Primary Care

Prevention (including immunizations) and health promotion/counseling (including injury prevention)
Prenatal care
Infant, child, adolescent, and adult preventive and health promotion; principles of development
Nutrition counseling
Family planning
Genetic counseling
Screening procedures: Pap tests, skin cancer screening
Death and dying counseling
Knowledge of community and public health principles
Knowledge of community resources
Continuity of care
Coordination of care
Comprehensiveness of assessments
Patient education skills
Knowledge of management of undifferentiated problems
Knowledge of occupational/school-related problems
Knowledge of the benefits of teamwork
Knowledge of the principles of cost-effective care
Knowledge of the basics of medical ethics
Competence in use and management of computerized information
Critical appraisal of literature skills
Practice management skills
Risk management skills

Adapted from Rivo et al (1994).

A *facilities-based* approach to assessing range of services compares the services available in various types of health plans or health care organizations and the office equipment available to handle the range of services. In addition, assessment should consider the competence of the staff to deal with a broad range of problems or the existence of a systematic approach to obtaining the services elsewhere if they are not provided in the facility.

The crux of the evaluation of comprehensiveness requires determining the frequency of health needs in the population to be served, setting the range of services to meet those needs that occur frequently enough for primary care physicians to maintain competence in dealing with them, and then providing those services when the needs occur. As will be noted below in the section on attainment of comprehensiveness, there is little evidence in the literature that bears on these issues.

Measurement of the recognition of needs

At the *population level*, the attainment of comprehensiveness is reflected by the extent to which the health services address evident needs of the population. Failure to recognize these needs is manifested by a systematic underdiagnosis of problems that are common in the population or by evidence of lack of receipt or provision of indicated services in the population of patients seen in primary care settings.

One approach suited to the assessment of comprehensiveness of care at the population level was developed by investigators at the Indian Health Services program in Arizona (Schorr and Nutting, 1977). The approach was concerned with the extent to which the health system adequately addressed certain recognized needs of the population and traced the care for the problems through its successive stages. The investigators identified seven health problems (hypertension, adult-onset diabetes, tuberculosis, urinary tract infection, head lacerations, infant gastroenteritis, and acute otitis media) and determined the extent to which there was adequate case finding (problem recognition) for the conditions, along with adequate diagnostic procedures, therapy, and follow up.

This type of approach to assessing comprehensiveness is particularly well suited to situations in which the needs of the community are known from prior studies of mortality and morbidity.

An alternative approach to judging the adequacy of the range of needed services in a community assumes that different communities should have approximately equivalent health, particularly for conditions that are responsive to medical care. If services are adequately comprehensive, there should be parity across communities in the frequency and severity of those illnesses where medical care is effective in prevention or treatment of illnesses.

The potential of this method in identifying areas where improvement in comprehensiveness was needed is demonstrated by two studies, one in the United States and one in Canada.

In a study in the United States, Woolhandler and colleagues (1985) compared death rates at different ages among whites and blacks for conditions in which death can be prevented by medical care to rates for all causes of death. At all ages below 60 years, the ratio of black to white preventable death rates was greater than the ratio of black to white deaths from all causes, indicating that at least some of the excess deaths were due to a failure of the health system to prevent deaths from these conditions. The disparity in death rates associated with preventable causes was particularly striking for youths and young adults. If the problem were simply greater susceptibility to life-threatening illness among blacks, the ratio for preventable conditions would be equal to the ratio for all causes. Unequal ratios suggest a problem with adequacy of health services that might be disparities in access to health services or in the breadth of services available to the two types of populations.

In Canada, Wilkins and Adams (1983) used data from vital statistics and health surveys in five regions differing in both population size and income levels to calculate life expectancy and quality-adjusted life expectancy of males versus females. There were systematic differences in both measures of health status in areas differing in family income. Because the Canadian health system is designed to reduce financial barriers to access to services, the differences are not likely to be due to differences in access to services; rather, they are likely to be due at least in part to the services being insufficiently broad to meet the health needs of the less affluent population.

At the *facilities level* one empirical approach to measurement depends on the availability of information on the types of problems and diagnoses that are seen and managed in different facilities and by different providers. In the absence of differences in population needs, there should be general parity in the frequency of conditions seen by different practitioners or seen by different groups of practitioners who purport to provide comprehensive care. For example, facilities that differ in their rates of diagnosis of adult depression or childhood behavior problems are likely to differ in their comprehensiveness of care unless it can be shown that their populations differ in the actual frequencies of these conditions.

Data from the National Ambulatory Medical Care Survey (see Chapter 4) provide information on problems and diagnoses in a representative sample of office-based practices of different specialists (and, more recently, in hospital outpatient facilities as well) in the United States. The data can be used to compare the distribution of problems and/or diagnoses in the practice of various primary care specialties to determine if they differ in their comprehensiveness. If data are obtained from all types of facilities in a community or country, the results are tantamount to a population-based method for comparing comprehensiveness across types of physicians.

In a normative approach to assessing comprehensiveness, a standard is set and facilities are measured according to their attainment of the standard. The Institute of Medicine (1978) checklist for primary care includes seven questions in its section on comprehensiveness. Four of the seven addressed the availability of a range of services, but they can be reframed to capture the actual provision of services by determining if the facilities accomplish the activity:

Is the practice unit willing to handle, without referral, the great majority (over 90%) of the problems arising in the population served (e.g., general complaints such as fever or fatigue, minor trauma, sore throat, cough, and chest pain)?
Are the practitioners in the unit willing, when appropriate, to admit and care for patients in hospitals?
Are the practitioners in the unit willing to admit and care for patients in nursing homes or convalescent homes?
Are the practitioners in the unit willing, when appropriate, to visit the patient at home?

Following are the three questions that directly address the process aspect of comprehensiveness:

Are appropriate primary and secondary preventive measures used for those people at risk, such as immunization for tetanus or polio, early detection of hypertension, and control of risk factors for coronary disease?
Are patients encouraged and assisted in providing for their own care and in participating in their own health care plan such as instruction in nutrition, diet, exercise, accident prevention, family planning, and adolescent problems?
Do the practitioners in the unit provide support to those agencies promoting community health such as health education programs for the public, disease detection programs, school health and sports medicine programs, and emergency care training?

Although this approach was designed for use at the facilities level, it can also be adapted to services organized at the population level. For example, do all practices in an area handle the great majority of problems in the population? Are appropriate primary and secondary preventive services used for people at risk?·

A third approach to measuring comprehensiveness is based on the extent of recognition of the needs of patients. Repeated studies have shown that practitioners often fail to recognize problems that patients express when they seek care. The deficiencies are particularly pronounced when the problems are of a psychological or psychosocial nature. To assess the extent of recognition of patients' needs, there has to be a mechanism to independently ascertain the nature of problems presented by patients. One technique is to have patients write their complaints and concerns while waiting to see the practitioner or to have the receptionist or equivalent person question the patient upon appearance at the facility. These complaints are then compared with those identified by the practitioners on a special data collection form or written in the medical record.

A fourth approach, which can be used either at the population level or the facilities level, assesses the proportion of individuals in the population or practice population who are seen in one year by specialists. If there is no reason to believe that one population has greater need for specialist services than a reference population, a higher proportion of patients who are seen by specialists indicates that the primary care practice is insufficiently comprehensiveness in its coverage of problems. Although norms for this proportion should be easily obtainable from a variety of health plans and health centers, few reference data exist. Synthetic estimates suggest that no more than one-fourth of individuals in a population should require clinical services other than those provided in primary care in a year. These estimates are based on guesses as to the proportion of patients (or people in the population) who have uncommon disorders or uncommon complications of disorders (and who therefore would be expected to need the care of specialists) and the proportion of patients who require short-term referral for the purpose of providing advice to primary care physicians or short-term interventions requiring specialist skills (such as major surgery or complex laboratory investigations and procedures). Countries, geographic areas within countries, or populations in different health facilities or centers that vary widely in the proportion of individuals seen by specialists should prompt investigation into determining whether this is a result of greater health needs or inadequacy of comprehensiveness of primary care. Reasons for this inadequacy may lie in insufficient training of practitioners, excessive patient loads leading to inadequate time to deal with certain types of problems, inadequate resources to deal with them, or perverse incentives to refer individually or in combination.

Other methods for assessing the comprehensiveness of services provided are presented in Chapter 13 in the context of assessments of primary care in general.

What Is Known About the Attainment of Comprehensiveness

A neurologist I know is frequently asked by patients whether he will make sure their heart exam is alright, "while he's at it." He replies, "Certainly, if you remind me where your heart is."   Dr. K., a pediatric resident

Comprehensiveness has been assessed in two ways. In some studies, the availability of a *range* of services was ascertained while in others the *extent* to which needed services were provided was determined.

There is little information that provides a basis for deciding what can be appropriately diagnosed and managed by the primary care physician and what requires referrals to other levels of care. Some types of referral are short term and largely for the purpose of obtaining advice, guidance, or a second opinion. Lawrence and Dorsey (1976) categorized such reasons for referral as follows:

1. A need for a specialized diagnostic or treatment procedure that the primary care physician does not provide. These types of referral are characterized by a relatively clear perception by the patient, the primary care physician, and the specialty physician as to what is to be done; the duration of the referral is brief, and the patient never leaves the area of the primary care physician.
2. Reassurance to the patient or physician regarding a second opinion in cases where the patient or a third party payer has some doubt about a suggested course of action, where there is reason to suspect that criteria other than medical justifiability might be operating such as financial incentives or threats of malpractice, or where there is legitimate uncertainty about a proposed course of action for a medical problem.
3. For more extensive or more general evaluation, as in situations where the patient's problem is complex and unclear. In these situations, the consultant is more likely to take greater initiative, and the period of consultation may be somewhat longer than for the two previously mentioned types of reasons for referral.

In each of these situations the referral is for purposes of consultation, the period of referral is relatively brief, and there is a clear expectation that the patient will return to the primary physician within a period of time that can generally be prespecified.

In contrast, some types of referrals are relatively long term and may involve significant disruption or even abandonment of their roles by primary care physicians. The reasons for this type of referral are of two types:

• For unusual or serious chronic conditions where management requires technical knowledge present only in major medical centers, where involvement in research provides the most current information about new therapies and interventions.
• For logistic reasons, convenience, or feasibility, such as the availability of financial resources that pay for services only if provided in particular types of facilities. This category of referrals should be minimized if relative predictability is desirable in a system.

As noted in the next chapter, there is an increasing trend for many referrals to retain a role for the primary care practitioner, even for the management of problems engendering the referral. Thus there are four types of referrals:

1. Consultative: short term shared care
2. Joint management: long term shared care

3. Temporary transfer: short term management
4. Extended transfer: long term transfer for management.

The indications for referral for individual conditions are part of the basic structure of chapters in only a few textbooks (e.g., Dershewitz, 1988; Stein, 1998). In these textbooks, the indications specified are almost all related to the presence of certain symptoms or signs rather than to the presence of diagnoses, suggesting that more referrals are for diagnostic or therapeutic advice than for ongoing care. Several other types of indications also suggest a need for short-term consultation rather than for long-term referral. These include confirmation or diagnosis; elucidation of etiology; routine assessment requiring specialized skills such as monitoring, social services, or supportive therapy; and advice on medication dosages. Another type of indication, refractory or recurrent problems, might require either long-term referral or short-term consultation, depending on the problem and the management strategy.

Very little is known about the relative frequencies of referrals for the different types of reasons. One study of 1,014 encounters reported by 40 family physicians provided some information on the issue; 90% of encounters were managed in the primary care setting, 7% were categorized as "shared" care in which a consultation only was requested, and 3% were referrals for "supportive" (referral) care (Taylor, 1981). But this was a relatively small study of an unrepresentative group of primary care physicians. Several large national studies in the United States underway at the time of this writing should shed additional light on this important aspects of primary care.

Some examples of the assessment of comprehensiveness are listed below. Some use the availability of range of services, while the others use the extent to which services are provided. All studies use the empirical approach rather than the normative approach.

1. In a facilities-based study of a representative sample of practitioners in a large U.S. city, the proportion of practices that were able to provide a breadth of services to their regular patients was determined. The services were sigmoidoscopy, electrocardiogram, audiometry, pelvic examination, superficial biopsy, minor suturing, tonometry, pulmonary function tests, blood hematocrit/hemoglobin determinations, counseling of more than 45 minutes, immunizations, and complete physical examination. A comprehensiveness index was created from six of the above measures. Internists, pediatricians, and family practitioners ranked highest, or most comprehensive, on the index; psychiatrists and surgical subspecialists ranked lowest; and other types of specialists were intermediate. The relatively high variability for medical subspecialists indicated the great variability in achievement of comprehensiveness by these types of physicians (Weiner, 1981; Weiner and Starfield, 1983).

2. National data derived from logs kept by physicians (such as in the National Ambulatory Medical Care Survey) have been used to assess the range of services provided by various types of physicians. One such study (Starfield et al., 1984)

ascertained the distribution of all visits made by children, including teenagers, according to the type of physician. It revealed the following:
- While about one-third of all outpatient visits made by children were to pediatricians, only about one in eight visits for minor surgery were made to them.
- Family physicians and general practitioners, on the other hand, saw approximately the same proportion of child visits for minor surgery as the proportion of children they saw overall, suggesting that they are more comprehensive in their care, at least with regard to the performance of minor surgery.
- Pediatricians also were under-represented in the extent to which they dealt with psychosocial problems; they provided less than one-fifth of the care for such problems, although they were the regular source of care for over one-third of children.
- Family physicians and generalists, on the other hand, provided approximately the same proportion of care for child psychological problems as for the proportion for whom they were the regular source.

These findings suggest that generalists may provide greater comprehensiveness of care directly to children than do pediatricians, who focus relatively heavily on preventive care and on care for medical illnesses. Additional confirmation of the belief that there is greater comprehensiveness in family practice derives from the finding that both family physicians and general practitioners saw relatively more young people for obstetric problems, as well as for environmental or economic problems.

A more recent study using data from the National Ambulatory Medical Care Survey from 1985 through 1992 examined the correlates of referrals made to internists, family physicians, and general practitioners during visits by adults. Regression analyses revealed that being a male patient (except in HMO practices); having fewer medications prescribed, a new problem (never having been seen before for the problem), longer visits, or less physician concentration in specific types of diagnoses; and being a female physician *all* independently increased the likelihood of referral. Moreover, practices with a larger proportion of HMO patients had higher referral rates, even when the HMO patients were removed from the analysis. Thus, even patients who are able to refer themselves because they have no "gatekeeper" requirements were more likely to be referred if they were in practices with a high proportion of HMO patients. However, it should be noted that HMOs during the time of the study were different from the managed care organizations more common during the ensuing decade, which undoubtedly imposed more disincentives and barriers to referral than was the case in the earlier time period (Franks and Clancy, 1997).

3. A facilities-based study of a national sample of recent graduates of residencies in internal medicine and family practice now in office-based practice used questionnaires and logs of all their encounters with patients for 3 days. Family physicians had relatively more patients with sprains and strains and relatively more patients with psychosocial problems. They saw more than three times as many adult patients with trauma and many more patients for prenatal and postnatal visits than did internists. The latter saw more patients for chronic illnesses, especially for young and middle-aged patients (Cherkin et al., 1986). These

findings suggest that family physicians provide a greater variety of types of care than do general internists, whose focus is relatively greater on the management of chronic medical illness.

4. A facilities-based study conducted in five types of facilities in different geographic areas found widely discrepant rates of diagnosis of certain types of problems among children (Starfield et al., 1980). Rates of diagnosis of psychosocial problems varied from 5% to 15% with no consistency by type of practice. The variability between the two multispecialty group practices was as great as that between multispecialty groups and the pediatric group and the family practice group. However, the rates of diagnosis of psychosomatic conditions, all of which had a somatic manifestation, was highly consistent (at about 9%). These findings suggested that comprehensiveness, at least as manifested by the extent to which facilities dealt with psychosocial problems in children, varied across facilities, probably as a result of factors other than the type of organization or primary care specialty.

   A study of adults in several types of health care facilities in three U.S. cities reached similar conclusions. A standard diagnostic test for depressive disorder was given to patients, and the results were compared with visit-report forms completed by the clinicians who saw the patients for the problem under care. Only about one-half of all depressed patients seen by their internist had their depression diagnosed; the proportion varied from 46% to 51% depending on the type of facility (Wells et al., 1989).

5. In a study comparing prepaid group practice with fee-for-service practice, 1,580 adult and children were randomly assigned to receive care free of charge from either a fee-for-service physician of their choice or a prepaid group practice. Patients receiving their care from the prepaid group practice had higher rates of preventive care than patients receiving care from fee-for-service physicians. This study indicated that comprehensiveness, at least as reflected in preventive care, can differ according to the type of organization in which care is received (Manning et al., 1984).

6. A facilities-based study of the extent to which professional guidelines for preventive procedures were met found that there was no consistent difference between generalists (family physicians and general internists) and subspecialty internists. However, patients who had a complete physical examination were more likely to have the indicated procedures. The most salient determinant was the extent to which the physician believed the procedure to be important. Patients whose physicians believed the procedure to be important were more likely to have them performed. This study indicates the importance of individual professional practice patterns in the achievement of comprehensiveness of care in situations where there are no particular mechanisms within the facility to ensure the performance of indicated procedures (Dietrich and Goldberg, 1984).

Both adults and children who make more visits are more likely to receive indicated preventive procedures (Benson et al., 1984; Fontana et al., 1997). However, those with a symptomatic common chronic illness, especially those who report poor health status, are less likely than comparable individuals to receive a wide variety of indicated preventive procedures, at least according to one study of over 4,000 adults of aged 52–64 years cared for by 42 primary care group practices (Fontana et al., 1997). That is, comprehensiveness appears to suffer when a primary care practitioner focuses on management of a disease rather than on total patient needs.

Adherence to guidelines for comprehensiveness cannot be assumed. For this reason some medical facilities have adopted computerized systems to remind physicians that certain procedures are indicated for individual patients. To further improve the performance of these procedures, stamped postcards addressed to the patients may be given to the physicians with the reminders. Better adherence to the guidelines results when these mechanisms are put in place (Schoenbaum, 1990).

A study of care provided to 10,608 adults from panels of 60 family physicians, 245 general internists, and 55 subspecialty internists indicated that there were very small but statistically significant differences in comprehensiveness as measured by receipt of preventive or health-promoting services, with general internists doing slightly better. The scores for the former were 84.1 and 86.6, respectively, and for the latter 47.1 and 49.0 (on a 0–100 scale) (Grumbach et al., 1998).

A study of all pediatricians in the state of Texas (Feigin et al., 1996) ascertained the frequency with which selected procedures were performed in a year. Table 10.5 lists these procedures according to whether they were common in the practices of

Table 10.5. Common and Uncommon Procedures in Pediatric Practice

Common procedures with significantly greater likelihood of performance in rural areas
    Bladder catheterization
    Debridement of second-degree burns
    Endotracheal intubation
Uncommon procedures with significantly greater likelihood of performance in rural areas
    a. More than 75% of pediatricians perform the procedure
        Blood culture
        Debridement/treatment of third-degree burns
        Drawing arterial blood gases
        Treatment of clavicular fractures
    b. Fewer than 75% of pediatricians perform the procedure
        Bone marrow aspiration
        Chest tube insertion
        Treat digital fractures
        Thoracentesis
Uncommon procedures with equal likelihood of performance in rural and urban areas
    Arthrocentesis (few pediatricians perform it)
    Drain subungual hematoma (few pediatricians perform it)
    Would debridement (most pediatricians perform it)
Common procedures with equal likelihood of performance in rural and urban areas
    Lumbar puncture
Common procedures with higher likelihood of performance in rural areas
    Umbilical artery catheterization
    Umbilical venous catheterization
    Venous cutdown

Source: Feigin et al. (1996).

the pediatrician (set at twice per month on the arbitrary assumption that this frequency would be required to maintain reasonable competence) and whether there were significant differences in rates of performance in rural areas (where the availability of specialists to perform needed services might be limited) versus urban areas.

The findings made it apparent that the availability of other specialists determines the comprehensiveness of primary care practices. In no case were pediatricians more likely to perform a procedure in an urban area. The findings also raise the issue of whether some pediatricians (particularly those in rural areas) should be performing procedures that they are now performing, considering the low frequency with which they are required. That is, it may be that the maldistribution of specialists is not only compromising comprehensiveness of primary care but also resulting in potential for poor quality of care in some primary care practices.

A study of 161 general practices selected randomly from the 5,825 practices in the Netherlands examined referral rates for 27 different types of procedures. Referral rates were well under 50% for 18 of the 27 procedures and over 80% only for 9. These primary care practitioners themselves took care of over 75% of stitching open wounds, dealing with ingrown toenails, shoulder and elbow injections, bandaging sprained elbows, inserting or adjusting intrauterine devices, adjusting pessaries, examining vaginal discharges, carrying out diagnostic testing for fungal skin infections, and treating varicose and pressure ulcers. They did between one-half and three-fourths of sebaceous cyst excisions, excisions of skin nevi and lipomas, incisions of abscesses, drainage of knee and elbow bursae, treatment of corneal injuries, audiometry testing, removing foreign bodies from ear, nose, or throat, and biopsies of skin. Those procedure performed less than half the time included hydrocoele punctures (6%), conservative treatment of fractures (26%), conservative treatment of dislocated toes, elbows, and shoulders (39%), mammary cyst drainage (2%), proctoscopy (9%), tonometry and fundoscopy (17%), paracentesis (1%), testing for infertility (6%), and allergy testing (4%) (Delnoij, 1994).

There is at least some evidence that encouraging primary care physicians to expand the range of services that they offer can have the effect of encouraging patients to come forward for intervention when they otherwise would not have done so and when it is not necessarily desirable that they do so. Increased availability of equipment for diagnostic testing and therapeutic interventions is known to increase the rate of performance of many procedures above and beyond what would be deemed necessary (Coulter, 1995; Rink et al., 1993).

Thus, comprehensiveness requires knowledge of the frequencies of problems and needs in the specific area in which practices are located (see Chapter 14). Because medical education does not necessarily train practitioners to practice in specific areas, continuing education must bear the burden of ensuring that competence is maintained for services that should be provided in primary care.

An international comparison of referral rates conducted in primary care practices (general practice) in 15 countries provides indirect evidence of differences in comprehensiveness in the different countries. Figure 10.3 indicates the extent of differences in percentages of visits resulting in a referral to a non-primary care specialist. Overall, the percentages range from 1.5 in Portugal to 45.7 in Belgium, with the preponderance of percentages between 5 and 20. In general, higher per-

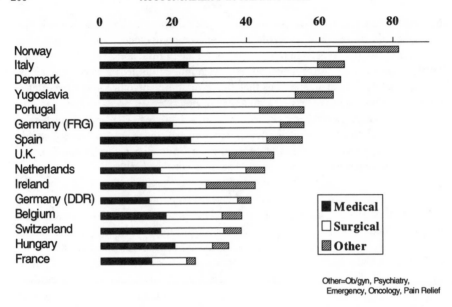

Figure 10.3. Referrals Per 1000 Consultations. Source: Fleming (1991).

centages reflect higher percentages to medical, surgical, and other types of specialists, but there are notable exceptions: Portugal's low referral percentage is due to low referrals to medical specialists only; in the United Kingdom, referrals to other types of specialists are relatively high; in Germany, referrals to surgeons are especially high. In this study, countries with high visit rates to general practitioners were also countries with higher percentages of consultations resulting in a referral, but this relationship did not hold for individual doctors within countries (Fleming, 1991). A limitation on the interpretation of the data, however, is the calculation of percentages on the basis of visits rather than on people seen. Countries with high referral rates might be those countries in which individuals make fewer visits to primary care, whereas countries with low percentages of visits resulting in a referral may also have high visit rates by individual patients. If either or both of these are the case, rates of referral for individual patients will be less variable than they appear in this comparison.

In northern Norway, one-third of people see at least one specialist in the period of a year, in a health care system that requires referral from a generalist to visit a non-primary care specialist and has no financial barrier to such visits. Areas with higher general practitioner/population ratios and those with a hospital had higher proportions of people who saw a non-primary care specialist; educational level and poorer health status each independently was associated with higher referral rates (Fylkesnes, 1993). In comparison, a study in 183 practices in Nottinghamshire, England, found that 22% of individuals were referred in a year: 14% for medical reasons and 8% for surgical needs (standardized for proportions of elderly vs. nonelderly people in the practice). Rates of referral were higher among solo practices and in low-income areas (Hippisley-Cox et al., 1997), demonstrating the imperative to consider the extent of health needs and related sociodemographic characteristics when interpreting differences in referral rates.

In the Netherlands, referral rates were calculated on the basis of proportion of episodes of care that resulted in a referral to a non-primary care specialist. Rates of referral declined from 16% in 1971 to 11% (standardized for changes in age and gender) in 1994, despite an increase in the number of non-primary care specialists; the decline was most notable from 1980 to 1985, especially in the case of referrals to surgical specialists, which in 1994 comprised about half of all referrals. These findings suggest that primary care may have become more comprehensive in this 20-year period in that country (Van de Lisdonk and Van Weel, 1996).

A study of referral rates among 121,958 visits to 242 general practitioners in Spain revealed wide variability that was associated with several patient, physician, and practice characteristics. Higher rates of referral were found for male patients, physicians over age 65 years, female physicians, large list size, smaller number of consultations per week, urban area of practice, perceived pressure from patients, and *not* working in a primary care team. The statistical significance of the regression model in predicting the referral rate in the practices was very high (García Olmos et al., 1995).

Summary

Table 10.6 summarizes the nature of comprehensiveness. Comprehensiveness of services requires that the scope of services be explicit and that there be recognition of situations where their application is appropriate. Thus, it should be assessed by examining the range of services available (a structure feature) and recognition of needs (a process feature). The range of services that are available should consist of a core that would apply to every population and additional services that should be available to meet special needs that are common in the population served. Fail-

Table 10.6. Summary of Comprehensiveness

	Capacity	*Performance*
Description: Availability and provision of services to meet all but uncommon population needs		
Involves	Specification of range of services available	Range of services provided considering population needs
Problem-related	Yes, based on frequency and distribution of needs	Yes, based on recognition of frequency and distribution of needs
Personal relationship required	No, but personal relationship probably facilitates recognition of needs	
Time dependent	Yes, recognition of needs should be timely, given current standards of care	
Specific measures	Benefit package specification	Population/patient survey
	Breadth of coverage of practice	Range of diagnoses made*
		Range of services covered*
		Percent of patients referred*

*Considering population needs.

ure to recognize needs and problems is manifested by a systematic underdiagnosis of problems known to be common in the population of patients or by evidence of lack of receipt of indicated services in that population.

Deciding on the appropriate locus of services is not straightforward. For preventive services, consideration of likelihood of risk as well as the nature of organizational features of clinical services influences decisions as to the relative advantages of public health versus clinical medicine approaches.

Practice or facilities-based studies can provide information concerning the extent to which a full range of services is available and even provided to patients who receive care within it but cannot provide the information necessary to determine whether the facility meets the needs of the population for which it assumes responsibility.

Assessment of the adequacy of comprehensiveness is compromised in the absence of an accepted terminology for specifying needs. When there are no well-validated standards for specifying the range of services, population differences in the frequency of conditions amenable to medical care serve to identify inadequate comprehensiveness.

Although primary care physicians generally provide more comprehensive care than other specialists, there are persistent disparities in comprehensiveness among the primary care specialties, and even within them.

Referral rates vary widely, both across countries and within them. This suggests either differences in population needs or differences in the comprehensiveness of primary care services.

The policy imperative related to comprehensiveness concerns the differences in the extent of the "benefit package" provided by various insurers, governments, and health services organizations. At present, these benefits vary widely. In the future, approaches employing considerations of population needs, the frequency of these needs in the population, effectiveness of various types of interventions on health status and health outcomes, and costs of the interventions will provide a more consistent and rational approach to the definition of the range of services to be made available.

References

Alpha Center. Program Update No. 10. Washington, DC: Alpha Center, June 1990, p 9.

American Academy of Pediatrics. Guidelines for Your Family's Health Insurance. Elk Grove Village, IL: American Academy of Pediatrics, 1989.

Battista R, Banta HD, Johnson E, Hodge M, Gelband H. Lessons from the eight countries. Health Policy 1994; 30: 397–421.

Benson P, Gabriel A, Katz H, Steinwachs D, Hankin J, Starfield B. Preventive care and overall use of services: Are they related? Am J Dis Child 1984; 134:74–8.

Bodenheimer T. The Oregon health plan—Lessons for the nation (first of two parts). N Engl J Med 1997; 337:651–5.

Cherkin D, Rosenblatt R, Hart L, Schleiter M. A comparison of the patients and practices of recent graduates of family practice and general internal medicine residency programs. Med Care 1986; 24:1136–50.

Coulter A. Shifting the balance from secondary to primary care: Needs investment and cultural change. BMJ 1995; 311:1447–8.

Crabtree BF. Individual attitudes are no match for complex systems. J Fam Pract 1997; 44(5):447–8.

Delnoij D. Physician Payment and Cost Control. Utrecht: NIVEL, 1994.

Dershewitz R (ed). Ambulatory Pediatric Care. 3rd Edition. Philadelphia: Lippencott-Raven, 1988.

Dietrich A, Goldberg H. Preventive content of adult primary care: Do generalists and subspecialists differ? Am J Public Health, 1984; 74:223–7.

Eddy DM. Benefit language. Criteria that will improve quality while reducing costs. JAMA 1996; 275:650–7.

Feigin R, Drutz J, Smith E, Collins C. Practice variations by population: Training significance. Pediatrics 1996; 98:186–90.

Fleming D. The European Study of Referrals From Primary to Secondary Care. Report of Project. Birmingham, England: The Concerted Action Committee of the Committee of Health Services Research for the EEC, 1991.

Fletcher R, O'Malley M, Earp J, Littleton T, Fietcher S, Greganti A, Davidson R, Taylor J. Patients' priorities for medical care. Med Care 1983; 21:234–41.

Fontana S, Baumann L, Helberg C, Love R. The delivery of preventive services in primary care practices according to chronic disease status. Am J Public Health 1997; 87:1190–6.

Forrest CB, et al., in preparation.

Franks P, Clancy C. Referrals of adult patients from primary care: Demographic disparities and their relationship to HMO insurance. J Fam Pract 1997; 45:47–53.

Fylkesnes K. Determinants of health care utilization—Visits and referrals. Scand J Soc Med 1993; 21(1):40–50.

García Olmos L, Gervas J, Otero A, Perez-Fern ndez M. Variability in GP's referral rates in Spain. Fam Pract 1995; 12:159–62.

General Medical Services Committee. Defining core services in general practice—Reclaiming professional control [a discussion paper]. BMJ 1996.

Grogan CM. Deciding on access and levels of care: A comparison of Canada, Britain, Germany, and the United States. J Health Polit Policy Law 1992; 17(2): 213–32.

Grumbach K, Selby J, Schmittdiel J, Quesenberry C. Quality of primary care practice in a large HMO according to physician specialty. unpublished manuscript, 1998.

Hickson G, Stewart D, Altemeier W, Perrin J. First steps in obtaining child health care: Selecting a physician. Pediatrics 1988; 81:333–8.

Hippisley-Cox J, Hardy C, Pringle M, Fielding K, Carlisle R, Chilvers C. The effect of deprivation on variations in general practitioners' referral rates: A cross sectional study of computerized data on new medical and surgical outpatient referrals in Nottinghamshire. BMJ 1997; 314:1458–61, 315:884.

Institute of Medicine. A Manpower Policy for Primary Health Care: A Report of a Study. IOM Pub. No. 78–02. Washington, DC: National Academy of Sciences, 1978.

Kohn R, White KL. Health Care: An International Study. London: Oxford University Press, 1976.

Lawrence R, Dorsey J. The generalist–specialist relationship and the art of consultation. In Noble J (ed): Primary Care and the Practice of Medicine. Boston: Little, Brown & Company, 1976. pp 229–45.

Manning W, Leibowitz A, Goldberg G, Rogers W, Newhouse J. A controlled trial of the prepaid group practice on use of services. N Engl J Med 1984; 310:1505–10.

Pierzchajlo RPJ, Ackermann RJ, Vogel RL. Colonoscopy performed by a family physician. A case series of 751 procedures. J Fam Pract 1997; 44:473–80.

Rifkin S, Walt G. Why health improves: Defining the issues concerning "comprehensive primary health care" and "selective primary health care." Soc Sci Med 1986; 23:559–66.

Rink E, Hilton S, Szczepura A, Fletcher J, Sibbald B, Davies C, Freeling P, Stilwell J. Impact of introducing near patient testing for standard investigations in general practice. BMJ 1993; 307(6907):775–8.

Rivo ML, Saultz JW, Wartman SA, DeWitt TG. Defining the generalists physician's training. JAMA 1994; 271:1499–504.

Rodewald LE, Szilagyi PG, Holl J, Shone LR, Zwanziger J, Raubertas RF. Health insurance for low-income working families: Effect on the provision of immunizations to preschool-age children. Arch Pediatr Adolesc Med 1997;151:798–803.

Rose G. The Strategy of Preventive Medicine. Oxford: Oxford University Press, 1992.

Russell L. Is Prevention Better Than Cure? Washington, DC: The Brookings Institution, 1986.

Schoenbaum S. Implementation of preventive services in an HMO practice. J Gen Intern Med 1990; 5(suppl) S123–7.

Schorr G, Nutting P. A population-based assessment of the continuity of ambulatory care. Med Care 1977; 15:455–64.

Sickle Cell Disease Guideline Panel. Sickle Cell Disease: Screening, Diagnosis, Management, and Counseling in Newborns and Infants. Clinical Practice Guidelines No. 6. AHCPR Pub. No. 93-0562. Rockville, MD: Agency for Health Care Policy and Research, Public Health Service, U.S. Department of Health and Human Services, April 1993.

Silver G. Child Health: America's Future. Germantown, MD: Aspen Systems Corp., 1978.

Simpson L, Korenbrot C, Greene J. Outcomes of enhanced prenatal services for Medicaid-eligible women in public and private settings. Public Health Rep 1997; 112(2):122–32.

Starfield B, Gross E, Wood M, Pantel R, Allen C, Gordon B, Moffatt P, Drachman R, Katz H. Psychosocial and psychosomatic diagnosis in primary care of children. Pediatrics 1980; 66:159–67.

Starfield B, Hoekelman R, McCormick M, Benson P, Mendenhall R. Moynihan C, Radecki S. Who provides health care to children in the United States? Pediatrics 1984; 74:991–7.

Starfield B, Vivier P. Population and selective (high risk) approaches to prevention in well child care. In Solloway MR, Budetti PP (eds): Child Health Supervision: Analytical Studies in the Financing, Delivery, and Cost-Effectiveness of Preventive and Health Promotion Services for Infants, Children, and Adolescents. Arlington, VA: National Center for Education in Maternal and Child Health, 1995, pp. 274–306.

Stein J. (ed). International Medicine. 5th Edition. St. Louis: Mosby, 1998.

Tallon JR, Jr. A health policy agenda including the poor. JAMA 1989; 261:1044.

Taylor RB. Categories of care in family medicine. Fam Med 1981; 13:7–9.

U.S. Preventive Services Task Force. Guide to Clinical Preventive Services: Report of the U.S. Preventive Services Task Force. 2nd Ed. Baltimore, MD: Williams & Wilkins Co., 1996.

Van de Lisdonk EH, Van Weel C. New referrals, a decreasing phenomenon in 1971–94: Analysis of registry data in the Netherlands. BMJ 1996; 313:602.

Walsh J, Warren K. Selective primary health care: An interim strategy for developing countries. N Engl J Med 1979; 301:967–74.

Weiner J. An Analysis of Office-Based Primary Care in Baltimore City. Dissertation. Baltimore: Johns Hopkins University, 1981.

Weiner J, Starfield B. Measurement of the primary care roles of office-based physicians. Am J Public Health 1983; 73:666–71.

Wells K, Hays R, Burnam A, Rogers W, Greenfield S, Ware J. Detection of depressive disorders for patients receiving prepaid or fee-for-service care: Results from the medical outcomes study. JAMA 1989; 262:3298–302.

Wilkins R, Adams O. Health expectancy in Canada, late 1970s: Demographic, regional, and social dimensions. Am J Public Health 1983; 73:1073–80.

Woolhandler S, Himmelstein D, Silber L, Bader M, Harnly M, Jones A. Medical care and mortality: Racial differences in preventable deaths. Int J Health Serv 1985; 15:1–22.

World Health Organization. Primary Health Care. Geneva: World Health Organization, 1978, p. 25.

— 11 —

Coordination of Care: Putting It All Together

I've been to so many doctors in the last few months, I need a doctor to put it all together.   A patient in an emergency room (early 1990s.)

Coordination, the fourth component of care, is essential for the attainment of each of the other features. Without it, longitudinality would lose much of its potential, comprehensiveness would be made difficult, and the first-contact function would become purely administrative. Descriptions of primary care from the physician's vantage often refer to the primary care professional as the patient's advocate (Robinson, 1977) or in terms of the primary care physician's commitment to people (McWhinney, 1975; Draper and Smits, 1975). To accomplish what these terms imply, the primary practitioner must be aware of all of the patient's problems in whatever context they arise, at least insofar as they relate to health. Enlargement of the scope of practice from individual offices to group sites and as part of integrated health systems provides both new challenges as well as better opportunities for coordinating services.

Coordination is a "state of being harmonized in a common action or effort." This definition expresses, in a formal way, what more down-to-earth descriptions imply. The essence of coordination is the availability of information about prior problems and services and the recognition of that information as it bears on needs for current care.

The term *case management*, which has recently been used to describe efforts at cost containment, may overlap with the idea of coordination of care, but there is little agreement on a standard operational definition of case management. In this book, case management is considered to be a function of care deriving from the presence of a regular source, that is, longitudinality (see Chapter 8).

The following account illustrates the challenges of coordination.

A 41-year-old woman is under care in a "primary care clinic" for mild hypertension. This vignette contains information about her care from one visit in the clinic to her next scheduled follow-up, a period of approximately 3 months. For purposes of assessing coordination, interest is on the extent to which the primary care practitioner recognized information relevant to the woman's care that arose in the interval of time between the initial visit and the follow-up visit.

- At her "index" visit in the primary care clinic, the physician noted that the patient had a "cold" and had signs consistent with this diagnosis. The physician ordered a chest x-ray and symptomatic therapy. At follow-up 3 months later, the practitioner made reference to the respiratory infection in his notes, but made no mention of the results of the x-ray and whether the patient had taken the medication or felt any relief from it.
- Two weeks after the index visit the patient appeared without appointment in the same clinic still complaining of symptoms of the respiratory infection. A prescription for an antibiotic was given but the primary care practitioner made no reference to it in his follow-up note.
- Two weeks later the patient appeared unexpectedly in another clinic in the same facility, with the same type of symptoms; the practitioner noted that she took Valium regularly and smoked. He recommended discontinuing smoking and additional symptomatic therapy.
- At the follow-up visit in the primary care facility, the practitioner made no mention of this visit or the therapy or advice in his notes in the medical record.
- One month later (and 1 month prior to the scheduled primary care follow-up visit), the patient was seen in the emergency room after an apparent suicide attempt. Again, there was no reference to this visit or to the associated problem in the primary care physician's note at follow-up.

Review of the patient's medical record for the period prior to the index visit revealed that she had been suffering from headaches for several years and was being followed in the neurology clinic where no abnormalities were found on repeated tests. At one visit, mild hypertension was noted, and she was referred to the primary care clinic, where she had been seen every 3 months to follow the progress of the mild hypertension. On at least one prior occasion, 1 year earlier, she had attempted suicide through an overdose of her medication. Despite this history, the patient's serious mental health problems were not integrated into her primary care. There was little or no coordination of care for this patient by the primary care physician.

Starfield et al., 1977

Knowledge about the extent of the challenges of coordination and about the relative impacts of different ways of achieving it is extremely sparse. The development of organized systems of health services, with integration of care across different levels of care and loci of services both heightens awareness of the absence of a sound information base as well as the need for more systematic attempts to develop one.

Not all needs can be satisfied within primary care (see Chapter 10). This means that people have to go elsewhere for various aspects of their health needs. Sometimes they do so with the explicit recognition of the primary care clinician through the processes of consultation and referral. At other times or in other circumstances they may seek such services on their own (direct access or "self-referral"). In addition, there is a need, within primary care itself, to integrate or coordinate services provided by different members of the team of practitioners.

In spite of the fact that I warned him, a surgeon gave a 550-pound patient of mine his regular insulin and a 2,500-calorie diet when he was admitted for an elective surgical procedure. The patient became comatose from hypoglycemia. I knew that the patient ate large quantities of food at home (far more than the 2,500 calories) and that the regular amount of insulin could be a problem. His normal breakfast was a liter of coke, 2 pounds of bacon, 2 dozen eggs, and a loaf of bread. I guess that the surgeon had trouble believing me.

Figure 11.1 provides a schematic representation of the challenges of coordination. It depicts primary care in relationship with care provided by non-primary care specialists. Path 1 reflects situations in which patients seek care directly from the other professionals. Other pathways reflect first contact with primary care and subsequent care by other types of professionals. Path 2 indicates referrals made within primary care for administrative reasons, such as requirements for certification; the patient may not even be seen by the primary care practitioner before the referral.

Path 3 shows referrals as a result of the primary care practitioner's uncertainty or inability to resolve a problem to a diagnosis, and the referral is made for the purpose of getting advice, guidance, or confirmation from the another specialist. Path 4 occurs further along in the processes of care, when a diagnosis has been made but advice, guidance, or second opinion is required about appropriate therapy. Path 5 occurs when patients needs ongoing reassessment and management that primary care practitioners are unable to provide either because of lack of resources or lack of knowledge to deal with an unusually complex or rare problem.

Paths 6–9 represent return of patients from other specialists to primary care. Path 6 occurs when specialists are unable to ascertain the nature of the patients's problem and believe that the primary care physician is in a better position to sort

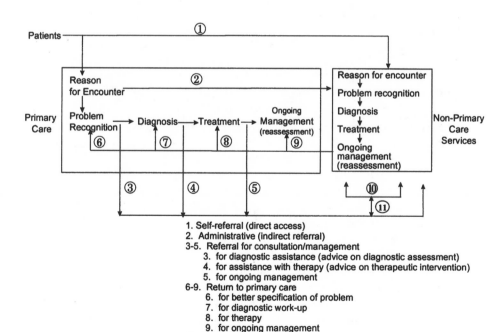

1. Self-referral (direct access)
2. Administrative (indirect referral)
3-5. Referral for consultation/management
    3. for diagnostic assistance (advice on diagnostic assessment)
    4. for assistance with therapy (advice on therapeutic intervention)
    5. for ongoing management
6-9. Return to primary care
    6. for better specification of problem
    7. for diagnostic work-up
    8. for therapy
    9. for ongoing management
10. Cross-referral
11. Primary Care involvement in decisions about cross referral

Figure 11.1. Challenges of coordination.

this out. In paths 7 and 8, patients are returned to primary care with advice about how to make a diagnosis or what treatment to institute, respectively. In path 9, treatment has been instituted and patients are returned to primary care for continuing management. In paths 10 and 11, patients are referred from one specialist to another, either without the knowledge of the primary care physician (path 10) or with it (path 11).

Thus, the challenges of coordination are threefold:

1. Within the primary care setting, when patients are seen by various members of the team and information about patients is generated in different places (including laboratories)
2. With other specialists called on to provide short-term advice or interventions
3. With other specialists who care for a particular patient over a long period of time becasue of the presence of a specific disorder.

> A friend of mine, a 45-year-old woman with a strong family history of breast cancer, was told by her gynecologist that she had a lump in her breast at the site of a previous biopsy and that it should be further evaluated. When the patient went to see the surgeon, whom she visited annually after the original biopsy, he dismissed the new lump as scar tissue from the biopsy. The following year, the gynecologist was dismayed to find out that nothing had been done and insisted to the patient that the scar could be masking some other process going on inside the breast. My friend returned to the surgeon, who then made a diagnosis of cancer. At some point, the surgeon asked her, ''Why didn't you alert me to this lump last year?'' despite the fact that she had.
>
> My friend, the wife of a prominent workmen's compensation lawyer, never wanted to blame the doctors. She developed metastatic disease last year, 5 years after diagnosis, and is now recovering from a stem cell transplant. Her husband views her as having been very unlucky, but not as a victim of medical malpractice. She is so accustomed to going to multiple different specialists for her medical care rather than a good primary care physician that she does not appreciate that the system, with its lack of a mechanism for coordinating care among specialists, failed her.   Dr R., a physician

An excellent case can be made for a "deliberative" model of patient–primary care practitioner relationship that views the physician as analogous to a listening teacher who then advises the patient on health-related matters. This bilateral "model" is extended to a trilateral one when another specialist is involved in the care of the patient. The special role of the primary care practitioner is to temper the tendency toward dominance in patients' decision-making, avoid unnecessary duplication of tests and procedures, and minimize expression to the patient of insignificant differences in judgment with the other practitioner who is involved. The special role of other specialists is to do only what is asked of them and to defer to the primary care physician's ultimate judgment (made in conjunction with the patient) about the need for other interventions. Both professionals keep the patient's confidences from the other physician if the patient wishes it and it does not interfere with the patient's ultimate welfare (Emmanuel, 1994).

> A dermatologist prescribed oral steroids for a patient with a few small (in my perception) sarcoidosis lesions around her eyes, resulting in a loss of control of her

diabetes. She wanted the lesions cured, the dermatologist wanted to cure them, and I wanted her diabetes controlled.

The complexity of the referral process and the multiplicity of reasons for referrals complicate study of the reasons for the great variability in referral rates that has been observed across different populations, different geographic areas, and even different countries, as described in the previous chapter. Salem-Schatz and colleagues (1994) demonstrated that patients' characteristics, including age, gender, and case mix (measured by the Ambulatory Care Group method of characterizing morbidity burdens in patients—see Chapter 3) accounted for fully half of the variability in referral rates in one large health maintenance organization (HMO) with 52 physician practices and almost 38,000 patients in a 1-year period. Once these characteristics were controlled, differences in physician age, practice tenure, site of practice, and extent of laboratory test ordering no longer had any relationship to referral rates. Sullivan (1992) found that the specific diagnosis was the most important predictor of the likelihood that a referral would be for long-term care rather than short-term care in adults; patients with rheumatoid arthritis or peripheral vascular disease were more likely to continue with a specialist beyond the initial visit than patients with osteoarthritis, psoriasis, or eczema.

Thus, the challenges of coordination vary with the reasons for referral and the nature of patients' needs. The rest of this chapter deals with the nature of the challenges to coordination that are present in primary care, how they are met, how they and the methods of dealing with them are measured, and the policy issues that are involved in bridging the gaps between different practitioners involved in the care of patients.

> One of our local gastroenterologists scopes every patient he sees. To me, many of these must not be indicated. To him, the patient has been sent because they are not well and need a complete work-up.

Benefits of Coordination

Until recently, there were no studies that specifically examined the benefits of coordination of care. Benefits accruing from coordination depend on the type of coordination that is required. When consultation is needed for short-term advice, guidance, or intervention, communication to the primary care practitioner need only summarize the nature of the recommendations or care given, with any special instructions that are required for the primary care practitioners to resume ongoing care. When the consultation is part of ongoing management of the particular problem by the other specialist, the challenge of coordination is greater because it requires a process of ongoing dialogue between the two levels of care to resolve any misunderstanding or to avoid absence of information that would interfere with best management practices.

> One of my patients, an elderly married male, was discovered to have colon cancer after having a screening test. He had surgery but developed metastases to the lungs about 4 years later. The surgeon told him there was not much to be done, and the

patient did not want much done. The surgeon continues to see the patient every 6 months and orders a CT scan of the chest (which verifies that he has continued growth of the metastases). I think the surgeon wants to do something; I care more about the outcome which is not going to be changed by the CT scans. After phoning the surgeon, he stopped ordering the scans, although he continues to want to see the patient even though I am the one who handles his medical and cancer-associated problems.

In a large survey of British general practitioners, Coulter et al. (1989) found that referral was sought for particular treatments or surgical procedures (36%), specific diagnostic investigations (35%), management advice (15%), reassurance of the generalists or patient (4%) and long-term transfer of responsibility from primary care to other specialty care (10%). Thus, the vast majority of referrals are for short-term consultation and care, with the patient expected to return directly to primary care.

Coordination requires both a means of information transfer (the structural or capacity component) and recognition of information (the process or performance component) (Fig. 11.2).

Shared care is a means of enhancing information flow from primary care physician to other specialists and back. As is noted below in the section on Policy Implications, shared care is an increasingly used mechanism of interchange of in-

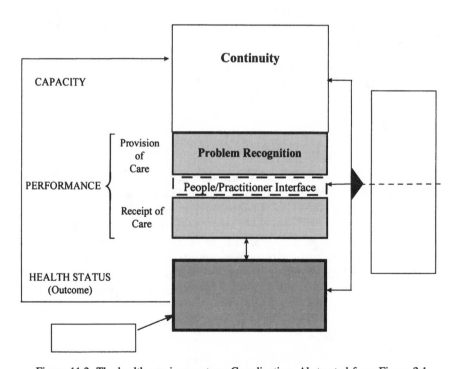

Figure 11.2. The health services system: Coordination. Abstracted from Figure 2.1.

formation about patients with ongoing problems. Shared care, however, can also be used to enhance the benefits of short-term referrals.

A Dutch study included 12 general practitioners with patients aged 10–75 years with orthopedic problems for whom the physicians were considering referral because of uncertainty about the diagnostic or therapeutic management. Patients were randomly assigned to joint consultation sessions with an orthopedist or to "usual" care in which they were left to refer or not as they decided. A year later the patients were evaluated by an orthopedist not involved in the care. There were significantly fewer referrals and diagnostic actions in the shared-care group, without negative effects on subsequent outcome. In fact, more patients were symptom free at 1-year follow up in this group than in the usual-care group (Vierhout et al., 1995).

A U.S. study explored the potential of collaborative management to achieve treatment guidelines for adult patients with depression. Patients of 22 primary care physicians were randomly assigned to one of two groups. Patients in the intervention group alternated visits to the primary care physician and psychiatrist, with verbal consultation between the two types of physicians. Patients in the comparison group were managed according to the primary care physician's discretion. Evaluation of outcomes at 1 month and 3 months revealed better adherence to therapy in the intervention group and better resolution of patient's problems, but the latter benefits accrued only in the patients with major depression (Katon et al., 1995).

More conventional (although not necessarily easier) methods of improving information transfer involve enhancements in continuity of practitioners or practitioner teams, medical records, or computerized information systems.

Several studies indicate that recognition of information about patients can be enhanced by improving the mechanisms of continuity. For example, continuity of practitioner results in better recognition of patient information. In a series of studies conducted in six different primary care facilities, continuity of practitioner improved the extent of recognition of various types of information, particularly with regard to clearly identified problems and therapies. Continuity of practitioner did not, however, facilitate practitioner recognition of visits elsewhere (Starfield et al., 1976; Simborg et al., 1978).

The addition of problem lists to medical records results in improved problem recognition. Studies in the six clinics indicate that such improvements in medical records facilitated recognition of information. Problem lists improved recognition of patients' problems especially if the duration between visits was long and if there was a different practitioner at each one (Simborg et al., 1976). Similar benefits accrued from the insertion of computerized printouts of information. This resulted in improved physician recognition of patients' previous problems and therapies, but did not improve recognition of visits made elsewhere between one visit to the primary care facility and a subsequent follow up. The improvements occurred whether or not there was continuity of practitioner from one visit to the next in the primary care facility (Starfield et al., 1977).

Computerized feedback of certain types of information also enhances patient care by facilitating coordination. Improved continuity in the form of a computerized summary in the medical records in a clinic lacking continuity of physicians can improve various aspects of care. One study consisted of a randomized controlled trial involving patients who were followed in three medical specialty clinics. A summary contained updated information about the patient and included a problem list, medications, and results of laboratory tests and suggested actions concerning the process of care. Those patients whose physicians were given the summaries were more likely to have indicated procedures and referrals actually carried out, greater implementation of indicated diets, and more discovery of both new and resolved problems. These patients also spent fewer days in the hospital on average (Rogers and Haring, 1979).

Improved continuity in the form of a computerized profile of drugs also can result in more effective use of information. In one study, the computer generated an updated summary of each patient's current and past medications whenever a drug was dispensed from the pharmacy. Using a random sample of patients seen in an outpatient setting, this profile was inserted within 24 hours into their the medical record. The duration of drug interactions experienced by patients was shorter for these patients than it was for those without the recorded profiles. The profiles also were associated with a reduced number of visits over a year of study, presumably due to a decrease in the number of visits for drug prescription renewals.

The recognition of important information by practitioners also can be improved by various other methods. For example, the presence of an observer during the practitioner–patient interaction can heighten a practitioner's sense of accountability to the patient so that the practitioner may inquire about problems of importance to the patient. One study demonstrated this effect by showing that the presence of an observer enhances the recognition of problems thought by the patients to require follow up (Starfield et al., 1979a).

In studies such as those summarized, the effect is probably a result of improved recognition of patients' needs by practitioners and therefore of greater agreement between patients and physicians concerning the patient's problems. When patients and practitioners agree on the patients' problems, the problems are more likely to improve than when only the patient or only the physician notes their existence. This has been found to be the case whether improvement in the patient's health was judged by the physician (Starfield et al., 1981) or by the patient (Starfield et al., 1979b).

Although most of the evidence cited above has been available for many years, it is not widely recognized and it is not self-evident that many subspecialists welcome opportunities to improve interaction with primary care physicians. At least some specialists do, however. In Canada, a survey of oncologists in one tertiary care medical center indicated their desire to have family physicians maintain a role in the care of patients with cancer in remission. Specific suggestions included developing guidelines, informal seminars to enhance the likelihood of sharing information, better mechanisms for flow of information, explicit policies to include family physicians in discussions of treatment plans, and shared roles in ongoing management, with the family physician as part of the team (Wood and McWilliam, 1996). However, the interests of other specialists in better coordination with primary care physicians may vary in degree. In the United States, where primary care physicians have not had a recent history of centrality in patient care, other specialists assign lower values to receiving information from primary care physicians than do primary care physicians in sending it, and both types of physicians rate the value of definition of roles and specific monitoring procedures lower than other aspects of the consultation process. Both types of physicians rate highly the value of initial verbal communication followed by written reports, and both rate highly the value of information about current medications, health beliefs and attitudes of the patient, drug sensitivities, matters that patients are not likely to discuss with the consultant, reasons for referral, chief symptoms and chronology, referring physician findings, and referring physician diagnosis (Williams and Peet, 1994).

Better communication between primary care practitioners and other specialists may lead to situations in which there is disagreement regarding the appropriate course of action. Specialists will tend to favor strategies that improve the patient's problem whereas primary care physicians should focus more on the overall situation of the patient. Sometimes these goals may be in conflict. Under such circumstances, it is the patient or patient's delegate who should ultimately make the decision after being provided with the alternatives and their rationale.

Policy and Research Implications of Coordination of Care

The management of illness is becoming increasingly complex. As technology advances, there are greater possibilites for diagnosis, intervention, and more specialization of personnel to provide the new services. The nature of illness is also changing: The aging of the population and the increased survival of individuals with complex and disabling conditions place an everincreasing burden on the health care system for coordination of care. Support of the coordination function depends on the development of better means of information transfer and patient management, especially when patients receive care from the variety of sources to which they have been referred.

> An outstanding figure of twentieth century medicine and a former editor of a prestigious medical journal developed an adenocarcinoma. After a successful operation that restored his ability to swallow, he was faced with a difficult choice: to undergo questionably effective and highly uncomfortable chemotherapy and radiation for possible but not detectable metastases or to forgo these therapies. Ironically, the area in which the cancer developed was one to which the eminent physician has devoted much attention in his career as a researcher. As he attempted to decide what plan to follow, he received from professional colleagues all over the country "a barrage of well-intentioned but contradictory advice." As a result, he and his family (including a son and a daughter who were both physicians) became increasingly confused and distraught. Finally one wise physician friend said, "What you need is a doctor." When that advice was followed, he reported that his family and he "sensed immediate and immense relief. The incapacity of enervating worry was dispelled, and I could return to my usual anxieties, such as deciding on the fate of manuscripts." Reported by S.J.R., The Pharos (Winter 1995)

Because referrals require patients to see different practitioners, continuity cannot be achieved by having the same practitioner. Other mechanisms are needed.

Historically, medical records have provided this mechanism, but standard medical records are not adequate for the task. Most of them serve solely as aids to memory recall and are useful primarily to the practitioner who wrote them; other practitioners are much less likely to use the information even if available.

Some improvements in medical record systems are designed to facilitate other purposes, such as billing and reimbursement, documenting the process of care, reviewing quality, monitoring, or legal functions. They do not improve recognition of information from referral visits or those made elsewhere on the patient's initiative.

The imperative for coordination is increasing rapidly as a result of major policy shifts in the financing and organization of health services, as by the "fundholding" approach in the United Kingdom, and by the expanding coverage of capitation payments to include specialty care in HMOs and "integrated" health systems in the United States. In these systems, primary care practitioners (in the United Kingdom) and managed care organizations (in the United States) are at risk for coverage of services delivered outside of primary care; if their budgets are exceeded by referrals to these services, they have less capital available for expansions or enhancements in their practice, and they may be even further at risk of not having their contracts renewed.

Thus, a variety of mechanisms to improve the likelihood of coordination have been developed in the most recent few years. These range from the development of formal guidelines, to outreach services by subspecialists, to the increasing use of telemedicine, to shared care between primary care physicians and other specialists.

Formal computerized guidelines are under development in some places. These guidelines operate in the form of programs that help primary care physicians know when it is appropriate to refer, what tests and procedures are appropriate to perform *before* the referral, what tests are inappropriate to perform because they may be unnecessary, and what information to provide to the other specialist. These programs are usually developed on the basis of informed judgements made by panels of specialist "experts"; optimally these panels should also include primary care physicians. No evaluations of the impact of this approach to improving coordination are known.

One of the more widely used strategies, especially in the United Kingdom, is the "outreach clinic" in which a specialist team provides a diagnostic or treatment service in primary care settings rather than in consultant settings such as hospitals. Bailey and colleagues (1994) evaluated the extent and nature of these efforts by means of telephone interviews with 50 hospital managers, 96 specialists, 88 general practitioners, and an additional 122 general practice fundholders in England. Most (60%) of the hospitals were involved in these outreach activities, and 32 fundholders identified an additional 61 outreach clinics covering surgical specialties, medical specialties, and mental health services (in that order of frequency). The most commonly reported benefits were, for patients, ease of access and shorter waiting times; for practitioners, improved communication was most commonly mentioned as a benefit. However, problems associated with these efforts were also reported, the most common of which were the 5%–10% of specialists who reported problems arising from increased time demands (Bailey et al., 1994).

Shared care is an effort to improve coordination by making explicit the responsibilities of primary care physicians and other specialists in the care of patients. It has been most extensively evaluated in the case of care for patients with diabetes. Greenhalgh's review (1994) of these evaluations stands as a model for a more extensive and far-reaching assessment of their potential value. The results of early studies of failures in coordination focused attention on the "unequivocal failure of unstructured care by general practitioners to produce acceptable levels of process and outcome," the "potential for high standards of care when structured care from a primary care team was accompanied by a high degree of support and enthusiasm from the specialist," the finding that "these extremes of quality can co-exist within local areas and even within a single shared care scheme," and the importance of the "three Rs: registration, recall, and regular review." Greenhalgh judged all three randomized controlled trials of shared care published since 1991, as well as most of the later longitudinal studies and descriptive accounts, as producing generally favorable results. He catalogued the various forms of shared care as follows: electronic mail requiring a common database with multiple access ports; computer-assisted shared care with an agreed upon dataset to be collected; shared record cards, which can be either patient-held or mailed back and forth between primary care physicians and specialists; liaison meetings (used most frequently for mental health and substance abuse problems); regular communication by letter or standard record sheet; community clinics, where a consultant physician or specialized nurse conducts clinics in primary care settings; or (and more radically) sharing of resources wherein consultants do not see the patients but provide education, support, and strategic planning to the primary care physician. Successful sharing of care has even been demonstrated for difficult pediatric problems and for targeted efforts such as retinal screening.

> The pediatrician and orthopedic surgeon scheduled their appointments back to back so that I would not have to make two separate visits. They shared a file, saving me the responsibility of relaying incomplete information. Appointments were scheduled—without my having to call each one independently—with a physiotherapist, an occupational therapist, a speech therapist, an ophthalmologist, and a psychologist. Information was shared between team members so that the speech therapist, for example, knew that the psychological assessment did indicate the possibility of a learning disorder.   W. Sibbald, The Medical Post (January 23, 1996)

Telemedicine is one form of a technique that could provide such support. Although advantages were demonstrated as long ago as the 1970s (Dunn et al., 1977), it is not clear that coordination of care would be enhanced by its greater use (Wyatt, 1996). The active participation of the patient may be reduced in the preoccupation with the technology, and there is no assurance that active interaction between primary care physician and consultant would be enhanced. Moreover, the range of specialists available for consultation may be reduced, leaving the primary care physician and patient less choice. Logistical problems in getting patients and physicians together, as well as costs of the technology, may also interfere with its widespread use, even where appropriate.

Unfortunately, the absence of a clear distinction between the secondary (consultative) care and tertiary (referral) care impedes the development of information systems tailored to specific needs. At least one study has shown that secondary clinics can be distinguished from tertiary clinics; both continuity of practitioner and coordination of care within the facility are higher in clinics characterized as tertiary than in clinics characterized as secondary. Despite these differences, specialists working in these clinics were unable to specify whether patients were under their care only for short-term advice and guidance or whether they perceived a long-term role involving the assumption of responsibility for more comprehensive care than specialists generally provide (Mawajdeh, 1988).

An understanding of the relative responsibilities of primary care physicians and other specialists can facilitate care of patients, as was demonstrated in a study of problem drinkers referred to a special alcohol clinic by their general practitioners in Great Britain. After an initial session in which they received advice and counseling in the clinic, the patients were randomly allocated either to a group that received continuing care from the clinic or to a group that returned to their general practitioner who was contacted and supported by the specialists from the clinic. After 6 months, patients cared for by their general practitioner had improved at least as much if not more than those cared for by specialists. Those seen by specialists made many more visits to the clinic whereas those cared for by general practitioners made more visits to the more convenient general practitioner's office. In this case, clearly defined responsibility for short-term care by specialists with continuing advice to the primary care physician served to improve the efficiency without any sacrifice in effectiveness of care (Drummond et al., 1990).

The challenge to development of policy regarding coordination of care depends on the development of more knowledge about the process of referral, the transfer of information deriving from referrals, and the extent to which primary care physicians recognize this information. Policy issues include the development of at least some standards for referral that can be taught during the process of medical education and that can be used for monitoring the quality of various components of medical care. New methods of information transfer are required to facilitate the recognition of information generated in visits to physicians other than the primary care physician. Client-held records, or "medical passports," may be a fruitful approach that is being implemented in various places and is part of national health policy in France as of 1997. It is also likely that better coordination will require more explicit recognition at the health systems level of the relative roles and responsibilities of primary care, secondary care, and tertiary care.

The coordination between these three sectors is known as *regionalization*. With regionalization, there is a well-established linkage between primary care, secondary care, and tertiary care. Services are organized according to the needs of the population and are designed so that there are enough practitioners and facilities at each level to take care of, but not to exceed, the needs at that level.

The need for resources at each level may be calculated either empirically on the basis of the experience of existing health systems or by estimating the number of required practitioners and facilities at each level from theoretical calculations based on existing needs or demands.

In many countries, care is organized so that there is generally one primary care practitioner for each 1,000–3,000 patients, depending on the age and illness level of the population and its geographic distribution. Community hospitals serve as a resource for consultations and for uncomplicated hospitalizations. Tertiary care hospitals are generally affiliated with medical teaching institutions and serve as a place to refer patients with unusually complicated or rare problems.

Theoretical calculations of the need for resources at each level may be based on professional judgements about what services should ideally be provided. The "needs-based" assessment was used by Lee and Jones (1933) and subsequently by a group at Yale University (Schonfeld et al., 1972) in the early 1970s. A panel of experts developed estimates of the average number of visits required to render primary care for specific acute and chronic conditions for different age groups.

In the Yale estimates, each acute condition was judged to require one and one-half visits per year on average; non-elderly adults with chronic conditions and those over age 65 years with chronic conditions were judged to require three and seven visits per year, respectively. Data from the U.S. National Health Interview Survey were used to determine the prevalence of acute and chronic conditions in the different age groups. The next step in the process of estimation required judgements concerning how many visits the average physician could handle. From these estimates the number of physicians required was calculated.

Practice-based surveys (such as the National Ambulatory Medical Care Survey in the United States) provide data on the number and type of visits that are managed by physicians so that professional estimates are no longer required for this step in the calculations. The Graduate Medical Education National Advisory Committee (1978) provided greater precision to the estimates made by the earlier efforts. Just substituting the actual visit rate for the theoretical visit rate increased the estimate for the number of required physicians by 20%–40%, depending on the specialty.

Estimates based on demand for services use information such as in the National Health Interview Survey in which respondents are asked about the number of visits they have made to physicians. Corrections can be made for anticipated changes that will influence utilization (such as expanded health insurance) or for changes in the anticipated balance between non-physician and physician practitioners. Using these types of procedures, the Graduate Medical Education National Advisory Committee developed estimates of the number of physicians that would be needed in both primary care and other physician specialties. In general, demand-based estimates are considerably lower than need-based estimates.

As noted in Chapter 4, the experiences of mature integrated health systems can provide estimates of the number of primary care practitioners and other specialists. However, differences in population characteristics and health care needs make adoption of any of these hazardous without careful evaluation of such differences. On the other hand, studies of the reasons for variability across different systems can provide important clues as to the most effective modes of delivering primary, consultative, and referral services particularly with regard to the relative roles each should play in achieving optimum care with minimum resources. Moreover, the remoteness of the primary care practice will certainly influence the nature and mode of interaction between primary care clinicians and other specialists.

The main challenges to coordination of care when different practitioners are involved differ according to the type of situation. Where several practitioners are involved as a result of patient-initiated visits, coordination will occur only if patients themselves serve as the conduit of information transfer or if there is a shared medical record. If a referral is involved, the challenge will depend on whether it is for short-term care or for long-term care. In the former instance, the major concern is with the timely feedback of information to patients and the referring practitioner. Mechanisms must be in place to ensure that the patient and all involved practitioners are aware of abnormalities and recommendations for intervention. In contrast, the challenges for coordination when the patient is in long-term speciality care arise from potential compromises to longitudinality of care. That is, when the majority of care is focused on management of a particular illness, there must be a mechanism to ensure that needed care unrelated to that illness (such as indicated preventive services) is provided. As the next section indicates, few studies have focused on this latter aspect of coordination.

Measurement of Coordination

The achievement of coordination on the population level can be assessed by aggregation of measures at the individual level. As is the case with each of the other three attributes, the assessment of coordination at the individual level requires consideration of a structural element of care, which provides the capacity for the achievement of the attribute, and a process feature, which provides the performance counterpart (Fig. 11.2).

The structural element essential to coordination is continuity of care; there must be a mechanism that makes the practitioner aware of problems wherever they arise so that possible interrelationships can be detected and managed. Continuity is generally achieved by having the same physician or other health professional care for the patient from one encounter to another. But there are other mechanisms for achieving continuity such as a team of individuals whose communication channels permit them to convey important information about patients to one another or by a medical record containing accurate and complete information about the patient, or by a computer that contains information about the patient, or by records carried by patients themselves.

The performance element paramount to coordination is the process of problem recognition or recognition of information about the care of problems. Only when problems are recognized can practitioners act on them. Because there can be no treatment without initial recognition of the existing problem, this step is most critical. When physicians do not act on information, it constitutes an error of omission rather than an error of commission. That is, the problem arises from a failure to recognize the existence of information rather than a failure to act on it.

Measuring continuity

To achieve coordination of care, there must be a mechanism to transfer information about a patient's problems or the care received for these problems. Continuity, in the context of the measurement of coordination, involves the presence of such a mechanism to ensure an uninterrupted succession of events between visits. Longitudinality and continuity differ in that in the former the succession of events is time-bound and occurs across the full spectrum of potential problems or reasons for visits. For continuity, the important issue is the succession of events between visits regardless of where they occur and for what reason. Many studies on the subject of continuity have been published, but most fail to distinguish between the separate concepts of longitudinality (the presence and use of a regular source of care over time) and continuity (the sequence of visits in which there is a mechanism of information transfer). Because the use of the same term to connote different phenomena impedes the process of research and of knowledge accumulation, it is important to distinguish between the concepts of longitudinality and continuity (Starfield, 1980). Table 11.1 compares longitudinality and continuity and, in addition, distinguishes these concepts from first contact.

Patients often lack an identifiable source of care that achieves longitudinality yet achieves continuity of care for particular problems. That is, it is possible to have continuity without longitudinality. For example, a complete medical record may be available to all practitioners while patients may see a different practitioner or go to a different facility for each visit. In this situation there is continuity but no longitudinality.

Conversely, patients may have a regular source of care in which longitudinality is reasonably well achieved, yet lack continuity for events that occur in sequence. For example, a patient who sees the same practitioner each time achieves longitudinality but there may be no mechanism, apart from human recollection, for information transfer. Furthermore, continuity of care may be a feature of tertiary care as well as primary care in the sense that individuals who are followed by tertiary care specialists for their rare or complex conditions may achieve a high degree of continuity. For example, there was no difference in continuity of care by generalists and by subspecialists for patients with chronic illness seen in a study of middle-aged and elderly adults in Quebec (Beland, 1989) or in one for patients in large, private multispeciality practices in California (Goldberg and Dietrich, 1985).

There are several methods of assessing continuity of practitioner and others for evaluating continuity achieved by alternative means:

- GINI and CON (Standardized Index of Concentration) (Shortell, 1976): These two measures of continuity have their roots in international economics where they are used to assess the concentration of resources. They are only useful when applied at the population level. Shortell (1976) applied them to assess the source of utilization during an episode of illness involving at least five visits. The measures cannot, however, distinguish patterns of use (e.g., seeing one

Table 11.1. Summary: Longitudinality Vs. Continuity Vs. First Contact

	Longitudinality	*Continuity*	*First Contact*
Type of Feature	Structure/process	Structure	Structure/process
Measured by	Utilization over time of the regular source of care	Continuity measure	Accessibility to the regular source and use of that source for each patient-initiated visit
Problem oriented?	No. Essence is use of the regular source of care, regardless of the nature or type of problem, in which a personal relationship is established and maintained	Yes. A mechanism to provide information follow-up of problems or types of problems	No. Most problems would be expected to be new, recurrences of old problems, and often undifferentiated
Personal relationship required?	Yes	No. Could be achieved by other means	No
Time specific?	Yes. A relationship over time	No. Relates to information generated in a series of two or more visits	No. Specific to a particular event in time
Person oriented?	Yes	No. Problem oriented	Yes
Shorthand summary	Over time, personal relationship	Episodes of illness (or chronic illness)	Single event
Suggested measures	UPC (Breslau and Reeb, 1975) COC (Bice and Boxerman, 1977) LICON (Steinwachs, 1979) "k" index (Ejlertsson and Berg, 1984	SECON (Steinwachs, 1979) LISECON (Steinwachs, 1979) "s" index (Smedby et al., 1984)	Population or patient interview

physician for several visits and another physician for other visits would result in the same index as patients who alternated physicians for the total number of visits). Thus, the measures cannot capture the succession of events within a sequence of care.

- Sequential Continuity (SECON): This measure is the fraction of sequential pairs of visits with the same practitioner. It ranges from 0 to 1, with an expected value of 1 divided by the number of available practitioners if care-seeking and scheduling are random (Steinwachs, 1979).
- Likelihood of Sequential Continuity (LISECON): This measure is the likelihood that SECON (sequential continuity) is greater than would occur if distribution of practitioners across sequential visits were random (Steinwachs, 1979):

Both SECON and LISECON are probability measures that control for the level of use and the number of practitioners available.

- "s" Index: In this method (Smedby et al., 1986), the patient is identified at a particular visit. This measure considers whether the practitioner seen on that occasion is the same practitioner who was seen at the previous visit to the facility. It has a value of 1 if the practitioner is the same and a value of 0 if not. Values can be aggregated by averaging over the visits of each person.
- Closed-loop referral rate (Holmes et al., 1978): This method measures the availability of information concerning one specific aspect of care (e.g., referrals). It is based on information in medical records and ascertains the percentage of referrals that resulted in a return of information about the referral.

  All of the above measures are empirical (i.e., relative measures). Because they do not yield standards for adequate continuity, their use is primarily for comparison between one facility or practitioner and another or between one population group and another. The measure developed by the Institute of Medicine, on the other hand, is normative, that is, it has a definable standard against which measurements can be graded.
- The Institute of Medicine measures: The Institute of Medicine (1978) checklist contains three questions concerning continuity. Can a patient who desires to do so make subsequent appointments with the same practitioner? Are complete records maintained in a form that is readily retrievable and accessible? Are relevant items or problems in the patient's record highlighted, regularly reviewed, and used in planning care?

Of the six measures of continuity, only the last two address mechanisms of continuity other than that of continuity of personnel. Two of the Institute of Medicine criteria explicitly recognize the importance of medical records. Their role in achieving continuity has been demonstrated by several studies. For example, Martin (1965) showed that patients are more likely to keep appointments when the follow-up dates are written in the medical record. Another study (Zuckerman et al., 1975) showed that patients are more likely to have information about their care (e.g., drug dosage and drug actions) if the information is in the record.

For records to serve as a mechanism of continuity, they must contain important information about patients. There are no standards for medical records, for computerized information systems, or for records kept by patients themselves, except for the most general categories including diagnosis and therapy. Not all types of information are equally well recorded in medical records. For example, Thompson and Osborne (1976) conducted an extensive nationwide study of pediatric practitioners and showed that there were many items of information that were widely considered as evidence of high-quality care but were not recorded. Items that were consistently recorded included certain routine measurements in infancy and childhood, symptom history in children with an acute recurrent condition, drug therapy and a program for continuing treatment in children with allergy, chief complaints, symptoms, as well as some types of diagnostic tests. The approach to assessing the adequacy of medical records for purposes of achieving continuity compares actual occurrence with what was recorded and is ascertainable. This involves several techniques:

- Interviewing patients and physicians: To obtain information by this method, both patients and physicians should be queried because they do not always agree on the events related to the visit. In fact, studies have shown that (1) patients and their physicians agree on the nature of the patient's problem in only half of all visits; (2) in one-fourth of the visits, a problem is mentioned only by the patient; and (3) in one-fourth of the visits a problem is mentioned only by the physician (Starfield et al., 1979b, 1981; Romm and Putnam, 1981).
- Audiotaping and videotaping the encounter (Zuckerman et al., 1975).
- Having an observer record the content of a visit and comparing it with the medical record (Starfield et al., 1979a).

Innovations in medical records can improve their usefulness for purposes of continuity. Problem lists inserted at the front of the record do improve practitioners' recognition of problems under care. Computerized summaries also achieve the purpose for some but not all aspects of care. Highlighting of information, either in a handwritten note (Williamson et al., 1967) or by computer (Barnett, 1976), achieves the same purpose. (Chapter 16 supplies more detail on information systems.)

Evaluation of the extent of information transfer is a conventional approach to assessing the structural aspects of coordination. A standardized and well-tested instrument for assessing the adequacy of the communication between primary care physicians and other specialists would make this approach more useful in judging both the relative and the absolute achievement of standards for such communication. Although no such instrument currently exists, there have been several initiatives that suggest directions for its content.

In 1996, the Welsh Secretary of Health (1997) set 20 health targets, among them targets for improving information transfer from primary to secondary care: The results of all diagnostic tests (except for sexually transmitted diseases) should be received by the patient's general practitioner within 2 working days, and all information regarding the clinical management of the patient should be received by the general practitioner within 24 hours of discharge from the hospital.

The College of Family Physicians of Canada and the Royal College of Physicians and Surgeons of Canada (1993) jointly proposed guidelines for information transfer, including the following:

- Referring physicians should involve patients in the decision to refer, the choice of specialist, and the proposed management plan, including follow up and continuity of care; should communicate clearly to specialists/consultants the purpose and problems for which help is needed and send specialists/consultants the results of findings and investigations, including radiologic films, to be available at the time of consultation; and should participate in peer and system review of the consultation/referral process.
- Patients should understand the need for and purpose of the referral; demonstrate courtesy for both physicians; understand the time and place of the consultation and what to bring to it and advise both physicians if unable to attend; understand

that the results will be communicated to them by the specialist/consultant; understand that the results of tests will be reported to them by the physician ordering them; understand that they should return to the referring physician for continuing care and advice as a result of the referral; participate in peer and system review of the consultation/referral process.

- Specialists/consultants should provide ease of access to their services; provide consultation at appropriate times or assist referring physicians to find appropriate alternatives; demonstrate courtesy and respect for patients and referring physicians; communicate clearly and promptly the results of consultation to the referring physician and patient; promptly report the results of laboratory tests to patients in the appropriate clinical context; advise referring physicians promptly about patients' admission to hospital and provide prompt reports on discharge; recognize referring physicians' concerns about lateral or cross referrals; return patients to referring physicians for continuing care at the appropriate time and, when ongoing care for some complex or specific problem is required, to involve the patient and the primary care physician in the decision; and participate in peer and system review of the consultation/referral process.

Measuring recognition of information requiring follow up

Five methods have been used to assess the recognition of information concerning patients' problems or the care provided for them.

1. Institute of Medicine (1978) measures are based on answers to several questions that serve as a normative measure of the achievement of coordination. Each deals in some way with the transfer of information to facilitate integration of care, although none actually assesses the recognition of the information. The questions are as follows: (a) Do the practitioners in the unit furnish pertinent information to other practitioners serving the patient, actively seek relevant feedback from consultants and other practitioners, and serve as the patient's ombudsman in contacts with other practitioners? (b) Is a summary or abstract of the patient's record provided to other physicians when needed? (c) Do the practitioners in the unit develop a treatment plan that considers the ability of the patient to understand it? (d) Do the practitioners use a variety of tactics to ensure that the patient will cooperate in the treatment? (e) Does the plan of treatment reflect the patient's physical, emotional, and financial ability to carry it out? The first two questions facilitate coordination by improving the likelihood that practitioners will recognize important information. The last three questions are more related to the quality of care than to the process of coordination itself.

2. The University of North Carolina method (Fletcher et al., 1984) assesses coordination more directly. Coordination is defined as written evidence that the specialist is aware of the primary care physician's involvement with the patient and that either the primary physician arranged the visit or knew about it beforehand. Alternatively, coordination is achieved if the primary physician was aware of a visit that a patient already made to another physician.

3. The assessment of coordination of care was further refined by the Dartmouth

Primary Care Cooperative Project (COOP), a collaborative practice-based network in northern New England. Care was considered to be coordinated only if the primary care physician was aware in advance of visits elsewhere. This could occur either when the primary care physician arranged for a visit elsewhere or when the physician discussed the need for it before the patient made the appointment, or when the physician knew in advance of visits that patients planned elsewhere on their own initiative. Information about visits was obtained from periodic phone calls to patients who kept diaries recording all of their contacts with physicians, hospitalizations, non-physician ambulatory visits, and filling of drug prescriptions. Coordination was present for 75% of ambulatory physician visits, 81% of nonemergency hospitalizations, and 78% of all drug prescriptions, but for only 33% of visits to non-physician practitioners (Dietrich et al., 1988).

4. In another approach to assessing coordination, patients are asked where and for what reason they have gone for care. Providers are asked if the patient has been seen elsewhere and, if so, where and for what. Alternately, information systems may be used as the source of information as to where patients went and for what reason. This alternative is useful primarily where the information system contains data on all visits made by patients; if claims forms are obtained for all visits, the database containing these would be a suitable source of data. Recognition of the information by practitioners is assessed either by querying them as to their knowledge of these visits and their content or by reviewing their records for evidence of recognition of the information. This is the method used in the study that provided the case history earlier in this chapter (Starfield et al., 1977).

5. Certain aspects of information recognition can be obtained directly from the medical record. For example, is there a mechanism for practitioners to sign off on laboratory results and to indicate that they have notified patients, as well as other involved physicians, of abnormalities? Are the mechanisms to ensure that patients know that they need a follow-up appointment or procedure implemented and recorded?

All of these methods pertain primarily to the challenges of coordination resulting from short-term referrals. Newer methods of measuring recognition of information requiring follow up are presented in Chapter 13 in the context of overall evaluation of primary care. Assessment of the adequacy of coordination when referrals are long term primarily focus on evaluations of the adequacy of recognition of patients' needs that are unrelated to the particular problem under long-term care. Consistent with the great preponderance of the short-term referral, most studies of the achievement of coordination focus on it.

What Is Known About the Attainment of Coordination

T.M. is an adolescent who reported having seen seven practitioners in seven different health plans. He also disclosed that he had so many goals to reach with these seven physicians that he chose not to deal with any of them because he was overwhelmed.   A case worker

Many primary care as well as specialty care facilities lack high levels of continuity. Studies described below provide evidence of this.

Early studies of the referral process and associated information transfer were conducted in England. After the 1948 reorganization, the hospital outpatient departments became the center to which a general practitioner could refer a patient for a specialist's opinion. Several studies were conducted in individual hospital clinics to determine the type of patients that had been referred by practitioners. The findings of these studies (Chamberlain, 1965) were as follows:

- Almost 10% of letters from practitioners accompanying patients were less than 15 words; only 15% had more than 100 words.
- There was a marked association between length of letter and social class for people who lived near the hospital. The higher the social class, the longer the letter.
- Less than half of the letters requested that the patient see a specific consultant. The largest proportion of referrals contained no tentative diagnosis but merely requested that the consultant "see and advise."
- The quality of the communication between doctor and consultant was poorer for doctors who lived closest to the hospital.

In the 1950s, the now classic studies of Williams and his colleagues in North Carolina examined the process of referral and the characteristics of information associated with them. In these studies, referring physicians and their referred patients were interviewed, and the medical records were reviewed. Adequacy of the referral process was judged according to the following five criteria (Williams et al., 1961).

- Definition and specification of the need and purpose of referral, including mutual understanding between patients and physicians
- Adequate communication of purpose to consultant
- Attention to purpose by consultant
- Adequate communication of findings and recommendations to the referring physician
- Clear understanding by patient, referring physician, and consultant of responsibility for the patient's continuing care (Williams et al., 1961).

Specification of the purpose of the referral was determined for 99% of the referrals. Only one-fourth of the time was the purpose specified; a nonspecific medical reason was given in another one-third of referrals. The most common reason (39% of the time) was "in response to a patient's request." About 1 in 25 referrals was related to an inability of the patient to afford medically needed services.

The reason for the requested consultation was specified in a communication in only 4 of 10 instances; it was more likely to be found in the written communication when the physician had stated it clearly in the interviews.

In only one of six instances was the reason for referral mentioned in the communication from the consultant back to the general practitioner.

Criteria concerning communication back to the referring physician was a policy of the medical center and was achieved 100% of the time. However, subsequent communications were never sent for 24% of patients for whom they were warranted.

Responsibility for continuing care of the patient was studied by examining the medical record and by interviewing the patients and referring physicians as to whether the patient had returned to them. Patients were more likely to return to the referring physician when the medical record clearly specified such an intent. In total, 62% of patients returned to their general practitioner, but the percentage was 79% if the note was clear and only 42% if the note was unclear as to the disposition (Williams et al., 1961).

More recent studies in Great Britain confirm the findings of the earlier studies. A substantial proportion of referral letters omit such information as details of prior drug therapy and illnesses. The adoption of fixed format letters has not been widespread, even though they more consistently contain needed information. Letters from consultants to primary care physicians are often unresponsive or at best unclear in aiding the primary care physician and are often considerably delayed (Wilkin and Dornan, 1990). General practitioners, patients, and consultants have different perceptions of the reason for referral, and these differences are generally not explicit. In such situations, it is difficult, if not impossible, to judge the appropriateness of the referral, the nature of the information transferred, and the procedures for the referral and for return to the primary care physician (Grace and Armstrong, 1987).

> I am sure that the patient remains somewhat confused, but this letter to you is an attempt to make the position clear. She does not need another appointment to the hospital clinic.   A British family physician's letter to a hospital specialist

Deficiencies in the transfer of information from consultants back to primary care physicians seem to be a problem in many countries, even those with very different primary care characteristics. A study of 340 referrals by 20 general practitioners showed wide variability in referral rates (from 1.6%–10.0%); letters were received from consultants in only one-third of instances, even when the referral resulted in a change of medication or diagnosis (Haikio et al., 1995).

Giving the *patient* written information may be very important. In a survey of 300 consecutive consultations carried out in England, both patients and physicians were asked what advice was given to them about the need for a return visit. Physicians and patients agreed less than half the time about what advice was given. Patients were especially likely to disagree with their physician when no specific advice was given during the physician–patient encounter; in these instances, patients were much more likely to indicate that a return visit was necessary (Armstrong et al., 1990).

One study, conducted in a major HMO in the United States, confirmed the importance of written information; if a written form was given for an appointment to return to the referring physician, the patient was much more likely to return to that physician than if the information was provided verbally. Also, patients were more likely to return to their physician if they considered the physician to be their family doctor (Lawrence and Dorsey, 1976).

Another study showed that consultants communicate their findings to referring practitioners in only 55% of the consultations. If the patient was given a return appointment to the primary care physician, the physician was more likely to know the result of the consultation (McPhee et al., 1984).

In a study conducted over a period of 7 months in six different facilities (three pediatric, three adult), there was wide variability in the percentage of patients seen by the same practitioner on two successive visits in which the second was a follow-up for the first. Percentages in five facilities ranged from 46% to 79%, and in only one was it above 90% (93%). Despite the fact that approximately one in nine patients in each facility made a visit elsewhere on recommendation of their own practitioner and even more made a visit on their own, medical records of these patients often did not contain information about the occurrence of these visits (Table 11.2) (Starfield et al., 1976).

Smedby et al. (1984) calculated sequential continuity rates in visits for nine different problems in a primary care facility. The percentage of visits in which there was continuity of practitioner ranged from 10% in the case of obstructive lung disease to 28% for diabetes. Continuity rates were higher for scheduled visits than for unscheduled ones and for those in which the patient was seen by a physician who had served at the facility for longer periods of time. Overall, continuity was only 22%.

Holmes et al. (1978) compared the closed-loop referral rate for patients of family physicians who had a family practice residency with patients of general practitioners whose knowledge was derived only from their practice experience. The two types of physicians did not differ in their closed-loop referral rate, which was about 80%.

There are few studies of the extent to which improved continuity of practitioners or information is associated with improved recognition of information important to adequate patient care.

In one study of the extent of coordination between the internal medicine primary care facility and other facilities at the University of North Carolina, the percentages of visits that were coordinated ranged between 22% for specialty clinics

Table 11.2. Continuity of Care by Medical Records: Percent of Charts Containing Content of Intervening Visits (Number of Charts in Parentheses)

	Suburban Group	Urban Group	Hospital Clinics
Scheduled visits			
Adult	96% (25)	92% (13)	87% (39)
Pediatric	77% (22)	100% (10)	82% (33)
Unscheduled visits			
Adult	81% (164)	63% (96)	32% (244)
Pediatric	83% (100)	36% (39)	54% (39)

Source: Starfield et al. (1979a).

and 47% for ''walk-in'' visits (Fletcher et al., 1984). Coordination for visits to the emergency room was 28%. In contrast, the percentage of hospital admissions for which there was coordination with the primary care facility was 75%. Overall, only about one-third (35%) of instances requiring coordination achieved it.

A poor thirty-ish woman has panic disorder for which she is receiving treatment. She works part-time, has no insurance, and her husband is disabled with back injury and psychiatric illness. Because of her monetary difficulties, she gradually began to space her medications at wider and wider intervals. One night at midnight she developed chest pain and shortness of breath. Her sister, who had never seen this before, rushed her to the emergency room where she had a large work-up and a bill of $2,500. I called the emergency room physician. Why all this workup for a panic attack? He felt her chest pain fit his protocol for ruling out myocardial infarct and had not determined what medications she was on nor that she had a history of panic disorder. This patient is paying off the emergency room visit, $10 at a time, but now she will have even less money for her medications.   Dr. M.

Another study of the attainment of coordination was conducted in six different primary care facilities, three internal medicine and three pediatric, all affiliated with a large medical center. It involved patients who were given an appointment for a follow-up visit within 6 months after a previous visit and who were identified at the follow-up visit. Before their second visit, their records were reviewed to ascertain the information generated in the first visit as well as that generated in subsequent visits elsewhere either on referral by the primary care facility or self-initiated. In all facilities, the recognition of information generated within the primary care clinic, whether or not the patient was seen by the same practitioner as in the initially identified visit, was much greater than the extent of recognition of information generated in visits made elsewhere. Table 11.3 shows this to be the

Table 11.3. Effect of Provider Continuity on Recognition of Information

Type of Information	Provider Continuity	Percentage of Instances in Which Information was Recognized
Clearly identified problems	Yes	75.3
	No	62.3
''Problem-in-text''	Yes	58.2
	No	52.7
Therapies	Yes	52.2
	No	43.0
Tests done	Yes	31.0
	No	22.7
Scheduled intervening visits	Yes	47.2
	No	41.8
Unscheduled intervening		17.3

Adapted from Starfield et al. (1976).

case for all types of information: (1) clearly identified problems, that is, those highlighted in the medical record because they were recorded as chief complaints or diagnoses; (2) problems mentioned in the text of medical record notes; (3) therapies prescribed; or (4) tests done (Starfield et al., 1976). The extent of achievement of coordination for visits occurring elsewhere was similar to that obtained in the University of North Carolina study.

Despite the high salience of the referral process from both the viewpoint of increasing need for referrals and the high costs of associated care (Glenn et al., 1987), there are few more recent studies in the United States concerning information transfer and coordination of care.

Jenkins (1993) developed and applied an 11-item questionnaire for 39 specialists to assess the quality of the referral letter. Specialists were instructed to compare the information in the letter with information obtained from the patient by history and clinical examination. Nine of the 11 questions concerned important aspects of clinical information (errors or omissions of clinically relevant data), one reflected absence of appropriate interventions prior to the referral, and one concerned the quality of the writing of the letter. Between 5% and 28% of the 705 letters had errors of omission (depending on the type of information), and 23% reflected absence of a relevant pre-referral investigation. The rates of both types of inadequacies were greater for referrals to medical specialists than to surgical specialists. Although accuracy of the specialists' decisions about appropriateness of the referral was tested against an independent judgment by a noninvolved general practitioner, neither the validity nor the reliability of the judgments about completeness and accuracy was tested. Nevertheless, the study shows the potential of such a method for determining the adequacy of information that is necessary for coordination of care.

Further evidence of deficits in coordination comes from a study of the immunization status of children in tertiary care for spina bifida (Raddish et al., 1993). Although it is clear that such patients require ongoing care from a specialist because of their rare and complex condition, it is apparent that this care does not substitute for, nor is it coordinated with, primary care. In this study of 120 children in a tertiary referral center, all but one child had an identified primary care physician. However, immunization delay increased from 20% to 50% from the first in the series of indicated immunizations to 18 months of age; at school entry, only one-fourth of the children were up to date on immunizations.

Another study of care provided to 10,608 adults from panels of 60 family physicians and 245 general internists found that patients of general internists rated their physicians higher on coordination (as measured by reports that the physician knew about other doctors or health professionals being seen) than did patients of family physicians (Grumbach et al., 1997).

The advent of "managed care" (see Chapter 6) might be expected to improve coordination because of the greater likelihood of modes of integration within an organized health system. Data from a survey of 84 general internists on the staff of a large teaching hospital in Washington, DC, did not provide cause of optimism. Forty-one of the physicians who participated in both managed care and nonmanaged care plans reported that their patients in managed care were referred more often to an unknown specialist, spoke personally with the specialist less often, and sent a written summary to specialists less often (Roulidis and Schulman, 1994).

Summary

Table 11.4 summarizes the nature of coordination. Achieving coordination is a challenge for primary care practitioners because of both the multiplicity of types of reasons for referral and the technical difficulties in transferring and recognizing information generated in different places. Patients frequently make visits elsewhere, either on the recommendation of their physician or at their own discretion, and information transfer about these visits or what occurred in them is often lacking.

Continuity of practitioner facilitates recognition of information concerning the care of patients within the primary care facility but does not improve the recognition of information about visits elsewhere.

Currently available improvements in medical records and other technologies facilitate the recognition of information generated about patients and improve the care provided to patients, but they do not extend to recognition of information that occurs elsewhere either upon referral or on the patient's initiative.

The greater the recognition of patients' problems by practitioners, the more likely the patients are to show subsequent improvement.

In most studies, coordination of care is judged to be poor. There are several methods for assessing the impact of coordinating care. Systematic attempts to apply them could provide an opportunity to detect systematic deficiencies and institute mechanisms to overcome them.

New policy implications are leading to exploration of a diversity of new approaches, including sharing of care between primary care physicians and specialists. Informed policy decisions concerning coordination of care require more research on differences in needs depending on the type of referral, the employment of measures to clearly distinguish between the concepts of continuity and coordination in

Table 11.4. Summary of Coordination

	Capacity	*Performance*
Description: Integration of all health-related services, wherever received		
Involves	Coordinating mechanism (persons, information system)	Awareness of services provided elsewhere or by others
Problem oriented	Yes, for each problem/need	Yes, for each problem/need
Personal relationship required	No	No
Time dependent	No (episode dependent)	No (episode dependent)
Specific measures	Provider survey	Provider survey
	Patient survey	Patient survey
	Medical record/information system audits	Medical record/information system audits

the context of both consultative (short-term) and referral (long-term) care, and mechanisms of sharing care when appropriate.

References

Armstrong D, Glanville, T, Bailey E, O'Keefe G. Doctor-initiated consultations: A study of communication between general practitioners and patients about the need for reattendance. Br J Gen Pract 1990; 40:241–2.

Bailey JJ, Black ME, Wilkin D. Specialist outreach clinics in general practice. BMJ 1994; 308:1083–6.

Barnett O. Computer-Stored Ambulatory Record (COSTAR). NCHSR Research Digest Series. DHEW Pub. No. (HRA) 76–3145. Washington, DC: US Department of Health, Education, and Welfare, 1976.

Beland F. A descriptive study of continuity of care as an element in the process of ambulatory medical care utilization. Can J Public Health 1989; 80:249–54.

Bice T, Boxerman S. A quantitative measure of continuity of care. Med Care 1977; 15:347–9.

Breslau N, Reeb K. Continuity of care in a university based practice. J Med Educ 1975; 50: 965–9.

Chamberlain J, Acheson R, Butterfield W, Blancy R. The population served by the outpatient department of a London teaching hospital. A study of Guy's. Med Care 1965; 4:81–8.

College of Family Physicians of Canada and the Royal College of Physicians and Surgeons of Canada. The Relationship between Family Physicians and Specialists/Consultants in the Provision of Patient Care. Task Force Report, 1993.

Coulter A, Noone A, Goldacre M. General practitioners' referrals to specialist outpatient clinics. BMJ 1989; 299:304–8.

Dietrich A, Nelson E, Kirk J, Zubkoff M, O'Conner G. Do primary physicians actually manage their patients fee-for-service care? JAMA 1988; 259:3145–9.

Draper P, Smits HL. The primary-care practitioner—specialist or jack-of-all trades? N Engl J Med 1975; 293(18):903–7.

Drummond D, Thom B, Brown C, Edwards G, Mullan M. Specialists' versus general practitioners' treatment of problem drinkers. Lancet 1990; 336:915–8.

Dunn EV, Conrath DW, Bloor WG, Tranquanda B. An evaluation of four telemedicine systems for primary care. Health Serv Res 1977; 1:19–25.

Ejlertsson G, Berg S. Continuity of care measures. An analytic and empirical comparison. Med Care 1984; 22:231–9.

Emmanuel LL. The consultant and the patient–physician relationship. Arch Intern Med 1994; 154:1785–90.

Fletcher R, O'Malley M, Fletcher S, Earl J, Alexander J. Measuring the continuity and coordination of medical care in a system involving multiple providers. Med Care 1984; 22:403–11.

Glenn JK, Lawler FH, Hoerl MS. Physician referrals in a competitive environment. JAMA 1987; 258:1920–3.

Goldberg H, Dietrich A. The continuity of care provided to primary care patients: A comparison of family physicians, general internists, and medical subspecialists. Med Care 1985; 23:63–73.

Grace J, Armstrong D. Referral to hospital: Perceptions of patients, general practitioners and consultants about necessity and suitability of referral. Fam Pract 1987; 4:170–5.

Graduate Medical Education National Advisory Committee. GMENAC Staff Paper 1. Physician Manpower Requirements. DHEW Pub. No. (HRA) 78-10. Rockville, MD: U.S. Department of Health, Education, and Welfare, Public Health Service, Bureau of Health Manpower, 1978.

Greenhalgh PM. Shared Care for Diabetes. A Systematic Review. Occasional Paper 67. London: The Royal College of General Practitioners, October 1994.

Grumbach K, Selby J, Schmittdiel J, Quesenberry C. Quality of primary care practice in a large HMO according to physician specialty. unpublished manuscript, 1998.

Haikio J-P, Linden K, Kvist M. Outcomes of referrals from general practice. Scand J Primary Health Care 1995; 13:287–93

Holmes C, Kane R, Ford M, Fowler J. Toward the measurement of primary care. Milbank Q 1978; 56:231–52.

Institute of Medicine. A Manpower Policy for Primary Health Care: Report of a Study. IOM Pub. No. 78–02. Washington, DC: National Academy of Sciences, 1978.

Jenkins RM. Quality of general practitioner referrals to outpatient departments: Assessment by specialists and a general practitioner. Br J Gen Pract 1993; 43:111–3.

Katon W, Von Korff M, Lin E, Walker E, Simon GE, Bush T, Robinson P, Russo J. Collaborative management to achieve treatment guidelines. JAMA 1995; 273(13) 1026–31.

Lawrence R, Dorsey J. The generalist–specialist relationship and the art of consultation. In Noble J (ed): Primary Care and the Practice of Medicine. Boston: Little Brown & Company, 1976. pp 229–45.

Lee R, Jones L. The Fundamentals of Good Medical Care. Chicago: The University of Chicago Press, 1933.

Martin D. The imposition of patients from a consultant general medical clinic. In White KL (ed): Medical Care Research. Oxford: Pergam Press, 1965. pp 113–21.

Mawajdeh S. Levels of Care in Pediatric Speciality Clinics. Dissertation. Baltimore: Johns Hopkins University, 1988.

McPhee S, Lo B, Saika G, Meltzer R. How good is communication between primary care physicians and subspeciality consultants? Arch Intern Med 1984; 144:1265–8.

McWhinney I. Family medicine in perspective. N Engl J Med 1975; 293:176–81.

Raddish M, Goldmann DA, Kaplan LC, Perrin JM. The immunization status of children with spina bifida. Am J Dis Child 1993; 147:849–53.

Robinson D. Primary medical practice in the United Kingdom and the United States. N Engl J Med 1977; 297:188–93.

Rogers JL, Haring OM. The impact of a computerized medical record summary system on incidence and length of hospitalization. Med Care 1979; 17:618–30.

Romm F, Putnam S. The validity of the medical record. Med Care 1981; 19:310–5.

Roulidis Z, Schulman K. Physician communication in managed care organizations: Opinions of primary care physicians. J Fam Pract 1994; 39:446–51.

Salem-Schatz S, Moore G, Rucker M, Pearson SD. The case for case-mix adjustment in practice profiling: When good apples look bad. JAMA 1994; 272(11):871–4.

Schonfeld H, Heston J, Falk I. Numbers of physicians required for primary medical care. N Engl J Med 1972; 286:571–76.

Shortell S. Continuity of medical care: Conceptualization and measurement. Med Care 1976; 14:377–91.

Simborg D, Starfield B, Horn S. Physician and non-physician health practitioners: The characteristics of their practices and their relationships. Am J Public Health 1978; 68:44–8.

Simborg D, Starfield B, Horn S, Yourtee S. Information factors affecting problem follow-up in ambulatory care. Med Care 1976; 14:848–56.

Smedby O, Eklund G, Eriksson E, Smedby B. Measures of continuity of care: A register-based correlation study. Med Care 1986; 24:511–8.

Smedby B, Smedby O, Eriksson E, Mattsson L-G, Lindgren A. Continuity of care. An application of visit-based measures. Med Care 1984; 22:676–80.

Starfield B. Continuous confusion. Am J Public Health 1980; 70:117–9.

Starfield B, Simborg D, Horn S, Yourtee S. Continuity and coordination in primary care: Their achievement and utility. Med Care 1976; 14:625–36.

Starfield B, Simborg D, Johns C, Horn S. Coordination of care and its relationship to continuity and medical records. Med Care 1977; 15:929–38.

Starfield B, Steinwachs D, Morris I, Bause G, Siebert S, Westin C. Patient–provider agreement about problems. Influence on outcome of care. JAMA 1979b; 242:344–6.

Starfield B, Wray C, Hess K, Gross R, Birk P, D'Lugoff B. The influence of patient–practitioner agreement on outcome of care. Am J Public Health 1981; 71:127–32.

Starfield B, Steinwachs D, Morris I, Bause G, Siebert S, Westin C. Presence of observers at patient-practitioner interactions: impact on coordination of care and methodologic implications. Am J Public Health 1979a; 69:1021–25.

Steinwachs D. Measuring provider continuity in ambulatory care. An assessment of alternative approaches. Med Care 1979; 17:551–65.

Sullivan FM, Hoare T, Gilmour H. Outpatient clinic referrals and their outcomes. Br J Gen Pract 1992; 42(3):111–15.

Thompson H, Osborne C. Office records in the evaluation of quality of care. Med Care 1976; XIV:294–314.

Vierhout WPM, Knottnerus JA, van Ooij A, Crebolder HFJM, Pop P, Wesselingh-Megens AMK, Beusmans GHMI. Effectiveness of joint consultation sessions of general practitioners and orthopaedic surgeons for locomotor-system disorders. Lancet 1995; 346(8981):990–4.

Welsh Secretary of Health: Ron Davies as reported by: Dobson R. News: Wales is set 20 health targets. BMJ 1997; 314:1785.

Wilkin D, Dornan C. GP Referrals to Hospital: A Review of Research and Its Implication for Policy and Practice. University of Manchester: Center for Primary Care Research, July 1990.

Williams PT, Peet G. Differences in the value of clinical information: Referring physicians versus consulting specialists. J Am Board Fam Pract 1994; 7(4):292–302.

Williams TF, White KL, Fleming WL, Greenberg BA. The referral process in medical care and the university clinics' role. J Med Educ 1961; 36:899–907.

Williamson J, Alexander N, Miller G. Continuing education and patient care research. JAMA 1967; 201:938–42.

Wood ML, McWilliam C. Cancer in remission: Challenge in collaboration for family physicians and oncologists. Can Fam Physician 1996; 42:899–910.

Wyatt JC. Commentary: Telemedicine trials—Clinical pull or technology push? BMJ 1996; 313(7069):1380.

Zuckerman A, Starfield B, Hochreiter C, Kovasznay B. Validating the content of pediatric outpatient medical records by means of tape-recording doctor–patient encounters. Pediatrics 1975; 56:407–11.

— IV —
Patients and Populations

— 12 —

Quality of Primary Care Services: A Clinical View

Social systems must be accountable for their performance. In the health system, this accountability takes the form of quality assurance. This chapter describes methods of assessing the quality of care and ensuring quality of care in primary care settings.

What Do We Mean by "Quality of Care"?

In the context of optimizing effectiveness and equity, quality of care is the extent to which health needs, both current and potential, are being optimally met by health services, given current knowledge about the distribution, recognition, diagnosis, and management of health problems and health concerns. Thus, high-quality services take into account awareness of health problems in the population as well as characteristics of populations and subpopulations that create both threats to, as well as potential for, health in the future. High-quality health services are concerned not only with adequacy of services for disease diagnosis and management but also with adequacy of services that prevent future disease and promote improved health. Of course, quality of care is an issue for all levels of health services, including emergency services and specialty care; this chapter addresses issues of special relevance to primary care.*

The term *quality* has also been used in a broad sense to reflect not only the quality of care as defined above but also satisfaction with services, the costs of care, the qualifications of health services personnel, the safety and congeniality of the facilities in which services are provided, and the adequacy of the equipment (as in laboratories) that contribute to the provision of services.

> F.S., my wife's grandfather, received high-quality care. His physician took 3 days to travel with him to a noted clinic for diagnosis and treatment. Although he died

*In fact, little is known about the quality of consultative and referral care from the viewpoint of its organization, its activities, or its responsiveness to patients' needs.

245

soon after the trip, his expectations were met. He had trusted that medical care would do the best it could, had evidence that it tried, and accepted the result. Appropriateness was decided by his physician as unquestioned by anyone. More was always better.   R.H. 1996

Satisfaction with services is not, in itself, a measure of the quality of care as defined above. However, it may be indirectly related to quality because it may influence the seeking of certain types of services that themselves influence health status. Similarly, costs of care are indirectly related to quality because they influence what services are affordable. Because the monetary resources available for health services are not boundless even in wealthy countries, money spent on less effective services or on services to less needy populations leaves less money available for more effective services especially for populations in greater need of them. Thus costs of care are powerfully related to inequities in the distribution of the effectiveness of health services according to the "inverse care law" by which those in least need of services receive the most (Hart, 1971).

Quality of care can be viewed from a population perspective as well as a clinical (i.e., individual) perspective. Viewed from a clinical perspective, concern is focused on the impact of individual practitioners or groups of practitioners on the health of their patients. Viewed from a population perspective, concern is focused on the impact of health systems on populations and on reducing disparities in health across population subgroups. As the organization and delivery of health services has moved, over time, from a focus on patients to a focus on defined populations and, in some countries, to a focus on the whole population, the boundaries between quality as viewed clinically and quality as viewed from the population vantage have become less distinct. Nevertheless, the scope of concern of quality measurement differs according to the perspective. This chapter addresses the subject of quality of primary care as viewed clinically; Chapter 13 addresses the subject from a population perspective. Figure 2.1 informs the choice of subjects addressed in the two approaches; in the clinical perspective, it is patients who are the focus, whereas in the population perspective it is all people who are of concern.

Dr. S. was lecturing to a class of freshman medical students on the subject of quality of care. Halfway through the lecture, a student in the back of the room raised his hand and said: "Dr. S., I don't know why we need a lecture on the quality of care. We had to be pretty smart to get into medical school in the first place and we all must be about the best there is since we were accepted to *this* medical school, which is the best in the country. I don't think there is any question that the care we deliver will be of high quality, so why do we need a lecture on quality of care?"

Early Approaches to Quality of Care Assessment in the Ambulatory Sector

Historically, efforts to ensure the quality of care started in the hospital. As the scientific basis for medical practice developed, the adequacy of physician training became an issue. Early in the twentieth century, reforms instigated by Flexner in the United States made education the focus of activities aimed at improving the quality of medical practice. For the first half of the century, the only systematic attempts to improve quality of care consisted of the credentialing of medical schools and instituting state requirements that graduates pass a standardized examination before being licensed. Codman, a surgeon in Massachusetts, advocated evaluating the "end results" of hospital care by examining what happened to patients after they were discharged. Rebuffed by his colleagues, his approach lay dormant for over 50 years until revived as the "outcomes" movement in the last decades of the twentieth century.

At midcentury, interest in quality of care revived, but was primarily focused on inpatient care. Lembcke (1956), for example, used the medical literature to define "good care" for selected diagnoses and developed lists of criteria for judging care of patients with information in the medical record. He proposed that every hospital maintain an internal audit based on criteria from the literature. Later the Joint Commission on the Accreditation of Hospitals required that, as a condition for accreditation, hospitals have committees to conduct internal audits, but did not specify what had to be audited or require that deficiencies be corrected.

Cochrane's use of the new technique of the randomized controlled clinical trial (1972) opened the potential for evaluation of the effectiveness of interventions based on scientific evidence.

In the 1960s, attention shifted to quality assessment in ambulatory care because, in the United States, at least, publicly accountable agencies (government) began to pay for such care for certain population subgroups. Ensuring the quality of care is more of a challenge in the ambulatory setting than in the inpatient setting (Palmer, 1988). A hospitalization is a clear "episode" for which there exists a definable reason and which has a point of entry and a clear endpoint when the results of hospitalization can be described. The outcome is more clearly defined; patients either die or are discharged, and their status on discharge is relatively easily described. In the ambulatory setting, the "product" is difficult to define and even harder to measure.

In primary care, many problems of patients are so poorly understood that the nature of their course or progression is unknown. Therefore, it is difficult to determine what changes in conditions of patients are a result of therapy and what would have occurred in time without treatment. In contrast to inpatient care, contact with patients is limited to a few minutes at infrequent intervals. Therefore, health personnel are less able to observe changes in illness and have less control over the management of treatment than they have in the inpatient setting. The unit of care is often undefinable. Many health problems have an uncertain onset, and primary care physicians encounter illnesses at different stages in different patients. In addition, the resolution of health problems is usually gradual, without a clear endpoint, and some problems do not resolve at all but rather go through periods of waxing and waning. Time, rather than a visit, is a more useful unit of analysis for quality assurance in ambulatory than in inpatient care, although the appropriate period of time may be difficult to specify. Outcome measures that focus on levels of disability and mobility, as well as on physical and mental functioning, are at least as important as disease resolution and improvement in biological manifestations of illness. Measures that do not depend on specific diagnoses are part of the armamentarium because primary care considers the person foremost and the disease only as it influences the person.

Ambulatory care settings have been much more isolated from peer influence than in-hospital practice so that problems of quality may be more chronic and more ingrained than would be expected for hospital-based physicians. Furthermore, ambulatory data systems are not nearly as well developed as those in hospital care, despite major advances that have recently taken place. Ambulatory medical records are generally much less accessible and less complete than are hospital records.

These differences in ambulatory care complicate the challenges of quality assurance; approaches other than those used in hospitals are needed. In primary care, the challenges are even greater. The functions of primary care are sometimes to cure, but are more often to care for patients until their problems resolve, stabilize, or at least stop progressing. In either case, or even when neither is possible, making patients comfortable and able to function to the limits of their capacity challenge the primary care professional.

Methods for Assessing Ambulatory Care Quality: A Chronology

Early approaches to assessing the quality of care depended heavily on medical records; they also focused primarily on inpatient care, probably because these records were more accessible and more standard in format than those in ambulatory care. The techniques used by early investigators, however, are equally applicable to primary care. One technique uses "profiles of care" in which information on a variety of characteristics such as diagnosis, operations, laboratory tests, and consultations are abstracted from medical records and used to make comparisons among hospitals in a given area (Eisele et al., 1956). Another technique, the medical audit, relies on the a priori development of criteria for good care.

When government funding was instituted for certain segments of the population in the United States in the 1960s, medical record audits were mandated for government-funded ambulatory care service programs, and demonstration programs were supported to develop the procedures (Morehead and Donaldson, 1974). By and large, medical audit procedures were employed, although the choice of diagnoses differed from those used for inpatient care; common targets for medical audits included well-infant and well-child care, recognition and management of iron-deficiency anemia and asthma in children, hypertension, diabetes, and peptic ulcer in adults; high-risk pregnancies in obstetrics; and pelvic inflammatory disease or menopausal symptoms in gynecology. Aspects that were scrutinized included justifiability of the diagnosis, components of the physical examination, indicated laboratory or x-ray studies, acceptability of therapy, and follow-up procedures and visits.

Payne et al. (1984) used a similar technique in studies of the quality of care in five different types of facilities, which included gynecology, family medicine, internal medicine, and pediatrics. The five sites were a solo practice, two university teaching clinics, a fee-for-service multispecialty group practice, and a prepaid (capitated) multispecialty group practice. Ten conditions were chosen for review: periodic adult medical examinations, periodic gynecological examination, periodic pediatric medical examination, therapeutic use of drugs with major side effects, anemia, hypertension, chronic heart disease, vulvovaginitis, acute urinary tract infection, and chronic urinary tract infections. Criteria for good performance were set by physicians representing the five sites. These studies showed that (1) specialists performed better but only in their specialized area of training, (2) younger physicians performed better, and (3) board certification was not consistently related to good performance. A more recent study of practices in Canada confirmed the importance of residency training in family medicine in achieving good quality of care as assessed by medical record audit (for charting adequacy, preventive activities, assessment procedures, and prescribing of medications) (Borgiel et al., 1989).

The staging technique (Gonella et al., 1984) provides a method to characterize diseases according to how far they have progressed; the more advanced the stage, the less adequate prior care is assumed to have been. Judgements about adequacy of care are relative, depending on comparison of the stages of disease seen in one facility with those seen in another (Gonella et al., 1977).

The algorithm approach (Greenfield et al., 1981) is another technique suited to assessing the workup and management of problems as well as other aspects of care. In contrast to the other methods, the algorithm approach starts with the patient's problem rather than with the diagnosis. Flow diagrams start with a patient's problem (such as headache) and consist of a series of branchings depending on how subsequent questions from the patient's history and medical workup are answered.

In New York City, several hospital outpatient facilities incorporated this approach into ongoing care. The use of these specified directions for diagnosis and management of children with respiratory problems, acute otitis media, asthma, and gastroenteritis results in better documentation in the medical record, fewer nonindicated laboratory procedures, more appropriate antibiotic prescribing, and reduced overall charges for services. Improved management, as measured by more rapid and more complete resolution of symptoms in the facility, also was demonstrated, at least for asthma (Cook and Heidt, 1988).

In another approach, the *tracer* method (Kessner et al., 1973), patients are chosen from community surveys to detect individuals with certain types of problems. Their physician or physicians are identified, and their process of care is traced to determine the recognition, diagnosis, and therapy of the problem as well as the follow-up. Although this method is too costly and impractical for routine use, it could be carried out on a sample basis when combined with other surveys such as the ongoing National Health Interview Survey. In this way, the costs of initially identifying patients with problems could be obviated, leaving only those costs of follow up.

A similar approach was used on a large native Indian reservation in Arizona (Nutting et al., 1981, 1982). The process of care for each of nine conditions was traced from its prevalence in the community to screening procedures, diagnostic evaluation, treatment and monitoring, and the institution of ongoing management when needed. Not all conditions were suitable for surveillance at each stage; for example, only ongoing management was useful for seizure disorders. For most of the conditions (hypertension, prenatal care, infant care including immunizations, lacerations, streptococcal pharyngitis, and gonorrhea) at least three phases of care could be assessed. Systematic differences in performance among different health service units on the reservation were noted.

The advantage of tracer methods is their applicability to populations rather than only to patients in a facility; the assessment starts with the prevalence of a problem in the community and traces it through the processes of medical care to determine when and if poor quality of care exists.

Still another approach to improving quality of care starts with the assumption that it is impossible for physicians to recall all the information required to provide optimum quality of care. To surmount this problem, a computer provides reminders to do certain things under certain circumstances, for example, a reminder to order a laboratory test if a patient is taking a drug that causes electrolyte imbalance (McDonald, 1976).

Approaches to Assessing Quality of Primary Care

Most of the literature on quality of care, as defined and described above, has been focused on disease-oriented clinical performance and often even more narrowly on those aspects of care that reflect management of diagnosed ailments or on the prevention of some specific diseases predominately but not necessarily in primary care. As indicated by the definition provided above, the concept of "quality" is more appropriately viewed as a strategy that involves more than disease-focused prevention and management, particularly in primary care (which is inherently person focused). Four aspects are important in considering and evaluating *primary care services* from this broader perspective: resource capacity, services delivery, clinical performance, and health status assessments (Table 12.1).

1. Capacity for organizing primary care

Adequacy of resources for providing clinical care involves consideration of all of the aspects of structure as described in Figure 12.1, for example, the number of appropriately trained personnel for delivering primary care for the patients served, the number and type of facilities in which the services are provided, the adequacy of financing for primary care services and the range of services that they cover, arrangements to ensure accessibility, the adequacy of information systems for providing services and evaluating them, and the mechanisms of governance to ensure that facilities are designed and operated to meet population needs. Because most of these subjects are dealt with in other chapters of this book, they are not described further here.

In the United States, there are no governmental standards for organizing or providing primary care. The Joint Commission on Accreditation of Healthcare Organizations (1997), a private professional organization, historically accredited hos-

Table 12.1. Four Aspects Important to Quality of
Primary Care

Resource capacity
Services delivery
  Capacity
  Performance
Clinical performance
  Condition-specific
    Appropriateness
    Timeliness
    Adequacy
  Generic
Outcomes (health status assessment)
  Generic
  Condition specific
  Problem resolution

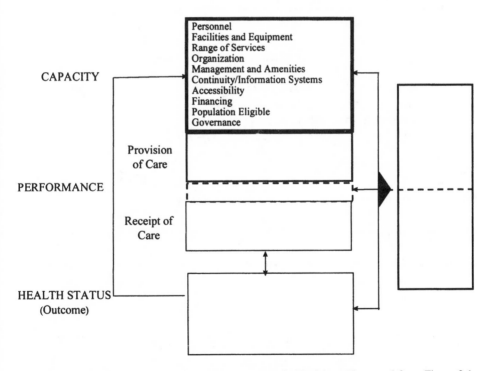

Figure 12.1. Quality of care. Capacity of system/facility/plan. Abstracted from Figure 2.1.

pitals and now conducts interviews and site visits of ambulatory care facilities for accreditation purposes. Various other approaches to quality assurance have been developed and employed by health facilities for their own purposes rather than accreditation. For example, the AmbuQual (Anderson et al., 1989) is designed to score 10 "parameters" of ambulatory care. These parameters address qualifications of the provider staff and support staff, mechanisms for achieving continuity of care, characteristics of information systems, patient risk management (quality control mechanisms), patient satisfaction, patient compliance, accessibility, appropriateness (services available), and cost of services (such as product monitoring), each weighted according to professional judgments of its relative salience in influencing health status. The system is designed primarily for internal assessments rather than for comparisons among facilities because both the method of collecting the data and ways of measuring them can vary from place to place. Furthermore, facilities can substitute the specific indicators with others that they believe more relevant to their situation.

Although there are many surveys of patients' satisfaction with various organizational aspects of their health care facility, such as ease of access and perceived competence of their practitioners, there have been few attempts to assess satisfaction in an objective way. An exception is a comparison of care provided in three managed care plans in a large western city of the United States (Borowsky et al., 1997). In this study, physicians were asked to rate various aspects of the capacity of their plan. The following are examples of the type of plan characteristics that physicians were asked to rate.

For personnel

Provides continuing medical education for physicians
Facilitates home nursing
Trains physicians to obtain authorization for care
Selects practitioners who do not overuse tests or procedures

For organization

Provides access to specialty care for patients who need it

For range of services

Usually includes needed care in the plan benefits
Includes mental health care

Management

Has effective reminder systems for preventive care
Provides enough time to see patients
Provides efficient authorization when needed
Authorization policies do not disrupt practitioner–patient relationships

Avoids providing conflicting information to patients and practitioners
Implements clinical guidelines

Financing

Avoids co-payments that interfere with seeking needed care

Information systems

Advises practitioner if patient
     Is receiving duplicate narcotics from different sources
     Needs preventive services
Provides profiles of care so that practitioners can compare their practices with
     others
Clearly communicates criteria used to evaluate practitioner performance
Uses fair and realistic criteria to judge practitioner performance
Provides high-quality educational material to patients about tests and procedures
     and about plan benefits

2. Services delivery component

This component focuses on the characteristics of services delivery that are important in achieving good primary care, as described in Chapters 7–11 and as noted
in Figure 12.2. Because the achievement of effectiveness and equity of health
services is dependent on a strong primary care system, the achievement of first-
contact care, longitudinality, comprehensiveness, and coordination is important in
assessing of the quality of services delivery in primary care. Evaluating the adequacy of primary care services involves both capacity and performance features of
the clinical facility or practices.

> Bob is a fourth-year medical student. During the first 3 weeks of his family
> medicine clerkship, he focused purely on medical problems. An elderly male patient
> suffering from end-stage chronic obstructive pulmonary disease tried repeatedly to
> get some reassurance and regularly asked Bob if he had a miracle with him that
> day. In the third week, the following exchange took place.
> Bob: Give me a call if you need me.
> Patient: I'm callin' you now.
> Bob: There's not a whole lot I can do.
> After the visit he commented: I'm going into radiology, medicine is too de-
> pressing.
> In the fourth week, the following exchange took place.
> Bob: If anything comes up, call me.
> Patient: What good can you do?
> Bob: We can talk
> Patient: That would be moral support.
> Bob: Sometimes moral support helps a lot.

In an early example of a study concerning children being seen in a tertiary
medical center, primary care pediatric practice was compared with office-based

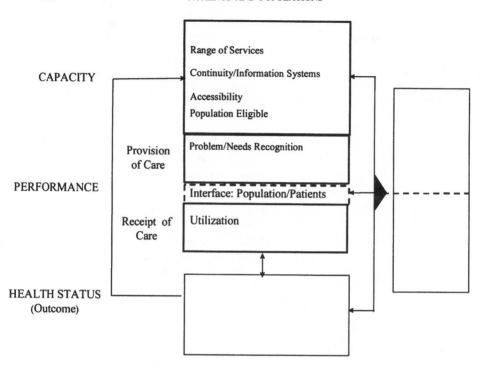

Figure 12.2. Quality of care. Services delivery assessment. Abstracted from Figure 2.1.

practices in the community to provide a basis for judging the relative adequacy of
performance with regard to achieving the ''longitudinality'' characteristic of primary care. In the facility under study, physicians kept encounter logs and patients
were asked four questions: Is this the child's first visit to the clinic? Did a doctor
from some place outside this hospital send you to this clinic? The last time this
child had a regular check-up, did the child go someplace else or come here? The
last time the child received medical care for a bad cold or flu, did the child go
someplace else or come here?

Answers to these questions served as a basis for categorizing encounters as
primary care, first-encounter care, specialized care, or consultative care. A score
was obtained and compared with scores obtained from office-based pediatric practices in the same community. The results of this evaluation indicated that the hospital clinic was equally as effective as office-based physicians in the extent of
provision of longitudinality of care (Wilson et al., 1989). In this study, the patient
was the unit of analysis, and the results were aggregated to characterize the clinical
facility.

Studies of the adequacy of services delivery in primary care settings can also
involve surveys of patients either in the facility or by taking a random sample of
users and contacting them by phone or mail. Parallel surveys can also be undertaken
of their practitioners or representatives of management of the facility or plan. When

practitioners and patients agree that there are inadequacies in services delivery, there is a clear case for modifying the organization of the resources. When they differ, it is necessary to explore the reasons for the discrepancies and to develop a mechanism that works toward resolving them to modify services delivery. The instruments for assessing adequacy of primary care are the same regardless of whether they are focused on patients or populations and are therefore described in Chapter 13.

3. Clinical performance

The third component of quality addresses the adequacy of the clinical component of service delivery, that is, the way in which health and health-related problems are met. Clinical performance measures are those in which the contribution of clinicians is identifiable (Conquest 1.0, 1996, p. 3). They may be focused on specific diseases or conditions or on more general aspects of people's health rather than on their specific disorder. The former are referred to as *condition specific* and the latter as *generic*.

Condition-specific measures of clinical performance. These may reflect preventive services, curative services, or rehabilitative services for specific diagnoses. Their adequacy involves first knowing if the services are appropriate given the current state of knowledge about indications for care, whether they are provided adequately or inadequately when they are indicated ("technical quality"), and their timeliness; services may be indicated and technically adequate but not provided at the optimal time. Figure 12.3 indicates that the aspects of the process that require consideration are recognition of problems and needs, diagnostic assessment, therapeutic interventions, and reassessments. Most of the vast literature on the quality of the processes of care addresses either the adequacy of the diagnostic process in arriving at the selected diagnosis or, even more commonly, the adequacy of the therapy given the presence of a diagnosis. But there is much more to the processes of care than this. Because most evaluations of the process of care start with the presence of a diagnosis, the entire process of diagnostic assessment, and particularly that aspect that addresses the adequacy of recognition of people's problems, is generally not considered.

An interesting study in a primary care setting provides graphic evidence of the variability in diagnostic assessment for 150 adults and children in three general practices presenting with the same complaint: abdominal pain. There were 15 different patterns of examination, nine different patterns of management, and 30 different diagnoses falling into five different types of diagnoses; an additional 36 diagnoses could be specified no more than "unknown" (21), "nonspecific viral" (9) or "other" (6) (Edwards et al., 1985). This study indicates how inadequate diagnostic assessments can be when they start with the diagnosis as the basis for assessing quality: They completely neglect consideration of the quality of care for those who present with a problem but do not necessarily receive a diagnosis for which quality of care is assessed.

The other aspect of condition-specific clinical performance, reassessment to

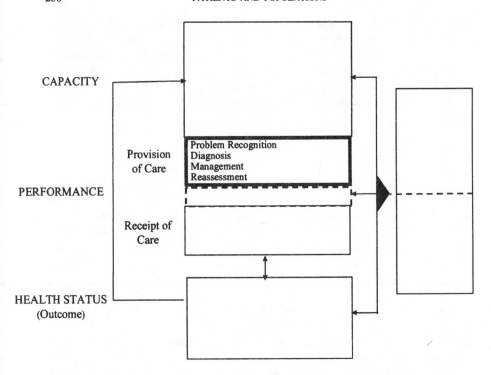

Figure 12.3. Quality of care. Clinical performance assessment. Abstracted from Figure 2.1.

ensure that expected outcomes have been achieved, has also been neglected. How-ever, its importance is increasingly recognized, largely through the development of approaches to determine whether practitioners have adequately monitored patients with chronic illnesses that require periodic follow up.

Adequacy of clinical performance at the facility or practice level is generally assessed using the conventional approaches developed over the past 50 years (as described earlier in this chapter).

Generic measures of clinical performance. Conventional condition-specific meth-ods are increasingly being supplemented with approaches that are less focused on diseases and more focused on patients' problems and on health viewed more broadly. Because this person orientation rather than disease orientation is more consistent with the focus of primary care, these generic approaches are especially relevant in the context of primary care. They are designated as generic because they do not relate to specific diseases, problems, or conditions, but rather apply to all patients regardless of their condition.

Louise was a 26-year-old student who was planning to specialize in family medicine. With considerable success, she sought to establish and maintain a doctor-dominated form of interaction in her home visits. Throughout her interview with patients she maintained her focus on strictly medical problems. When the patient asked for help, the response was medical.

In the following dialogue, Louise ignored the crucial item of information concerning the patient's sudden weight gain:

Patient: The more I try to get away from salt, the more I get. My wife gives me peanut butter with salt. I'm afraid I'll have to go to the hospital to get salt-free food.

Louise: Are you having trouble with your urine?

Patient: No, but it's uncomfortable. But what worries me is the salt.

As it turned out, but not evidently to Louise, long-standing animosity between the patient and his wife was exacerbated by his homebound condition and she was seeking retribution by giving him a high-salt diet, while he was helpless to do anything about it.

Table 12.2 shows the characteristics of an evaluation of a primary care clinic for adults (Barker et al., 1989). The practitioners in the clinic established a priori a level of performance that they considered appropriate. The performance of the primary care clinic was then assessed against these *absolute* standards.

Patients who were keeping an appointment for a follow-up visit were chosen for study if the follow-up visit took place within 6 months of the prior visit. Before the follow-up visit, records were reviewed to obtain all items of information from the prior visit. After the visit the records were again reviewed to ascertain recognition of the information.

The investigation showed that

- Recognition of problems identified at the index visit fell just short of the criterion level of 75%, but recognition was consistently better when the problem was on a problem list.
- Recognition of therapies that had been prescribed met the pre-set standards, but was better for major drugs (91%) and for minor drugs (70%) than for nondrug therapies (38%).

Table 12.2. Program Evaluation in a Primary Care Clinic for Adults: Aims and Mechanisms of Evaluation

Aims	Mechanism
Longitudinality	Patient identification with a specific doctor
Comprehensiveness	Knowledge of patient's social profile
	Recognition of psychosocial problems
	Attitudes toward/knowledge of preventive and psychosocial needs
Coordination	Recognition of information from visits elsewhere
Record keeping	Documentation of medications and compliance
	Problem lists/Problem-oriented medical record
	Preventive care
Communication skills	Review of videotapes
Quality of care	Control of hypertension

Adapted from Barker et al. (1989).

- Recognition of all tests scheduled at the prior visit (59%) did not reach the standards both for tests with abnormal results and for those with normal results.
- Recognition was also inadequate for intervening visits, both scheduled and unscheduled.

As a result of the evaluation, the clinic directors altered the encounter form to require the separate recording of all nondrug therapies as well as for intervening visits.

Another evaluation in the same clinic examined the recognition of patients' needs, as reflected by information in medical records (Kern et al., 1990). Sixteen items were used to assess recognition of needs: legibility, past medical history, presence of a problem list on the front sheet of the patient's medical record, completeness of the problem list, allergy history on front sheet, smoking and alcohol history on the front sheet, completeness of the social history on the front sheet, clarity of recording of functional status, and clarity of the medication regimen. Also assessed were recording of compliance, problem orientation of the visit notes, visit notes in SOAP format (see Chapter 16), use of a flow sheet for active problems, adequacy of care for active problems, documentation of patient education, and use of a flow sheet for preventive care.

Preventive care was assessed by the provision of diphtheria/tetanus vaccine within 10 years, pneumococcal vaccine in high-risk patients, yearly influenza vaccine in high-risk patients, rectal/prostate examination every 2 years in patients aged 45 years and above, stool occult blood examination yearly at age 45 years and above, cervical cancer screening at least every 3 years, physician breast examination yearly for patients aged 40 years and older, one serological test for syphilis, and one tuberculin test. The chart audit took place for 6 consecutive years and adequacy of performance was defined as recording of indicated procedures in at least 75% of the records; performance of less than 50% was considered a major inadequacy. Only 3 of the 26 items reached the standard of 75%; 15 had major deficiencies.

Improvements in performance occurred over the 6-year period. The items that showed the least improvement were documentation of functional status, patient compliance, patient education (both over 50% initially) and documentation of a few items of preventive care.

Generic measures of the processes of care were used successfully, in combination with condition-specific measures, in a comparison of the quality of care provided in different types of primary care facilities to the Medicaid population in the state of Maryland (Starfield et al., 1994). The condition-specific indicators were divided into three categories: access to primary care, technical quality, and appropriateness of care for several conditions or types of care—diabetes, asthma, and hypertension in adults (as well as routine adult care for people with these types of conditions) and asthma, otitis media, and well-child care in children. Access indicators (for all except routine care in adults) included visits for emergency services or hospitalization on the assumption that provision of accessible primary care should minimize these types of care. Technical quality indicators reflected current standards for procedures directed at medical diagnosis, treatment, and monitoring of patients with the specific conditions. Appropriateness indicators were those *not* indicated for patients with the conditions, for example, chest x-rays for people with an acute asthmatic attack. (One additional category of indicator, outcome, was represented by control of blood glucose among individuals with diabetes.)

The generic indicators were applied to all individuals, not only those with the particular conditions. They included the presence or absence of a problem list in the medical record, the presence of a medication list in the medical record, no recognition of visits to other practitioners (as reflected by no mention in the medical record of the visit or anything occurring in or from the visit), documentation of psychosocial problems (on the assumption that a finite proportion of patients should have a diagnosis of a psychosocial problem within 1 year if patients' problems are adequately recognized), and rates of hospitalization for ambulatory care–sensitive conditions (Chapter 14). In all, there were 21 indicators of the quality of care. Although not always statistically significant, there were differences in scores by type of facility for 19 of the 21 indicators. In 11 of the 19, patients receiving care in community health centers had the best scores, and in another 8 they had the second best. Patients receiving their primary care in hospital clinics had the worst scores for 10, and physicians in office-based practice had the worst scores for 9.

One type of generic approach to assessing performance in delivering services has received little attention in assessment of the quality of the processes of care: inappropriate or contraindicated tests, procedures, or different modes of therapy.

The potential for such an approach was demonstrated in a study in 133 physician groups who were part of a large health maintenance organization (HMO) in California. The medical or quality assurance director of each group was asked about the ways in which quality was monitored in the group. Indicators addressing possible overuse, and the percentage of groups that monitored them were cesarean section deliveries (92%), outpatient prescription drugs (70%), and angioplasties (57%). (In comparison, between 50% and 66% monitored possibly underused preventive services such as childhood immunizations, screening mammograms, follow up of abnormal Papanicolaou tests, influenza vaccination in the elderly, and patients aged 42–64 years with a physician visit in most recent 2 years.) Less frequent monitoring of potential underuse included follow-up treatment after myocardial infarction, annual retinal examination for diabetic patients, and annual follow-up examination for asthmatic patients; at least the first of these has been demonstrated to improve outcomes (Kerr et al., 1996).

> A man in his 50s went to his doctor complaining of chest pain. As part of a thorough examination, the physician examined the man's prostate. He though it felt abnormal and ordered a test to check for prostate cancer. The results were normal so the patient was referred to a cardiologist, who, without consulting the family physician, ordered the same test. When the results were reported as "borderline," the cardiologist ordered another; this time the results were abnormal.
>
> The cardiologist referred the patient to a urologist, who ordered a fourth test; the results were normal. The urologist booked the patient for ultrasound and biopsy of the prostate. The patient refused to undergo these procedures, as their necessity was unclear to him.

For example, many conventional studies of the quality of care examine the extent to which indicated (effective) medications are provided, but few examine the extent to which nonindicated medications are prescribed. A summary of 33 articles evaluating appropriateness of prescribing found a 43% overall rate of inappropriateness, well over half of which concerned an inappropriate indication for the medication or inappropriate choice of drug (Einarson et al., 1989). More information is available on inappropriate prescribing for the elderly; in general, about 5% of all elderly in a population received an inappropriate prescription in 1 year (Lexchin, 1998). In the United Kingdom, Spain, and Italy, improving quality of prescribing in general practice is an explicit objective. In the United Kingdom, for example, a system known as PACT (Prescribing Analysis and Costs) is a computerized review of all medications prescribed in general practice. It is used to help set budgets for prescribing, examining reasons for prescribing variability, and developing indications for prescribing specific medications. The system contains markers of both good and bad prescribing (Majeed et al., 1997).

There is, unfortunately, no available compendium of inappropriate indications for specific medications. The best current source of such information is contained in the book *Worst Pills, Best Pills* (Wolfe et al., 1993), which pertains particularly to the elderly. Because inappropriate prescribing is likely to be the most common evidence of compromised quality of care, it should be an important part of quality assessment and assurance efforts. Buetow et al. (1996) convened 10 experts to suggest criteria for appropriateness of prescribing. These experts suggested 19 indicators that were collapsed into five categories: invalid indication; inappropriate choice of drug, contraindication, or duplication; overdosing or excessive duration; inadequate drug history or inadequate prescription; and inadequate monitoring. Then, 62 studies were reviewed for appropriateness of prescribing. Although there is no assurance that the studies that were reviewed are representative of practices in general, they did cover the range of drugs prescribed for common long-term conditions such as asthma, hypertension, insomnia, and anxiety. The indicators that were developed are applicable to review of medical records or other practice-based information systems and could serve as an initial basis for monitoring the adequacy of performance as viewed generically. Another useful strategy examines actual prescribing against standard guidelines for prescribing, as represented by approved indications. Although the absence of such an indication could reflect the inadequacy of the standard (resulting from unavailable scientific evidence) rather than poor quality of care, consistent failure to adhere to standards could identify clinical performance at high risk of being inadequate. Such an approach has been used with Food and Drug Administration standards as the criteria (McKinzie et al., 1997).

The importance of inappropriate prescribing is highlighted by a study conducted by the Centers for Disease Control and Prevention (CDC). This study concluded that more than one-third of the prescriptions for antibiotics written annually are not needed. These include all the antibiotic prescriptions for the common cold; one-third of the antibiotics for children with a cold and middle ear fluid with no ear pain, eardrum inflammation, or fever; half of the antibiotics for sore throats (those not caused by streptococcal infections); 80% of the antibiotic prescriptions for bronchitis (those not due to a few specific infections or in patients without severe lung disease); and half of the antibiotic prescriptions for sinusitis (those without facial pain or swelling in the first 10 days of symptoms) (CDC, unpublished data, 1997).

Another important but neglected focus of generic clinical performance concerns the timely provision of information to patients. Although there is a wealth of anecdotal evidence of delay in providing information to patients, particularly concerning the results of tests, there has been no systematic attention either in research or in quality assessment activities to this aspect of care. The challenges to assessment involve consideration of information transfer to the practitioner, the recognition of the information by the practitioner and the length of time for it to occur, and the timeliness of and mechanism for conveying the information to patients. Thus this aspect of quality of performance is intimately tied to the coordination function of primary care and deserves much more attention than it has received in the past.

4. Outcomes of care component

Although health status and ''outcomes'' are conceptually equivalent, the former generally is used when the focus of interest is on populations or subpopulations whereas the latter generally applies to situations where clinical care of a group of patients is being assessed. Historically, outcomes of care were initially measured by mortality rates because they were generally available whereas other aspects of health status were not. The International Classification of Diseases (ICD) brought international standards to the effort to develop methods of coding causes of death so that they could be compared from area to area and country to country with regard to the occurrence of avoidable mortality. Decades later, a focus on morbidity was added to the armamentarium of clinical quality assessment. Revisions of the ICD added sections enabling the coding of conditions that were rarely if ever lethal; in the 1980s, a more primary care–friendly adaptation known as the International Classification of Health Problems in Primary Care was developed (World Organization of National Colleges, Academies, and Academic Associations, 1979). Clinical assessments of outcomes of care often focus on changes in morbidity as manifested by trends in laboratory values that are thought to reflect disease severity or stage. Growing recognition of the additional importance of physical function to health and well being of populations led to the development, by the World Health Organization (1980), of the International Classification of Impairments, Disabilities and Handicaps.

New ways of thinking about outcomes followed from the relatively recent realization that illness as defined by biophysiological characteristics is an inadequate representation of both impact of illness on people and impact of health services. The new focus is on the extent to which they are able to perform the activities of their lives and on health-related quality of life (HRQOL). Functional status is the representation of morbidity on the daily life of people. Thus, it considers how illness affects the way in which people perceive themselves and how it influences their professional and personal activities. HRQOL is a broader concept, taking into account how people feel about their lives and what they are able to do. In practice, most HRQOL assessments are forms of functional status assessments in which there is an overall score rather than a profile representing scores on different "domains" of health. One advantage of an overall score is that the health of different populations (as represented by the overall score) can be simply and directly compared.

Figure 12.4, which is adapted from work done by Wilson and Cleary (1995), represents the types of concerns that are involved in these approaches to outcomes assessment, and Figure 12.5 specifies the components of a multidimensional approach to health status assessment that has been used to characterize the health of youth aged 11–17 years, as described later in this chapter.

These new methods are particularly relevant to the assessment of outcomes of primary care. Because only a small minority of people in primary care settings will die within any period of time, mortality is inappropriate as a measure of outcome unless there is a suspicion of very poor care or malfeasance leading to death from iatrogenic causes. Levels of morbidity are also less relevant in primary care than in other levels of care (especially specialty care) because illnesses in primary care practice often cannot be attributed to specific diagnoses. However, morbidity can be an outcome of primary care in three types of instances: complications resulting from inappropriate therapy, inadequate efforts at prevention of preventable conditions, and inadequate recognition of the existence of problems that then progress to later stages of disease. Functional status or HRQOL measures, in contrast, are *particularly relevant to primary care* because of their focus on people rather than on their diseases.

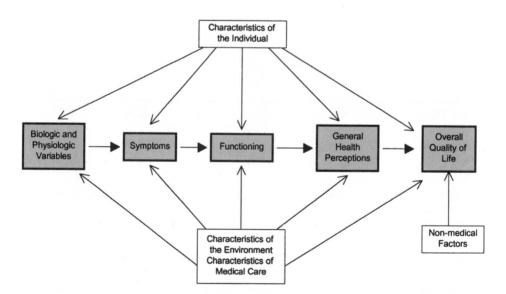

Figure 12.4. Relationships among different measures of patient outcomes. Adapted from Wilson and Cleary (1995).

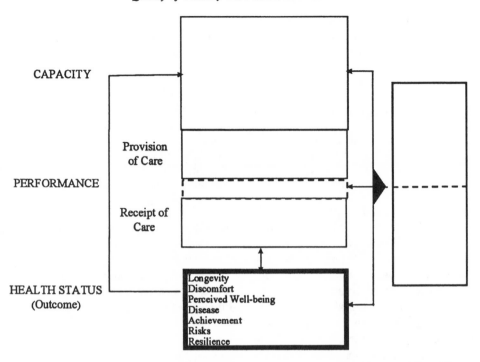

Figure 12.5. Quality of care. Outcomes/health status assessment. Abstracted from Figure 2.1.

Thus, outcomes assessments, like clinical performance assessments, can be viewed as condition specific (related to particular conditions) or generic (not specific to any particular condition).

Condition-specific approaches. Condition-specific measures are the conventional armamentarium of outcomes assessment in patients, consistent with the predisposition of physicians and other health care professionals to gravitate to measures of outcome that reflect improvement in disease status. Because of their relative ease of measurement and compatibility with biophysiological phenomena, the measures employed often are in the realm of laboratory results or findings on physical examination. Typical examples are blood levels of hemoglobin A1c as a manifestation of the effectiveness of control of diabetes or serial measurements of blood pressure as an effect of hypertension control. Because most preventive care is targeted at avoiding the occurrence of particular diseases (e.g., coronary artery disease in the case of cholesterol levels; cervical cancer in the case of Pap smears; breast cancer in the case of mammography screening), the adequacy with which people receive the procedures is sometimes a proxy for outcomes in cases where the linkage between receipt of responsiveness and the subsequent occurrence of the disease is strong. The U.S. Preventive Services Task Force (1996) document *Guide to Clinical Preventive Services* provides the scientific basis for establishing the linkage, as well as current evidence on the justification for implementing these interventions.

Generic approaches to outcomes assessment.

> I thought I was going to learn a lot about diabetes. I learned a lot more than I thought I would. This is very corny, but I learned a lot more about how you really have to look at the whole person because in fact management of diabetes is what I am supposed to learn, but it was such a minor part of the life of my patient. It was dealing with how it had limited her which I wasn't expecting. . . .
>
> D., a fourth year medical student just finishing her family medicine clerkship

The generic approach to outcomes assessment is the same regardless of whether the focus is on patients or populations; it views health status or outcomes as separate from any particular disease or type of disease and involves collection of information directly from patients. Information encompasses behaviors such as limitations on activities of normal daily living (work, play, school attendance, physical activities required for living independently) and may also encompass activities that are thought to reflect a propensity to enhance future health (e.g., physical fitness and prowess, or to reduce it, e.g., smoking and other substance abuse, bicycle or motor-bike riding without helmets).

For the most part, the measures are used individually; days of work missed due to acute illnesses, the extent to which there are limitations on ability to carry out normal daily activities or major activity, or percentage of the population that exercises regularly are examples. More recent additions to the armamentarium of these types of measures are batteries of questions that combine several items into a scale representing physical, emotional, and social functioning. The range of types of functional status or HRQOL scales is wide. These tools have been tested for their psychometric integrity (reliability and validity), and they generally provide scale scores in various domains (Stewart and Ware, 1992; Feeny et al., 1995; Landgraf and Abetz, 1996; McDowell and Newell, 1996).

The generic approach to assessing outcomes is particularly appropriate in monitoring for the adverse effects of interventions, where the nature of the effect might not be predictable. Several studies have shown that between 4% and 16% of patients admitted to the hospital suffer harm from treatment, as much as half of which is preventable (Brennan et al., 1991; Wilson et al., 1995). The frequency of adverse effects from outpatient management, particularly from adverse effects of medications, is unknown, but is likely to be substantial. Only generic measures of outcome would be able to detect the majority of problems due to medications that have no currently known specific side effect.

The potential for person-focused assessments of health status has been enhanced by the development of the concept of profiles. In contrast to more conventional health status assessments, which treat different aspects of health (e.g., physical, social psychological) as separate and independent, profiles make it possible to characterize health according to a pattern across domains of health. For example, the Child Health and Illness Profile—Adolescent Edition (CHIP-AE) (Starfield et al.,

1995) has six domains of health: Satisfaction with health status, Discomfort, Risks, Resilience, Disorders, and Achievement. Thirteen combinations of the first four of these domains comprise a taxonomy of profiles of health, and adolescents fall into one and only one of these profiles depending on whether their scores on the different domains are in the highest, middle, or lowest third of the distribution of the score distributions in populations of adolescents. Outcomes of services can be assessed according to whether individuals or populations of individuals move to profiles that characterize better health, move to worse profiles, or stay the same (Starfield and Riley, 1998; Riley et al., 1998). These profiles have been tested among adolescents in schools, in settings for the treatment of acute illnesses, in specialty clinics for the management of chronic illnesses, and among youth with mental disorders; they show how both expected and unexpected weaknesses and strengths of individuals are manifested and interact. Tools such as these are particularly suited to assessment of the impact of interventions targeted to improving the constellation of health, particularly in groups of individuals. Viewing health from the perspective of individuals rather than from the perspective of various aspects of individuals provides opportunities to tailor primary care in a way that is more appropriate to this constellation of needs, which are likely to interact in ways that make more conventional categorical approaches to interventions ineffective.

Resolution of patient-specific problems as a measure of outcome. An underused and potentially useful generic approach to assessing outcomes of certain aspects of clinical care is based on the idea that people seek care for perceived needs or problems and that effective care should ameliorate these problems. "Needs" or "problems" that people bring to health services include indicated preventive care, treatment for acute self-limited problems, and amelioration of the manifestations of chronic illness, impairments, disability, and handicap. The International Classification of Problems in Primary Care (see Chapter 16) makes it possible to categorize and code these needs and problems. Approaches to implementing this aspect of outcomes assessment require careful documentation of problems when they are presented to health professionals, either as the "chief complaint" or "reason for visit" or when they occur in the course of the patient–professional interaction. High-quality medical care should generally lead to resolution of problems or, at least, to reductions in their intensity, severity, or manifestations regardless of what the problem is or how it is manifested. Therefore, this approach elicits information from patients after a period of time that is considered adequate to achieve a response. Differences among health professionals, or among different health care facilities or systems, in the time to achieve amelioration of health problems can reflect differences in the effectiveness of services provided. In an early application of this method (Mushlin and Appel, 1980) patients were contacted several days after a visit to determine whether they still had symptoms, how much limitation of activity they were experiencing, and their understanding of the cause and prognosis of their problems. When these outcome assessments were compared with standard medical record audits, the assessments were more sensitive than the audits in detecting substandard care, at least as measured against overall expert judgements of the quality of care.

The Duke Severity of Illness Checklist (Parkerson et al., 1993) is a similar approach except that it judges severity of symptom levels, complications, prognosis without treatment, and expected response to treatment from the physicians' viewpoint. It was tested by 22 volunteer family physicians in nine countries for adult patients. The practitioners believed the tool to be useful primarily for older patients and those with chronic health problems (Parkerson et al., 1996). Because it requires a visit for the judgement to be made, it would not be useful to judge improvement for patients without a return visit unless it were adapted for telephone or mail use.

When systematically employed in facilities, this approach draws attention to the deficits or, conversely, successes in management of patients' problems or by particular practitioners or types of practitioners and thus serves as ongoing "continuing education" focused on outcomes of care. It also provides a basis for generating clinical research to determine why expected levels of problem resolution or amelioration have not occurred and for setting goals for improvement.

What Are the Determinants of High-Quality Care?

Studies have shown that there are three major determinants of quality of care: length of the physician's experience in managing the particular problem under study, the nature of the organization in which the physician works, and the length of postgraduate training in the subject being studied (Palmer and Reilly, 1979). More recent studies suggest the continuing salience of the characteristics of the organization. For example, capitated arrangements in which physicians work in groups rather than independently have better outcomes in role and physical functioning for depressed patients (Rogers et al., 1993). However, the widening of focus to more generic, person-focused aspects of care may make characteristics such as the nature of the physician–patient interaction much more important.

It is clear that different types of approaches to assessing quality may not always lead to the same conclusions. Services that excel in achieving the characteristics of primary care may not always provide the best quality of care as measured by specific clinical interventions and are not guaranteed to achieve the best outcomes at all times. Conversely, services of technically high quality may not be mirrored by adequate performance in modes of delivering services and may not always reach those in greatest need of them. Although little is known about the correlation in judgement of quality of care as measured by the different approaches, we know that judgements of the quality of care that are based on assessment of outcomes do not always agree with judgements made on the basis of a review of the characteristics of the care provided, even in the same patient. For example, Brook et al. used information from medical history questionnaires, screening examinations, insurance claims, and interviews with physicians and patients to judge the quality of ambulatory care (not necessarily limited to primary care physicians) for three chronic conditions in adults and four chronic conditions in children. Expert judges suggested that although approximately 70% of patients were receiving suboptimal care according to predetermined criteria, better care would result in more than minor improvement in fewer than half of the patients (Brook et al., 1990). Several studies have shown that practitioners who are substandard in one set of judgments are not necessarily substandard in others (Palmer et al., 1996; Brook et al., 1996).

If the purpose of medical care is to improve health and relieve suffering, assessments that directly address these characteristics are of greater value than assessments of the procedures that are intended to achieve them. A large-scale study conducted in physician practices in several cities in the United States provides an interesting example of the employment of both condition-specific and generic determinants of outcome for individuals with four chronic conditions (hypertension, noninsulin-dependent diabetes mellitus, congestive heart failure, and depressive disorder) seen in different types of organizational arrangements and by different types of practitioners, including family physicians, general internists, cardiologists, endocrinologists, psychiatrists, clinical psychologists, and other mental health professionals (Tarlov et al., 1989). Outcomes included clinical measures such as blood pressure; physical, social, and role functioning of patients in everyday life; patients' perceptions of general health and well being; and patients' satisfaction with treatment (Tarlov et al., 1989). There were no systematic differences either by type of organization or by physician specialty in the quality of care as measured by outcomes among patients with diabetes or hypertension (Greenfield et al., 1995). However, elderly and low-income patients (with any of the four conditions) had worse physical health outcomes than patients in health systems characterized by capitated payments; conversely, non-poor chronically ill elderly patients had better physical health outcomes under these circumstances. No consistent differences were found for mental health outcomes. The authors hypothesized that patients with fewer health and social resources are less able to take advantage of new types of health settings than individuals with greater resources (Ware et al., 1996). Other analyses from the study showed that, for the patients in general, most differences in functioning and in well being were not explained by the presence of specific chronic medical conditions in patients (Stewart et al., 1989). Moreover, all health status measures were worse if patients also had depressive symptoms (Wells et al., 1989). Thus it is clear that assessment of the outcomes of care for particular health problems must take into account both patient factors, such as the presence of other conditions ("co-morbidity") experienced by patients, and characteristics of the setting in which care is provided.

Because quality of care is a "successive re-definition of the unattainable," it will undoubtedly be impossible to set absolute normative standards for quality that will be invariant over time. At any one time, however, accreditation and regulatory agencies might want to set minimum standards in each of the four areas of quality assessment. Currently the main application of quality assessment is for internal management wherein individual facilities examine their quality according to goals they set for themselves and then devise mechanisms to improve what appear to be substandard performance. The advent of competitive managed care, in which quality is often defined as successful marketing and adequate return of profit to investors, has prompted efforts to develop quality assessments that are somewhat more consistent with the components of quality described in this chapter. Consistent with the "competitive" focus of the current health services system, adequacy of quality is derived primarily from comparisons among facilities and plans rather than directed at achievement of pre-set standards.

Sources of Information for Clinical Performance Measurement

Since primary care is now often covered by insurance plans or by governmental programs, in most countries, albeit incompletely in some (such as the United States), quality of care is a growing concern of these "third-party" payers. To maintain surveillance over quality of care, these agencies now require or encourage the collection of information for quality assurance activities. Some of this information comes from the same claims forms that are used for billing purposes, in places where fee-for-services payments are still common. One problem, however, is that information tied to billing purposes is sometimes displayed in a way to maximize reimbursement rather than to reflect clinical care. Computerized encounter forms serve the same purposes as claims forms and have similar limitations, that is, uncertain accuracy and completeness. However, they generally contain more information than claims forms, are easier to use, and are usually more available.

Judgements about the adequacy of clinical care may be based on either standards set a priori or by comparisons with other facilities. When facilities are compared, differences in quality of care are often difficult to interpret because they might be due to differences in the quality of care or in the extent or severity of illnesses in the populations in the various facilities. This is a matter of concern whether the focus of attention is on specific diseases or on generic measures of quality. In either case, comparisons of quality between two facilities are interpretable only if the extent of morbidity of their populations is the same. Some populations may be sicker than others and require a different type of care even for the same condition under investigation. If the degree of morbidity is not the same, the same criteria for adequacy of care may be inappropriate and cannot be applied to both.

Another approach to characterizing co-morbidity in ambulatory settings is the Ambulatory Care Group (ACG) method. This method characterizes patients according to the types of combinations of their health problems over a period of time rather than at individual visits. The ACG system predicts both concurrent and subsequent use of services and also distinguishes populations known to have different burdens of morbidity. It can also be used to examine reasons for variability in practice patterns across geographic area and among primary care physicians (Starfield et al., 1991). Techniques such as the ACG method are required in assessing the quality of care to characterize co-morbidity so that comparisons among different facilities can be more accurately interpreted.

Medical records are the most common source of data for research studies of quality of care that deal with clinical performance. Because of the expense of reviewing individual paper-based records, this approach is generally impractical for use in ongoing quality monitoring activities. Computerized claims forms or encounter summaries provide a more practical source; computerized medical records should eventually make the monitoring of quality of care more accurate and feasible.

However, since claims forms are easily available, they are a logical source of information about several aspects of the quality of care. Data from claims forms, especially when linked to "beneficiary files" to obtain information on demographic characteristics, are useful for quality improvement activities in enrolled populations (such as Medicare recipients in the United States) or patients in a health care organization. Weiner et al. (1990) recommended 60 indicators of quality that employ information obtained from claims forms and that one can use to monitor quality of care in such populations. Some are condition specific, whereas others are generic.

One category of these indicators reflects preventive care; it includes procedures that prevent disease and screening procedures that detect illness at an early stage. An example of this category is the percentage of children or adults receiving recommended immunizations at the appropriate time. Examples of criteria for screening include the percentage of persons receiving a recommended test (such as Pap test for cervical cancer for adult women) and the percentage of infants receiving the recommended number of well-child visits.

A second category of indicators concerns the adequacy of diagnostic procedures. One example is the percentage of persons with a given diagnosis who received the recommended diagnostic tests; another is the overuse of procedures or medications that needlessly expose individuals to iatrogenic problems.

A third category concerning treatment and management has the largest number of suggested indicators. Among the indicators are those concerning medications, such as rates of patients receiving inappropriate or contraindicated medications, and those concerning therapeutic surgical procedures, such as the rates of tonsillectomy or the extent to which criteria for performing tonsillectomies are met. Also included within this category are follow-up procedures, such as the percentage of patients lost to follow up. Indicators of continuity or of access to care include such elements as the percentage of all visits without a referral made to the patient's primary care practitioner, the percentage of patients who experienced delays in receiving indicated procedures, and the percentage of visits for emergency care that earlier contact with the primary care practitioner could have averted. Specialty referrals is another type of indicator in this category; one example is the percentage of patients over age 50 years with insulin-dependent diabetes who should be regularly examined by an ophthalmologist.

Yet another category of indicators are those that reflect general functions such as rates of hospitalization, re-admissions, and sentinel conditions, which should never or only rarely occur under conditions where health services are adequate. Additional categories of indicators reflect inpatient care that may be under the control of the primary care physician.

High or low rates of occurrence of indicators are the basis for interpreting some of the criteria, while for others the occurrence of specific untoward events signals a problem with quality. Indicators such as preventive activities reflect desirable events while others represent undesirable ones.

When information about quality of care is obtained from claims forms, it is limited to users of services who are not necessarily representative of those eligible to receive care. Another limitation of claims records is the relative paucity of information concerning details of clinical care. Furthermore, and like medical records, they are of little use in assessing the extent to which practitioners adequately recognize the concerns that bring patients to seek care. This latter facet of care is not yet a feature of most quality improvement activities. Assessment of other aspects of diagnosis, therapy, and reassessment requires additional information from sources other than claims forms to identify the nature and source of the lack of quality so that remedial steps can be undertaken. Surveys of people randomly selected from enrollee rosters (patient lists) rather than from among those who inconsistently make visits are more suitable for assessments that involve people eligible for care who do not use it, as well as those who do.

Monitoring of the outcomes of care resulting from clinical performance is challenging because data are often unavailable. Outcomes of care are infrequently reported in medical records and are never reported in claims forms or encounter records. Because of this gap in information, the National Committee on Vital and Health Statistics recommends that data on functional status be routinely reported for each encounter. Because there is no well-accepted method to assess functional status either in patients or in populations, implementation of this recommendation will not occur until the field of outcomes assessment advances further.

Several other techniques can facilitate quality improvement in the primary care setting. Periodic and systematic telephone surveys of patients are sources of information concerning patients' judgements of their care and their responsiveness to medical therapies. Patients can be questioned about the time it took for abatement of symptoms and about difficulties they may have had with the prescribed treatment. Employment of simulated patients on a regular basis can provide information about the way care is delivered and whether patients had concerns about any aspects of it.

As clinical facilities assume responsibility for defined populations over a period of time, the orientation of these patient-based approaches will move toward clinical performance measures that are more oriented toward people than to their diseases. The impetus toward this is explicitly recognized by the work of FAACT (Foundation for Accountability), a nonprofit organization established in 1995 by several consumer organizations, government agencies, and private employers in the United States to ensure the availability of reliable information to make health care decisions (Lansky, 1996). Although its aim is to expand interest to categories of concern other than specific diseases, so far its work has been limited to breast cancer, diabetes, major depressive disorder, and some health risks such as tobacco or alcohol use. It operates by compiling and analyzing existing information, which is reviewed by both expert and consumer groups for importance and relevance in three areas: ''steps to good care'' (aspects of care that serve as quality markers), consumer satisfaction with care received, and ''results'' (impact of care as determined by functional status and avoidance of preventable use of health services such as hospitalizations). For example, the diabetes portfolio consists of 11 quality measures; 6 rely on information from yearly patient surveys, and the remainder come from claims records, laboratory records, or medical records. Of the 11 measures, 6 relate specifically to "results," and 3 are outcome measures derived from yearly surveys, including how well patients cope with their disease, smoking cessation, and ability to maintain daily activities. FAACT's intention is to ultimately make its work more generic by developing a wide variety of portfolios that encompass the full range of health characteristics in enrolled populations.

Policy Issues Related to Improving Clinical Performance in Primary Care

Two mutually reinforcing types of approaches currently form the basis for development of policy concerning quality assurance activities: evidence-based medicine and self-improvement strategies.

Evidence-based medicine (Sackett and Rosenberg, 1995) is an approach to improving condition-specific quality of care through the use of information derived from systematic reviews of scientifically sound studies, usually randomized controlled clinical trials. Where such evidence exists, it provides a powerful tool for thinking about what is appropriate and inappropriate in delivering clinical services regardless of whether the service is primary care or specialty care. Unfortunately, the vast majority of medical practices have evolved without systematic evidence to justify them. This is particularly the case in primary care, since most medical research has been conducted in large medical centers dominated by specialists other than primary care physicians. The thesis that "evidence" should be the basis for medical practice provides the rationale for the development of clinical guidelines for the practice of medicine. Although thousands of guidelines have been developed by many professional, regulatory, and research groups, they are often inconsistent with each other even when they address the same clinical topic, thus indicating the incompleteness of the evidence on which they are based (Merritt et al., 1997; Dixon, 1990). Moreover, it is not clear that scientifically sound evidence could ever hope to inform the majority of clinical decisions that must be made in everyday medical practice. Randomized controlled clinical trials, by their very nature, require that the conditions of research be carefully specified and controlled, thus precluding the inclusion of populations who do not meet the criteria for inclusion in the trial. Thus, these trials often include relatively small subsets of people with the problem under study—a situation further exacerbated by failure of otherwise eligible people to volunteer to participate in the trial. Thus, many of the findings of randomized controlled clinical trials are not generalizable to ordinary practice with a variety of different types of populations because the conditions that had to be fulfilled in the trial are not applicable.

The extraordinary variability among people and their illnesses, which results from both biological and social characteristics (including the extent to which patients agree with and adhere to practitioners' recommendations), is further complicated by the variability that exists in the conditions of practice and the characteristics of practitioners. Assessment of the quality of care for the purpose of improving it must take into account the reasons for failure to meet standards or expectations. Is the problem with the practitioner's qualifications, training, or knowledge? Is it a result of the conditions under which the practitioners work, which limit the extent to which they can implement indicated practices or encourage inappropriate practices? Is it because their patients differ sufficiently in personal or disease characteristics from the typical patient so as to make the criteria for adequacy of practice inapplicable? The other limitation of judgments about the quality of care based on evidence is that they are useful only for the particular subject under evaluation, which is usually a specific problem or diagnosis. As noted above, there is no evidence that judgments about substandard care for one medical practice are generalizable to others.

Because of the myriad difficulties in specifying scientifically sound criteria for quality, many approaches to assessing and improving quality are based on the idea that techniques for self-assessment will, in the long run provide a better basis than insisting on adherence to norms for clinical care (Berwick, 1989; Oxman et al., 1995). These approaches take advantage of the variability across practitioners and facilities to examine possible reasons for differences in practices and thereby gain insight into which are associated with better outcomes or equivalent outcomes at lower costs than others. This approach to quality improvement has many advantages, among them allowing attention to the full range of clinical activities rather than being limited to only those for which scientific evidence has been accumulated. It also provides greater incentives for practitioners to make changes in their practice because the evidence is more immediately relevant to their own practices. It does, however, require the existence of good information systems deriving from patient care experiences (see Chapter 16) and concerted efforts of practitioners to systematically review these experiences as an important focus of their own continuing education.

One of the major challenges to clinical training is incorporating components that encourage the development of self-assessment skills. To accomplish this, training programs need a well-developed information system with which trainees can periodically and systematically review their own performance and compare it with that of their peers and with evidence in the scientific literature.

In general, the approach based on careful review of scientific evidence is most useful in identifying aspects of care that are *not* indicated. In contrast, the approach based on reviews and comparisons of practitioners' own experiences, especially when they are compared with those who have similar types of practices, holds greater promise for improving the overall level of services, especially in primary care where the basis for scientific decision-making is especially lacking. This type of approach has been called *population-adjusted clinical epidemiology*. It requires that practitioners join forces in a collaborative effort to systematically document the characteristics of their patients, their problems, the interventions provided to them, and their outcomes. It has its origins in the recognition that most of the evidence used to support "evidence-based medicine" comes from highly selected and unrepresentative populations. Experience, both nationally and internationally, with practice-based research networks has demonstrated how wrong conventional wisdom, based on research in academic medical institutions, often is.

The major challenge for the future of quality of care is relevance to population needs, not doctor's interests. In some provinces in Canada, particularly in Manitoba, administrative data from claims forms is successfully used to examine quality of care from a population perspective (Roos et al., 1995). There are many examples of its usefulness in highlighting clinical inadequacies; the approach can find much wider applicability in all health systems that collect claims on encounter forms with standard ways of collecting and recording clinical information. These approaches form the bases for many national strategies to assess and improve clinical performance.

National Approaches to Clinical Performance Assessment and Improvement

Growing concern about the utility of many medical interventions and the increasing availability of techniques to document and compare them in different settings and geographic areas has stimulated the development of activities on a scale larger than that in individual clinical settings.

For many years professional groups have engaged in setting standards for a variety of medical interventions against which professional practice patterns can be judged. For example, the American Academy of Pediatrics publishes a series of manuals that provide guidance to practitioners as to the components of well-infant and well-child care and the appropriate diagnosis and management of infectious diseases in children (American Academy of Pediatrics, 1997a, b). In addition, large health insurers, such as the Blue Cross and Blue Shield Associations, have been attempting to set guidelines for the appropriateness of many diagnostic and treatment services.

The Dutch College of General Practitioners has developed 45 guidelines for general practice; they cover such problems as noninsulin-dependent diabetes, sprained ankle, otitis media, and sleeping disorders (Grol et al., 1995). A comparable effort is underway in New Zealand, (Hadorn and Holmes, 1997), although with less emphasis on primary care problems than is the case for the Dutch guidelines. National governments also have become involved in setting guidelines. In the United States, the Agency for Health Care Policy and Research had an organized program of guidelines development that was abandoned in the mid-1990s, at least partly because of the many nongovernmental efforts.

In the United States, the advent of managed care has generated concern that emphasis on cost control will lead to the sacrificing of quality of care. In response, the National Committee on Quality Assurance (a group mostly sponsored by large employers and managed care organizations) proposed a set of performance measures for health plans to consider adopting and sharing their results. Five main categories comprise the HEDIS Health Employers Data and Information System (HEDIS): quality, access and satisfaction, utilization, plan management, and finance. The quality measures are primarily related to clinical performance measures of the processes of care for selected conditions and preventive care primarily using approaches to quality assessment that were devised in the 1960s for evaluating care in government-sponsored health facilities. HEDIS provides manuals containing directions for selection of patients for study and for ways of compiling and reporting data. For most indicators, minimum enrollment periods are required for patients to be eligible for inclusion in the quality analyses. Therefore, HEDIS is strictly a patient-oriented (rather than a population-oriented) approach to quality assessment because people who are not enrolled in the plan, who disenroll from it for any reason (including dissatisfaction or poor outcomes), or who recently joined it or left it are not represented in the quality assessments (National Committee on Quality Assurance, 1997).

In the United States, the government also plays a role in ensuring the quality of care. Government-mandated quality assurance activities were vested in "peer-review organizations" (PROs) created by Congress in 1982 to oversee health services paid for by federal funds (primarily those for the elderly in the form of Medicare). The Health Care Financing Administration, an agency of the Department of Health and Human Services, has the responsibility for these activities. The most recent program is entitled "Health Care Quality Improvement Initiative" (HCQII); it operates through peer-review organizations (organizations of physicians in local areas) to employ explicit, national uniform criteria to examine patterns of care and outcomes (Jencks and Wilensky, 1992). These PROs focus primarily on persistent differences between the observed and achievable rather than on occasional or unusual deficiencies in provision of care. The PROs are to identify the deficiencies and call them to the attention of practitioners, who are then to conduct more intensive study to identify causes and propose solutions. However, this program is primarily focused on in-hospital care and thus has limited application to primary care.

The Bureau of Primary Health Care (1995), an agency of the Health Resources and Services Administration in the U.S. Department of Health and Human Services, developed recommendations for measuring the impact of health centers on reducing gaps in health status between minority or low-income populations and the U.S. populations as a whole. The focus is primarily on assessing capacity, performance, and outcomes for a set of specific clinical conditions, including diabetes, cardiovascular disease, breast cancer, cervical cancer, infectious diseases (such as acquired immunodeficiency syndrome and gastroenteritis in children), immunization rates in children, asthma, and pregnancy outcomes. Table 12.3 provides examples of the approach for two of these conditions. In addition, it also includes assessment of hospitalization rates for ambulatory care–sensitive conditions (see Chapter 13).

A combination of governmental and nongovernmental groups has produced a "report card" for mental health services, some of which could be expected to be part of primary care services. This effort is the result of collaboration between consumer groups, the mental health advocacy groups, and the Substance Abuse and Mental Health Services Administration of the Department of Health and Human Services (Mental Health Statistics Improvement Program, 1966). It focuses on the consumer perspective, on outcomes, and on people with serious mental illness. Its activities are organized in domains, including access, appropriateness, outcomes, and prevention.

The ORYX system of the Joint Commission on Accreditation of Healthcare Organizations, a nongovernmental accrediting organization in the United States, is

Table 12.3. Examples of Measures for Assessing Primary Care

Condition	Structure	Process	Intermediate Outcomes	Ultimate Outcomes
Breast cancer	Presence of mammography services (directly or by referral)	Referral for/receipt of mammograms Follow-up of abnormal mammograms Aggressiveness of treatment	Downward shift in stage of disease over time	Reduced mortality
Immunization	Availability of age-appropriate immunizations Tracking system Reminder system	Fewer missed opportunities	Receipt of antigens in timely manner (can choose multiple endpoints)	Reduced incidence of immunizable disease

Source: Bureau of Primary Health Care (1995).

aimed at integrating the use of outcomes assessments and clinical performance measurement into the accreditation process. Facilities and health plans are permitted to choose among 60 systems for assessing care. None of these systems are capable of addressing the quality of primary care services delivery, however. Their focus is primarily (56 out of the 60) on clinical performance measurement; 17 also include assessment of "satisfaction," which might, in part, contain information relevant to achievement of the cardinal features of primary care. Because the vast majority of these instruments are proprietary and not in the public domain, their specific content, method of interpreting data, and applicability to primary care in particular are not known (Joint Commission on Accreditation of Healthcare Organizations, 1997).

None of these U.S. efforts at formulating national approaches to ensuring quality of clinical performance focuses specifically on primary care services. However, the centrality of primary care is implicitly recognized in all of them, and the indicators that have been chosen represent issues that are generally primary care issues. Moreover, they represent a spectrum of concerns about capacity and organization of services, clinical performance, and, to a much more limited extent, outcomes of care. The vast majority of indicators in the HEDIS effort concern capacity and performance, such as the performance of indicated procedures for specific conditions. Immunization rates among users of managed care organizations represent an attempt to include at least one measure of outcome under the assumption that immunization is directly related to avoidance of certain diseases. The Mental Health Statistics Improvement Program (1966) indicators involve outcomes assessment in 43%, process assessments in 23%, and assessment of structural characteristics in 34%.

Other countries are developing methods to improve quality of primary care services. For example, in Spain, the National Health Service (Insalud) sends to general practitioners each month a list of the medications they have prescribed, their cost, and indications of the quality of their prescribing as measured by the prescription of drugs with no known therapeutic valve (e.g., medications for varicose veins). These lists are personalized to the individual, with the age–sex considerations based on the physician's patient list, and are accompanied by a summary of the combined performances of the practitioners in the same health center so that practitioners can compare their performances with overall performance in the health center.

Public disclosure of information is an approach that may be increasingly used, especially in health systems with a market orientation. The assumption is that providing consumers with information about the performance of health care organizations will help them select physicians or facilities whose performance is better, thus encouraging all physicians and facilities to provide superior service. This potential approach was recognized by the Institute of Medicine (1981), which stated that "the feasibility and effectiveness of publicizing instances of persistent poor quality by individual practitioners should be explored." The Institute of Medicine also endorsed the policy of disclosing to the public all information except that which identifies specific patients. It recommended that information be available in a form in which institutions are identified and in a form that identifies specific physicians by unbreakable code but not name. It also recommended that quality-review organizations disclose to a requesting patient or patient-designee any data about the patient that has been derived from a medical record abstract (Institute of Medicine, 1981). Further development of approaches to specifying appropriate outcomes of ambulatory care could lead to public disclosure concerning this aspect of the performance of primary care physicians as well. It should be recognized, however, that this is a very indirect approach to improvement of quality of care because it would operate only through expressed widespread dissatisfaction leading to disenrollment in health plans with consequent incentives for plans to determine the reasons for the dissatisfaction.

Better information systems now are able to overcome many of the earlier difficulties in obtaining data on quality of care. New integrated health organizations are more likely to have information systems that are relatively accessible and relatively complete, at least as compared with records in most offices of individuals or small groups of physicians. Practices and plans that now involve patients in decision-making or in an advisory capacity could also develop prototypes for consumer participation in quality assurance. Primary care organizations with defined populations might also experiment with techniques to combine clinical and population-oriented measures to provide an improved basis for planning and policy formulation.

Thus, current attempts at assessing and ensuring the quality of care by accrediting bodies are beginning to move away from earlier foci on structural and performance characteristics to a focus on outcomes of care, to involving physicians in reviewing their own performance relative to others, and to involving patients not only in judging their own care but also as active participants making use of increasing amounts of data about quality of care to inform their own choices about care-seeking. Ethical principles demand consideration of autonomy, beneficence, malfeasance, and justice in health service delivery. The traditional concerns of effectiveness, efficiency, appropriateness, acceptability, and access primarily address autonomy and beneficence. More attention to inappropriateness will address the issue of malfeasance. Finally, a focus on evaluating the extent to which services are provided where they are most needed will bring attention to issue of justice, a conventionally neglected area of consideration in quality of care endeavors. Because a major limitation of all of these assessments is availability of data to support them, their success will depend heavily on forward movement in the development of methods to obtain information from practice-based information systems, from people themselves, and, ultimately, from community-based information systems that enable health facilities to move from a strictly patient focus to a population focus.

References

American Academy of Pediatrics. Guidelines for Health Supervision. 3rd Ed. Elk Grove Village, IL: American Academy of Pediatrics, 1997a.

American Academy of Pediatrics. Report of the Committee on Infectious Diseases. 24th Ed. Elk Grove Village, IL: American Academy of Pediatrics, 1997b.

Anderson J, Benson D, Schweer H, Gartner C, Jay S. AmbuQual: A computer-supported system for the measurement and evaluation of quality in ambulatory care settings. J Ambulatory Care Manage 1989; 12:27–37.

Barker L, Starfield B, Gross R, Kern D, Levine D, Fishelman B. Recognition of information and coordination of ambulatory care by medical residents. Med Care 1989; 27:558–62.

Berwick D. Continuous improvement as an ideal in health care. N Engl J Med 1989; 320: 53–6.

Borgiel A, Williams JI, Bass M, Dunn E, Evensen M, Lamont C, MacDonald P, McCoy JM, Spasoff R. Quality of care in family practice: Does residency training make a difference? Can Med Assoc J 1989; 1035–43.

Borowsky S, Davis M, Goertz C, Lurie N. Are all health plans equal? JAMA 1997; 278: 917–21.

Brennan TA, Leape LL, Laird NM, Hebert L, Localio AR, Lawthers AG, Newhouse JP, Weiler PC, Hiatt HH. Incidence of adverse events and negligence in hospitalized patients. Results of the Harvard Medical Practice Study I. N Engl J Med 1991; 324(6): 370–6.

Brook R, Kamberg C, Lohr K, Goldberg G, Keeler E, Newhouse J. Quality of ambulatory care: Epidemiology and comparisons by insurance status and income. Med Care 1990; 28:392–410.

Brook R, McGlynn E, Cleary P. Measuring quality of care. N Engl J Med 1996; 335:966–70.

Buetow S, Sibbald B, Cantrill J, Halliwell S. Prevalence of potentially inappropriate long term prescribing in general practice in the United Kingdom, 1980–95: Systematic literature review. BMJ 1996; 313:1371–4.

Bureau of Primary Health Care. Consensus Conference of Health Status Gaps of Low-Income and Minority Populations. Bethesda, MD: U.S. Department of Health and Human Services, Health Resource and Services Administration, 1995.

Cochrane A. Effectiveness and Efficiency: Random Reflections on Health Services. London: The Nuffield Provincial Hospitals Trust, 1972.

Conquest 1.0. A *C*omputerized *n*eeds-oriented *qu*ality measurement *e*valuation *sys*tem. (for

DHHS AHCPR) (R. Heather Palmer and colleagues). President and Fellows of Harvard College©, February 1996.

Cook CD, Heidt J. Assuring Quality Out-Patient Care for Children: Guidelines and a Management System. New York: Oxford University Press, 1988.

Dixon A. The evolution of clinical policies. Med Care 1990; 28:201–20.

Edwards MW, Forman WM, Walton J. Audit of abdominal pain in general practice. J R Coll General Practitioners 1985; 35:235–8.

Einarson T, Segal H, Mann J. Drug utilization in Canada: An analysis of the literature. J Soc Admin Pharm 1989; 6:69–82.

Eisele C, Slee V, Hoffman R. Can the practice of medicine be evaluated? Ann Intern Med 1956; 44:144–61.

Feeny D, Furlong W, Boyle M, Torrance G. Multi-attribute health status classification systems. Pharmacol Econ 1995; 7:490–502.

Gonella J, Cattani J, Louis D, McCord J, Spirka C. Use of outcome measures in ambulatory care evaluation. In Giebink G, White N, Short E (eds): Ambulatory Medical Care-Quality Assurance 1977. La Jolla, CA: La Jolla Science Publications, 1977.

Gonella J, Hornbrook M, Louis D. Staging of disease: A case-mix measurement. JAMA 1984; 251:637–44.

Greenfield S, Cretin S, Worthman L, Dorey F, Solomon N, Goldberg G. Comparison of a criteria map to a criteria list in quality-of-care assessment for patients with chest pain: The relations of each to outcome. Med Care 1981; 19:255–72.

Greenfield S, Rogers W, Mangotich M, Carney M, Tarlov A. Outcomes of patients with hypertension and non-insulin–dependent diabetes mellitus treated by different systems and specialties. Results from the medical outcomes study. JAMA 1995; 74: 1436–44.

Grol R, Thomas S, Roberts R. Development and implementation of guidelines for family practice: Lessons from the Netherlands. J Fam Pract 1995; 40: 435–9.

Hadorn D, Holmes A. The New Zealand and priority criteria project. BMJ 1997; 314:131–4.

Hart JT. The inverse care law. Lancet. 1971; 1(696):405–12.

Institute of Medicine. Access to Medical Review Data. Washington, DC: National Academy Press, 1981.

Jencks S, Wilensky G. The health care quality improvement initiative: A new approach to quality assurance in Medicare. JAMA 1992; 268:900–3.

Joint Commission on Accreditation of Healthcare Organizations. ORYX: The Next Evolution in Accreditation. Chicago: Joint Commission on Accreditation of Healthcare Organization, 1997.

Kern D, Harris W, Boekeloo B, Barker, Hoegeland P. Use of an outpatient medical record audit to achieve education objectives: Changes in residents' performances over six years. J Gen Intern Med 1990; 5(3):218–24.

Kerr E, Mittman B, Hays R, Leake B, Brook R. Quality assurance in capitated physician groups: Where is emphasis? JAMA 1996; 276:1236–9.

Kessner D, Kalk C, Singer J. Assessing health quality—The case for tracers. N Engl J Med 1973; 288:189–94.

Landgraf JM, Abetz LN. Measuring health outcomes in pediatric populations: Issues in psychometrics and application. In Spilker V (ed): Quality of Life and Pharmacoeconomics in Clinical Trials. 2nd Ed., Philadelphia: Lippincott-Raven, 1996.

Lansky D. Foundation for Accountability (FAACT): A consumer voice on health care quality. J Clin Outcomes Manage 1996; 3:54–8.

Lembcke P. Medical auditing by scientific methods. JAMA 1956; 162:646–55.

Lexchin J. Improving the appropriateness of physician prescribing. Int J Health Serv, 1998; 28:253–67.

Majeed A, Evans N, Head P. What can PACT tell us about prescribing in general practice? BMJ 1997; 315:1515–9.

McDonald C. Protocol-based computer reminders, the quality of care and the non-perfectibility of man. N Engl J Med 1976; 295:1351–5.

McDowell I, Newell C. Measuring Health: A Guide to Rating Scales and Questionnaires. New York: Oxford University Press, 1996.

McKinzie J, Wright S, Wrenn K. Pediatric drug therapy in the emergency department: Does it meet FDA-approved prescribing guidelines? Am J Emerg Med 1997; 15:118–21.

Mental Health Statistics Improvement Program. Consumer-Oriented Mental Health Report Care. Rockville, MD: Department of Health and Human Services, April 1966.

Merritt TA, Palmer D, Bergman D, Shiono P. Clinical practice guidelines in pediatric and newborn medicine: Implications for their use in practice. Pediatrics 1997; 99:100–14.

Morehead M, Donaldson R. Quality of clinical management of disease in comprehensive neighborhood health centers. Med Care 1974; 12:301–15.

Mushlin A, Appel F. Testing an outcome-based quality assurance strategy in primary care. Med Care 1980; 18(5)suppl:1–100.

National Committee on Quality Assurance. Health Employer Data and Information System. Washington, DC: National Committee on Quality Assurance, 1997.

Nutting P, Burkhalter B, Dietrick D, Helmick E. Relationship of size and payment mechanism to system performance in 11 medical care systems. Med Care 1982; XX:676–90.

Nutting P, Schorr G, Burkhalter B. Assessing the performance of medical care systems: A method and its application. Med Care 1981; 19:281–96

Oxman A, Clarke M, Stewart L. From science to practice. Meta-analysis using individual patient data are needed. JAMA 1995; 274; 845–6.

Palmer RH. The challenges and prospects for quality assessment and assurance in ambulatory care. Inquiry 1988; 25:119–31.

Palmer RH, Reilly M. Individual and institutional variables which may serve as indicators of quality of medical care. Med Care 1979; 18:693–717.

Palmer RH, Wright E, Orav EJ, Hargraves JL, Louis T. Consistency in performance among primary care practitioners. Med Care 1996; 34:SS52–66.

Parkerson GR Jr, Bridges-Webb C, Gérvas J, Hofmans-Okkes I, Lamberts H, Froom J, Fischer G, Meyboom-de Jong B, Bensten B, Klinkman M, de Maeseneer J. Classification of severity of health problems in family/general practice: An international field trial. Fam Pract 1996; 13:303–9.

Parkerson GR Jr, Broadhead WE, Tse CK. The Duke Severity of Illness Checklist (DUSOI) for measurement of severity and comorbidity. J Clin Epidemiol 1993; 46:379–93.

Payne B, Lyon T, Neuhaus E. Relationships of physician characteristics to performance quality and improvement. Health Serv Res 1984; 19:307–32.

Riley AW, Green B, Forrest CB, Starfield B, Kang M, Ensminger M. A taxonomy of adolescent health: Development of the adolescent health profiles. Med Care 1998 (in press).

Riley AW, Forrest CB, Starfield B, Green B, Kang M, Ensminger M. Reliability and validity of the adolescent health profile-types. Med Care 1998 (in press).

Rogers W, Wells K, Meredith L. Outcomes for adult outpatients with depression under prepaid or fee-for-service financing. Arch Gen Psychiatry 1993; 50:517–25.

Roos N, Black C, Roos L, Tate R, Carriere K. A population-based approach to monitoring adverse outcomes of medical care. Med Care 1995; 33(12 suppl):s127–38.

Sackett D, Rosenberg W. The need for evidence-based medicine. J R Soc Med 1995; 88: 620–4.

Starfield B, Powe N, Weiner J, Stuart M, Steinwachs D, Scholle S, Gerstenberger A. Costs versus quality in different types of primary care settings. JAMA 1994; 272(24):1903–8.

Starfield B, Riley A. Profiling health and illness in children and adolescents. In Drotar D (ed): Measuring Health-Related Quality of Life Assessment in Children and Adolescents: Implications for Research and Practice. Mahwah, NJ: Lawrence Erlbaum and Associates, 1998. pp 87–106.

Starfield B, Riley AW, Green BF, Ensminger ME, Ryan SA, Kelleher K, Kim-Harris S, Johnston D, Vogel K. The adolescent CHIP: A population-based measure of health. Med Care 1995; 33(5):553–6.

Starfield B, Weiner J, Mumford L, Steinwachs D. Ambulatory care groupings: A categorization of diagnoses for research and management. Health Serv Res 1991; 26(1):53–74.

Stewart A, Greenfield S, Hays R, Wells K, Rogers W, Berry S, McGlynn E, Ware J. Functional status and well-being of patients with chronic conditions: Results from the medical outcomes study. JAMA 1989; 262:907–13.

Stewart A, Ware J. Measuring Functioning and Well-Being—The Medical Outcomes Approach. Durham: Duke University Press, 1992.

Tarlov A, Ware J, Greenfield S, Nelson E, Perrin E, Zubkoff M. The medical outcomes study: An application of methods for monitoring the results of medical care. JAMA 1989; 262:925–30.

U.S. Preventive Services Task Force. Guide to Clinical Preventive Services: Report of the U.S. Preventive Services Task Force. 2nd Ed. Baltimore, MD: Williams & Wilkins Co., 1996.

Ware J, Bayliss M, Rogers W, Kosinki M, Tarlov A. Differences in 4-year health outcomes for elderly and poor chronically ill patients treated in HMO and fee-for-service systems. Results from the medical outcomes study. JAMA 1996; 276:1039–47.

Weiner J, Powe N, Steinwachs D, Dent G. Applying insurance claims to assess quality of care: A compendium of potential indicators. Qual Rev Bull 1990; 16:423–38.

Wells K, Stewart A, Hays R, Burnam A, Rogers W, Daniels M, Berry S, Greenfield S, Ware J. The functioning and well-being of depressed patients: Results from the medical outcomes study. JAMA 1989; 262:914–9.

Wilson IB, Cleary PD. Linking clinical variables with health-related quality of life. A conceptual model of patient outcomes. JAMA. 1995; 273:59–65.

Wilson M, Weiner J, Bender J, Bergsstrom S, Starfield B. Does a residents' continuity clinic deliver primary care. Am J Dis Child 1989; 143:809–12.

Wilson R, Runciman W, Gibber R, Harrison B, Newby LL, Hamilton J. The quality in Australian health care study. Med J Aust 1995; 163:458–71.

Wolfe S, Hope P-E. Worst Pills, Best Pills II. 2nd Ed. Washington, DC: Public Citizen Health Research Group, 1993.

World Health Organization. International Classification of Impairments, Disabilities, and Handicaps. Geneva: World Health Organization, 1980.

World Organization of National Colleges, Academies, and Academic Associations of General Practitioners/Family Physicians. ICHPPC-2, International Classification of Health Problems in Primary Care. 2nd Ed. Oxford: Oxford University Press, 1979.

— 13 —

Evaluation of Primary Care: A Population View

The subjects for evaluation of primary care systems and programs are the same as those for study of the quality of care with the exception that they are focused on populations rather than on patients. These subjects include resource capacity and services delivery as well as outcomes (health status of the population). However, sources of data are different and the focus is on the general population rather than on an enrolled population or a population of users of facilities. In the context of general populations, two aspects merit special consideration: adequacy of primary care services delivery and evaluation of outcomes that are particularly in the province of primary care. (The important issue of equity is addressed in Chapters 14 and 18.)

At the very least, evaluation of primary care systems and programs requires attention to the attainment of the features of primary care. In addition, primary care systems can be evaluated or compared according to the impact they have on health status of populations and people. This chapter opens by providing a summary of the attributes of primary care that can be evaluated and the sources of information that can be used in evaluations. It then turns to specific examples of four different approaches: from an educational perspective, from a practice population perspective, and from community population perspectives. The remainder of the chapter addresses evaluation of impact of primary care on designated conditions in the population.

Assessing the Attainment of Primary Care Characteristics

Three types of characteristics are involved in evaluating primary care programs: (1) unique features of primary care, (2) derivative features, and (3) essential but not unique features. Most evaluations of primary care will do more than focus on the unique features of primary care (first contact, longitudinality, comprehensiveness, and coordination) by incorporating their assessment with those of related characteristics. Table 13.1 summarizes the various characteristics, the type of in-

Table 13.1. Measuring the Attainment of Primary Care

Feature	Type of Information Needed	Source(s) of Information
The Unique Features		
First contact care	Accessibility of facility	Program design
	Access to care	Survey
	Use of facility as place of first contact	Claims forms/audit/interview
Longitudinality	Definition of eligible population	Age–sex register
	Knowledge of patient and patient's social milieu	Record audit/interview
	Use of the regular source of care	Claims/record audit/interview
	Length and strength of relationship with patients regardless of type of need for care	Interview/survey
Comprehensiveness	Spectrum of problems dealt with	Program design
	Primary and secondary preventive activities	Claims forms/record audit
	Recognition and management of health problems (including mental health) in the population	Program design (e.g. home visits)/record audit/interview
	Percentage of people managed without a referral	Clinical information systems
Coordination of care	Mechanisms for continuity	Program design (personnel; records)
	Recognition of information from prior visits	Record audit
	Recognition of referral/consultation visits (occurrence and results)	Program design/record audit
Essential but Not Unique Features		
Medical record format	Problem list	Record unit
	Completeness of the medical record	Record audit
Continuity of care	Percentage seeing same practitioner on follow up	Information systems
Practitioner-patient communication	Content/quality of interaction	Observation/tape recording
Clinical quality of care	Qualifications of personnel	Program design
	Adequacy, appropriateness, and timeliness of services	Record audit, observation, interview, simulated patients
Advocacy for patients	Awareness of community resources	Interview (personnel)
	Use of community services	Record audit/interview
Derivative Features		
Family centered	Knowledge of family members	Record audit/interview
	Knowledge of health problems of family members	Record audit/interview
Cultural competence	Arrangements to meet special needs associated with cultural characteristics	Program design (governance)
	Provision of special services to address cultural needs	Survey
Community oriented	Mechanisms to achieve knowledge of community health needs	Awareness of community statistics/interview
	Participation in community activities	Interview
	Community involvement in practice	Program design

formation needed to assess them, and the sources of information required for the purpose. To provide more detail than is given in Table 13.1, a brief description of each of the characteristics follows.

The unique features of primary care

Chapters 7–11 provided the theoretical bases for these characteristics of primary care and for ways of assessing them. The mechanics of assessment require specification of the characteristic as well as sources of and methods to obtain information.

First contact care. Three areas of information are required for assessment. The first involves accessibility of the facilities, which can be determined from the program design. Special characteristics of the evaluation involve (1) hours of availability, (2) accessibility to public transportation, (3) provision of care without requirements for payment in advance, (4) facilities for the handicapped, (5) after-hours arrangements, (6) ease of making appointments and waiting time to appointments, and (7) absence of language and other cultural barriers.

The second area of information concerns the people's experiences with access to care. This can be determined by interviewing patients or populations for their views of the temporal, spatial, organizational, or cultural characteristics as noted in the preceding paragraph.

The third area of information concerns the actual use of the facility as a place of first contact. Such information is obtained by interviewing patients and by auditing the medical records or claims forms to determine the place of visit for newly experienced problems or for health needs.

Longitudinality. Achievement of longitudinality requires that both patients and practitioners know they have a mutual relationship. This is generally achieved by some form of enrollment by the patient and the maintenance of a patient list in the practice. The mutual relationship can be tested by confirming that members of the enrolled population indeed know the place responsible for their care and that a patient list does exits. Assessment of longitudinality demands a knowledge of the patients in the program and their social milieu. This can be learned by interviewing patients and physicians and by examining the record for important information about them. Special characteristics to be considered are social history and exposures, work history and exposures, housing, diet, health history, family history, and genetic profile. Special characteristics to be determined from patients are identification with the regular source of care and experiences with the long-term relationship.

The regular source of care can provide information to evaluate longitudinality. Interview of patients for regularity of use for non-referred care and for their reports about the person-focused aspects of their interactions with practitioners are the key elements. Specific areas concern the degree to which patients always use the primary care source for visits including disease management, management of signs and symptoms, administrative purposes (need for certification of illness and health), test results, preventive care, need for and return from consultation or referral, and prescriptions for medications or other therapies. Characteristics of their interaction should focus on those aspects that are especially relevant to primary care: mutual understanding and appreciation of those aspects of the person that are related to their health overall.

A third type of information required for evaluation of longitudinality involves the length of relationship between a patient and a practitioner apart from specific disease management. Interviewing patients and examining the record can supply this information.

Comprehensiveness of care. Several types of information are needed for assessment. The first involves the range of activities the system is designed to handle. Such information can be determined by examining the adequacy of personnel, facilities, equipment and the supporting services. Specific areas for consideration include the ability to provide care for short-term, long-term, and recurring illnesses; health education; minor surgery; mental health; and referral to ancillary services. In particular, the primary care facility should be equipped to recognize and manage *all* common health problems in its population, regardless of their type.

A second type of information involves the performance of activities related to meeting the needs of the population. These include indicated primary and secondary preventive activities such as immunizations, health education, and indicated screening procedures as well as activities directed at detecting and managing health problems in the community served. They can be ascertained from medical records and claims forms.

A particularly relevant challenge involves recognition and management of problems existing in the population. Such information is available from the medical record, by interview of patient and physician, and from program design, such as the ability to make a home visit when one seems advisable. There are several techniques for evaluating this characteristic. For example, they include the rate of recording of diagnoses of the major conditions in each age group and determining whether it conforms with known rates in the population served; adequacy of recognition of conditions in comparison with the results of standard screening inventories administered to patients; and use of home visits for suspected social determinants of illness (allergies, poor heating conditions, poor sanitation, hazardous substances, and environments). A useful prototype for assessment concerns the recognition of psychosocial problems, which should achieve levels commensurate with the extent of their existence in the population.

A fourth way to examine comprehensiveness is to examine rates of referral. Where they are high, this may suggest lack of comprehensiveness for one or more categories of health needs.

Coordination of care. The first area to be examined is the mechanism for continuity. The program design and personnel records will supply this information. To be taken into consideration are continuity of practitioner or team, ready availability of records, and ease of retrievable information. Second, one should examine the record for recognition of information from prior visits. A third item of information concerns referrals for consultation or for ongoing care. This can be learned from the program design and record audit. Special characteristics are the use of an organized system for referral and for retrieval of information concerning the results of referral and documented recognition of the results of referrals.

The derivative features of primary care

A high level of achievement of the unique and of the essential qualities of primary care results in three additional aspects called *derivative features*. They are "family centeredness," "cultural competence," and "community orientation." Both theoretical and empirical analyses support this designation as "derivative."

Family centeredness results when the achievement of comprehensiveness provides a basis for considering patients within their milieus, when the assessment of needs for comprehensive care considers the family context and its exposure to health threats, and when the challenge of coordination of care confronts the limitations of family resources.

Family centeredness is evaluated by interviewing family members and by comparing the information with either interviews of physicians or with information from the medical record.

Knowledge of family members is evaluated by interviewing family members and by comparing the information with other interviews with physicians or information from the medical record. Areas of particular interest include awareness of intrafamily communication and support and an appreciation of family resources (including its educational levels and financial means) for dealing with patient's health problems.

A second aspect of family-centeredness requires a knowledge of the health problems of family members. This information can also be obtained by interviewing patients and physicians and by examining the record. Knowledge about the patterns of illness in families can shed light on possible mechanisms of etiology and response to therapy.

Cultural competence involves recognition of the special needs of subpopulations that may not be in the mainstream because of ethnic, racial, or other special cultural characteristics. If comprehensiveness, particularly the aspect of it that relates to problem recognition, is well achieved, these special needs should be recognized and addressed in designing the range of services and how well they are applied. Evaluation requires determining whether these are arrangements to identify the existence of special cultural needs and the extent to which special populations perceive their special needs as being met.

Community orientation, the third derivative feature, results from a high degree of comprehensiveness of general care. All health-related needs of patients occur in a social context; recognition of these needs often requires knowledge of the social context. Patients may not realize that they need health services either because they lack knowledge about the importance of a preventive strategy or because they do not realize that a problem has a medical basis or might be amenable to medical interventions. An understanding of the distribution of health characteristics of the community and of the resources available in the community provides a more extensive way of assessing health needs than an approach based only on interactions with patients or with the families of patients.

Evaluation of community orientation requires three types of information. The first is a knowledge of the health needs of the community, obtainable by interviewing physicians and comparing their responses with community statistics. Areas that might be examined are awareness and use of morbidity and mortality statistics, health surveys including disability levels as well as illnesses, and school or work absence rates. A second type of information is the extent to which practitioners become involved in community affairs, a facet ascertainable by interviews. Specific characteristics include knowledge about available social networks and support systems, including recreational, religious, political, or philanthropic resources. A third type of information involves the extent to which the practitioner involves the community in practice-related issues, such as provision for a community or patient advisory council or periodic surveys of patient satisfaction and suggestions for improvement.

Psychometric analyses of data from consumer questionnaires indicate that both family centeredness and cultural competence are related to comprehensiveness. Community orientation is too poorly achieved in most practice settings to examine its unique integrity or derivative character (Cassady et al., 1998). As discussed in the next chapter, this is a major challenge for primary care health systems.

The essential but not unique features of primary care

Several characteristics are important in primary care, although their importance is not limited to it; they are important in specialty care as well as in primary care. They include a responsibility to be organized and efficient in providing care; to understand, advise, and guide patients; and to provide advocacy for patients when it is needed. These characteristics are important at *all* levels of care.

In assessing the aspects of primary care that are essential but not unique to it, five areas merit investigation. They are (1) adequacy of medical records, (2) continuity of personnel, (3) practitioner–patient communication, (4) quality of care, and (5) advocacy for patients. Each one has its particular type of information source for information and its method for evaluating the characteristic.

Adequate records. Every record should contain an updated problem list that includes new problems and deletes resolved ones. Information concerning the problem list can be obtained from the medical record or from a computerized printout.

The format of the encounter notes also yields relevant information. Each facility may have its own style, including updated medication and allergy lists, preventive care or laboratory flow charts, timely entry of the results of pertinent laboratory tests or referrals, or a problem-oriented format for the encounter notes. Evaluation of all of these requires record audits, although these may need supplementation by other information in order to judge whether the record is complete.

As the components of records become more standardized (U.S. Department of Health and Human Services, 1996) evaluation of their completeness and adequacy increasingly will be possible.

Continuity of personnel. Continuity of personnel from one visit to the next can be learned from the medical record. The important factor is the percentage of patients who on follow up see either the same practitioner or a team member.

Practitioner–patient communication. This characteristic concerns the content and quality of interaction between the patient and the practitioner, in addition to those aspects that are unique in maintaining the interpersonal focus of primary care. Such information may be obtained from audiotapes and videotapes or by interviewing patients and physicians. Aspects to be assessed are agreement on the patient's problems, joint understanding of procedures for diagnostic assessment and management strategies, and the patient's satisfaction with the physician's approach to understanding the patient's needs. Evaluation of practitioner–patient communication might also involve indication that practitioners allow patients to play an active role in their care by responding constructively to their questions and their concerns and by seriously considering their suggestions for alternative approaches.

Clinical quality of care. Adequate qualification of personnel is the structural feature that facilitates quality of care. It is determined by reviewing program design and administrative records. Information concerning the processes and outcomes of care can be found in the record, by observation, by interviewing patients, or by using actors who pose as patients (simulated patients). Aspects of quality include performance of appropriate generic and disease-specific processes of care, including the adequacy of recognition of presenting problems, diagnostic and therapeutic procedures, and reassessment, monitoring, and surveillance for adequacy of biological, psychological, and social responses and functional status.

Advocacy for patients. Assessment of advocacy by a program is based on the degree of awareness and the extent of utilization of the many health, social, occupational, and fiscal agencies that have an impact on health and health services. Interviews of patients and physicians can determine their awareness of these agencies and of the resources they can provide. Aspects that characterize advocacy are securing needed improvements in housing, work conditions, neighborhood safety, and sanitation and in obtaining financial resources related to the improvement and maintenance of health.

Evaluation from an Educational Perspective

An approach to evaluation from an educational perspective uses the facility in which training occurs. One such study judged the extent to which a grant program funded by the federal government succeeded in enhancing the training of primary care physicians. One aspect of the evaluation entailed a detailed mail survey of all training programs in pediatrics and in internal medicine and dealt with the measurement of primary care. All program directors were asked whether they currently have a primary care training program or whether they had one in the past. A primary care training program was defined as one especially designed to train physicians for careers as generalists. In contrast, a traditional program was defined as one designed to provide training for physicians who will pursue careers delivering subspecialty medicine exclusively or in combination with generalist care. It further defined a primary care training program as one that devotes more time to ambulatory care training than does a traditional one, and this training emphasizes "continuity care" practice and training in settings in which residents provide continuous (not episodic) and comprehensive (not specialized) care (Noble et al., 1992).

Separate analyses compared traditional programs with primary care programs as to continuity scores, teaching comprehensiveness, and rotation comprehensiveness. Federally funded primary care programs were compared with nonfederally funded primary care programs for the three features of percentage of time spent in a continuity setting, comprehensiveness of teaching, and comprehensiveness of rotations; the extent to which other features were achieved was also assessed (Table 13.2). These other features included the extent of use of community training sites, faculty/trainee ratio, faculty breadth, minority recruitment, extent of internal evaluation of the programs, and attainment of features of primary care. The features particularly pertinent to primary care practice included (1) access (a component of first-contact care), (2) size of the panel followed over the time of the residency (a proxy for longitudinality), (3) the range of services provided (the structural component of comprehensiveness), (4) continuity (the structural feature of coordination), and (5) mechanisms to improve the recognition of information about patients (the performance feature of coordination). The following questions tapped these elements of primary care:

Access measure

- When the continuity practice is closed, as in the case of weekends or evenings, do patients have access to a physician member of the practice by telephone?

Longitudinality measure

- What is the average panel size of the trainees in the continuity practice (total number of patients) at the end of the third year of training?

Table 13.2. Comparisons of Training Programs

Continuity score*
Teaching comprehensiveness*
Rotation comprehensiveness*
Community training sites
Faculty/trainee ratio*
Faculty breadth*
Minority recruitment
Internal evaluation efforts
Primary care score: continuity site*
Summary score

*Components of summary score.

Continuity measure

- When the continuity practice is closed, how are patients handled if they need to be seen by a physician before the next scheduled practice day? Three choices were listed.
- What involvement are the primary care trainees expected to have with their continuity practice patients during hospital admission of these patients? Three choices were provided.

Comprehensive measures

- Who is responsible for ensuring the routine provision of primary and secondary preventive measures, such as routine immunizations, screening, health maintenance assessments for the patients of trainees?
- Are residents ever expected to make home visits?
- Are statistics compiled to profile the health problems of the patients served by the continuity practice?

Coordination measures

- What methods (if any) are used to ensure that the indicated primary and secondary preventive measures are undertaken for individual patients? Seven methods were listed.
- What mechanism is used in the continuity practice to make trainees aware of the results of recent laboratory test/procedures and referrals to consultants for their patients? Three choices were provided.

(An additional question was designed to ascertain the extent to which trainees were taught to manage a spectrum of problems without referral. The question ascertained the percentage of patients with the selected problems and sought to determine whether trainees handle them without referral to another health professional within or outside the continuity practice. The problems in pediatric practice were minor laceration, need for tympanocentesis, failure to thrive, and behavior problems. In internal medicine the problems included acute painful shoulder, rash, pelvic pain, and symptomatic depression. Unfortunately, a typographical error on the questionnaire rendered the answers useless.)

In both internal medicine and pediatrics programs there were large and statistically significant differences between traditional and primary care programs for percentage of time spent in a continuity site, for teaching comprehensiveness, and for rotation comprehensiveness, and hence, the summary score of the three (Table 13.3).

There were differences between federally funded primary care training programs and other primary care training programs in some areas of care and no differences in others. Areas with no differences included teaching comprehensiveness, rotation comprehensiveness, use of community training sites, faculty/trainee ratio, faculty breadth, minority recruitment, and efforts at internal evaluation of the program or of the trainees. There were, however, differences in attributes unique

Table 13.3. Differences Between Primary Care and Traditional Training
Programs

Dimension	Traditional	Primary Care
Results: Pediatrics		
Continuity score*	36.5	59.5
Teaching comprehensiveness*	75.4	84.6
Rotation comprehensiveness*	20.0	26.8
Summary score*	130.1	170.9
Results: Internal Medicine		
Continuity score*	28.8	57.3
Teaching comprehensiveness*	67.6	81.0
Rotation comprehensiveness*	13.9	32.5
Summary score*	109.5	167.9

* Significance at the 0.05 level with a one-tailed test. Higher scores reflect better performance.

to primary care. The continuity score was much higher for federally funded programs, an expected result because the programs were required by the terms of the training grant to achieve a certain level of continuity. In addition, however, the federally funded programs in both internal medicine and pediatrics had primary care scores that were significantly higher than those of other primary care training programs as indicated in Table 13.4. The summary scores, made up of the continuity index and the primary care score, were also significantly greater for the federally funded programs in both pediatrics and general medicine. That is, programs that operate under formal expectations for primary care perform better.

In a mail survey such as this one, responses to questionnaires may be distorted by intentional or nonintentional inflation of responses perceived to be desirable, a problem less likely to appear in a personal discussion and observation. Site visits made as a part of this study confirmed the results from the mail survey and, if

Table 13.4. Differences Between Primary Care Training
Programs, by Source of Funding

Dimension	Non-Federally Funded	Federally Funded
Results: Pediatrics		
Continuity score*	35.5	65.9
Primary care score*	61.1	68.4
Summary score*	296.5	344.5
Results: Internal Medicine		
Continuity score*	37.6	65.8
Primary care score*	50.6	61.2
Summary score*	283.9	330.3

*Significance at the 0.05 level with a one-tailed test. Higher scores reflect better
performance.

anything, suggested that the questionnaire findings underestimated the differences between the federally funded programs and the nonfederally funded ones.

Evaluation From Patient Perspectives

As a by-product of a larger study that examined the differences in experiences with care among adults with one or more of several chronic diseases who were being seen in fee-for-services settings or health maintenance organizations (HMO) settings by physicians of different specialities (family medicine, general internal medicine, endocrinology, or cardiology), an effort was made to evaluate the attainment of primary care by the physicians. Although the measures were not designed specifically to assess primary care, they were subsequently organized into scales that were thought to reflect primary care dimensions. Seven indicators were devised: financial and organizational accessibility, continuity, comprehensiveness, coordination, and interpersonal and technical accountability. The accessibility scales contained 8 and 11 indicators, respectively. The "continuity" scale had only 1 item: Is the doctor (who asked you to take part in the study) still one of your doctors? The comprehensiveness scale had 2 items addressing the number of doctors seen in 6 months and how many were with the doctor who asked the patient to be in the study. The coordination scale had 2 items eliciting information about visits made to other doctors and medications prescribed by them and whether the doctor who asked them to be in the study knows about them. The Interpersonal Accountability scale had 14 questions and the Technical Skills scale had 10 questions. The study indicated that patients in fee-for-service systems scored higher in some dimensions (organizational access, continuity, and accountability), whereas financial access was highest in prepaid systems. HMO patients had the highest scores for coordination and the lowest for comprehensiveness. From the viewpoint of primary care assessment, several limitations to this study should be noted; all patients had at least one chronic illness and hence are not representative of the diversity of patients in primary care settings. Second, the questions forming the scales were not developed specifically for the purpose of assessing primary care, and some of the scales do not address the concept they are purported to represent (Safran et al.,1994).

The PROSPER (Patient Reports on System Performance) is designed as a self-administered questionnaire that focuses on patients' reports about the process of care rather than on their ratings of services or satisfaction with them. It inquires about access to care, communication between practitioners (coordination), and receipt of conflicting information. It is completed by patients who have made a visit or been referred within the past 3 months. It has been validated on several groups of patients and is particularly useful when interest is on individuals with illnesses requiring the seeking of care from more than one physician. Thus, it is particularly suitable to evaluating primary care performance for that subset of patients who have ongoing health needs or chronic conditions requiring at least occasional care from a specialist (Zapka et al., 1995).

Evaluation From a Community Perspective

An evaluation of primary care conducted from the perspective of facilities serving an entire urban population was initiated by the Baltimore City Medical Society as a cooperative venture involving state, regional, and city health planners and faculty and students in a school of public health to study the extent to which primary care resources were available in an entire U.S. city. The study had two purposes: to provide data for local planning of the primary care delivery system and to provide information to complement national data on measurement of the extent of primary care in office-based settings (Weiner et al., 1982).

Data were obtained from all physicians in the area. A stratified random sample was also requested to complete an encounter log for each patient seen in 1 week.

Three methods were used to assess the extent of primary care in office-based practice. In the first method (the "empirical" method), an algorithm was used to distinguish visits that were first contact, visits for consultation only, visits for on-going nonreferral specialized services, and principal care visits. The last category included visits that were not for any of the other three purposes *and* when both the patient's last contact for a check-up and for care of a cold or the "flu" were to the doctor seen at the sample visit. The researchers developed an Empirical Primary Care Index (EPCI), a weighted index of these four types of visits in which principal care was given a weight of 3, first-encounter care was given a rate of 2, specialist care was given a weight of 1, and consultative care was given a weight of 0. Visits that did not fall into the above categories were assigned a weight of 2.

The second method of assessment of the extent of primary care had four components, three of which were related to the unique attributes of primary care while the fourth component concerned family-centeredness. The method is "normative" because the characteristics were judged against criteria that are assumed to be standards.

Comprehensiveness, it was assumed, would be greater if a certain defined set of services was available in the practice. Services included physical examinations, immunizations, pelvic examinations, electrocardiograms, blood hematocrit or hemoglobin determinations, and analyses requiring a microscope.

Accessibility of the practice was scored according to the availability of emergency appointments, willingness of the practitioner to make outside office calls (to home or emergency room), use of an answering service, and formal arrangements for after-hours coverage.

Longitudinal care was measured by the average duration of the patients' relationships with the particular physician seen and was controlled for the age of the patient.

The *family-centeredness component* was based on the percentage of patients in the practice who had at least one other immediate family member seen by the same physician.

The four separate scores were combined to develop the Normative Primary Care Index (NPCI).

In the third method of assessing the extent of primary care, the self-assessed primary care index (SAPCI), physicians were asked the question "What percentage of the visits at your main site would you estimate as being general medical care for patients for whom you maintain ongoing responsibility? Physicians with higher percentages were assumed to be providing more primary care than physicians with lower percentages.

The results showed that

- The percentage of principal care visits was higher for family physicians, general internists, and pediatricians than for all other physicians.
- The percentage of first-encounter visits was lower for psychiatrists and higher for medical subspecialists, but did not differ greatly for the other types of physicians.
- The percentage of specialized care encounters was high for obstetrician/gynecologists and medical subspecialists, low for family physicians and pediatricians, and intermediate for all others.
- The percentage of consultative care visits was low for pediatricians and family physicians; high for psychiatrists, surgical subspecialists, general surgeons, and medical subspecialists; and intermediate for the others.

Thus, EPCI, derived from the above scores appropriately weighted, was high for family physicians, pediatricians, and general internists; low for psychiatrists and surgical subspecialists; and intermediate for the others. The NPCI was highest for family physicians, pediatricians, and general internists; lowest for surgical subspecialists; and intermediate for the rest. The SAPCI was consistent with the results from the other two methods in indicating that internists, family physicians and pediatricians practice more primary care than do any of the other specialists.

The findings lend credence to the usefulness of the measures in distinguishing achievement of the various characteristics of primary care in a population of practices.

This study also involved an assessment of the availability and utilization of primary care services in the different areas of the city. Office-based visit rates were calculated by age, sex, race, and residency of patients within the areas. The measure of physician availability was visits per person. The study revealed that

- The residential area with the highest availability of physicians had 4.3 times the average number of visits as the area with the lowest availability.
- The percentage of the total ambulatory visits made to private offices varied from 41.6 to 96.5; overall, residents obtained only 37.5% of their office-based care within their home districts.
- The percentage of primary care visits to the four primary care specialties within their home districts was slightly higher (43.2%) than the percentage of all visits made within the home district.
- The use of office-based services varied markedly by race of the population: black residents made only 59% of the number of office-based visits as did white residents.

Using U.S. data as a standard, Baltimore residents had an adequate level of utilization of specialty services but a much lower level of primary care visits than the national average. In five of the eight areas of the city, average family income was more closely related to use of services than was availability of resources, whereas in the three other areas both income and availability of resources were equally associated with use. This implies that the presence of primary care resources in an area is a lesser factor in determining use of primary care services than is the average income of its residents. Residents in high income areas compared with those in lower income areas had relatively high utilization, regardless of the availability of care in their home areas. In areas of low family income, utilization was low even though office-based primary care facilities were sometimes available.

A means of assessing the usefulness of population-based measures to describe some aspects of primary care was provided by two unique and linked datasets in Manitoba, Canada. A study analyzed data from linked survey and claims data from all physician visits (Black, 1990). Two measures of primary care were developed: a measure of longitudinality and a measure of comprehensiveness. The measure of longitudinality was created by applying the continuity of care measure (COC) (see Chapter 8) to the first visit in each episode of care for an illness, regardless of the type of reason for the visit. The measure was validated by testing it against what was reported by survey respondents as their "regular source of care"; individuals who reported that they had a regular source of care had higher longitudinality scores. Comprehensiveness was measured by determining whether the individual received an immunization for influenza. Attempts also were made to assess both first-contact care and coordination of care; although both methods were judged as promising, they did not attain standards for criterion validity.

The study indicated that

- Individuals who had been referred for consultation to another physician had lower scores for longitudinality, while those who received a greater proportion of services from primary care practitioners had higher longitudinality scores.
- Comprehensiveness was significantly related to the volume of primary care services that individuals received.
- Among individuals who had referral visits, those for whom a greater proportion of their visits were with a primary care practitioner had greater comprehensiveness.
- In fact, the volume of primary care services was a greater predictor of attainment of comprehensiveness than was volume of total ambulatory visits.

This study demonstrated the potential for using data from claims forms to assess the attainment of at least two characteristics of primary care (longitudinality and comprehensiveness) on a population basis rather than from a practice perspective.

Another survey of adults in 41 counties in California in 1993 examined the relationship between perceived access to services and the strength of primary care received by the individuals in the survey. The strength of primary care was assessed by scoring four aspects, as follows:

Availability: A count of five features of care, including one or few days waiting time for an appointment when sick; 20 minutes or less waiting time in the office; after-hours telephone access telephone access during weekdays; and less than 20 minutes travel time (range of scores, 0–1; maximum score if all five answered affirmatively).

Continuity (longitudinality): Less than or more than 1 year coming to regular place (range of scores, 0–1)

Comprehensiveness: Would go to this place if had a new problem such as flu or sprained ankle; care for a flare-up of an ongoing health problem; for a checkup or vaccination or Pap test (score range, 0–1 for each item; range of scores for category, 0 or 1 [if score on all three = 1]).

Communication: Doctors at place take time to listen; doctors take time to explain; trouble talking with doctor because of a language problem (scored 0–2 on each item; range of scores for category, 0 or 1 [if all three scores = 2]).

The individual was considered to have optimal primary care if the highest possible score was achieved on all four characteristics. Of the 6,674 individuals in the study, only 18% achieved optimal primary care as defined by the researchers. It should be noted that the concept of comprehensiveness differs from the approach suggested in this book because it does not address the full range of services available and provided by the primary care practitioners but, rather, whether people sought to go to that practitioner when they experienced the particular type of problem. Moreover, the measure "communication" is part of the concept of "longitudinality" (person-focused care over time) as described in this book.

Another broad evaluation of primary care was carried out in a large region in Spain. In 1984, Spain initiated health care reform that focused on achieving better primary care. This reform was implemented incrementally, thus permitting the evaluation of the reform by comparing certain characteristics of primary care achieved in areas where it was implemented and areas in which it was not yet implemented. Although no specific plans were made to evaluate the reform, the collection of relevant information on various types of surveys permitted the assessment of some aspects of primary care. In the Basque region, a household interview survey in 1992 collected information that permitted the assessment of accessibility (as the structural component of first-contact care), comprehensiveness (in terms of the achievement of indicated preventive procedures), and longitudinality (in the context of the purchase of private insurance to allow the individual to seek care elsewhere, thus jeopardizing the building of long-term person-focused relationships). The region was divided into areas that had a good penetration of reform services and those that did not. Longitudinality of care was better in reformed areas, as measured by lower rates of purchase of private insurance. Accessibility was better in the reformed areas for people in the lower but not the upper social classes, indicating an improvement in equity of access but not in access overall. Rigidity in scheduling of appointments in the reformed facilities was thought to be responsible for the lower achievement of accessibility among chronically ill people in these areas. The failure to achieve better comprehensiveness of care was thought to be related to inadequacies of care-seeking behavior of patients as well as to the fact that two of the four preventive procedures depended more on speciality care than on inadequacies in primary care because the procedures (mammograms and Pap smears) are done by specialists other than generalists in the reformed system (Larizgoitia and Starfield, 1997).

In the United Kingdom, a statistical approach to assessment of the quality of primary care practices started with quality indicators that were assumed to be related to outcomes. The method (data envelope analysis) yields a measure of relative technical efficiency of practices in local areas (Family Health Services Authorities). Seven important indicators of quality were used: general practitioners per 10,000 patients; percentages of general practitioners not practicing single-handedly; percentage of general practitioners achieving high childhood immunization levels; percentage of females aged 35–64 years with an adequate Pap smear in previous 5.5 years; and percentage of practice facilities with minimum structural standards (wheelchair access, privacy of consulting rooms, fire precautions, and adequate waiting areas). Taking into consideration the illness ratio of the area (limiting long-term illness standardized for age and sex) and the unemployment rate in the area, the efficiency of primary care in the area can be calculated using the gross expenditure on general practitioner services per individual in the population (Salenas-Jiménez and Smith, 1996).

The relatively recent recognition of primary care as a distinct scientific discipline has brought new attention to the assessment of health system characteristics of particular relevance to primary care. Whereas earlier research cited above did not distinguish evaluation of primary care from health services in general, newer research differs by addressing those features of care that are of special relevance to primary care.

The Agency for Health Care Policy and Research, in conjunction with several academic researchers in the United States, developed and tested a tool designed for consumer assessment of health plans (Consumer Assessment of Health Plans, 1997). One section of the core adult questionnaire (mailed version) inquires as to whether the individual was able to find a personal doctor ("one who knows you best"), whether it was easy to do so, whether some other doctor had to be seen instead because the personal doctor was not available in the most recent 6 months, and an overall rating of that doctor on a 1–10 scale. It also inquires as to whether there is a requirement for a referral to see a specialist and how easy it was to get one. Questions abut phone access, ease of making appointments for routine and well-person care, waiting time in the office, helpfulness and courtesy of office staff, and various aspects of communication (explanations, respect shown, time spent, knowledge of patient's medical history, involvement of patient in decision-making, and overall rating of health care) in the most recent 6 months are included, but they reflect care in general rather than specifically for the primary care services. Thus, the instrument addresses some aspects of primary care (access to services for common needs, certain aspects of interpersonal communications important in primary care) but without specific relevance to the primary care experiences of patients. Adaptation of the questions could make it more useful for evaluation of specific aspects of adequacy of primary care. Because the purpose of the information is to help employers and (when they have the opportunity) consumers select a health plan, it has little to offer in providing an understanding of the way in which primary care services are designed and delivered or how they might be improved. Furthermore, it omits consideration of those aspects of care that relate to comprehensiveness or longitudinality of services with a primary care practitioner.

Franks et al. (1997) assessed the primary care orientation of visits included in the National Ambulatory Medical Care Survey, which includes information on visits made to a stratified representative sample of office-based physicians in the United States. Ten items of information were obtained from the data tapes from this survey in order to address first-contact care, comprehensiveness of care, coordination, and accessibility. The following describe the measures used to assess the primary care orientation of the different types of specialists in the survey.

Accessibility: The proportion of patients who are black, the proportion of patients with Medicaid insurance, and the percentage of physicians practicing in rural areas (on the assumption that better access would attract these population groups with generally poorer access)

First-contact care: The proportion of patient visits for which the patient was *not* referred by another physician

Comprehensiveness of care: Three measures were used. The first consisted of the Herfindahl index, which reflects the extent to which the physicians' diagnoses are concentrated in one or more diagnostic categories and therefore reflects a variety of type of diagnoses made. The second concerned the proportion of patients for which physicians reported obtaining a blood pressure measurement. A third measure was the average decade of life represented by the physicians' patients. (A fourth measure of comprehensiveness was also used, consisting of information on the proportion of patients seen previously for a different problem. However, its nature suggests a better fit with the concept of longitudinality because it addresses the seeking of care for a variety of types of problems from the same physician.)

Coordination: An item was formed from information on whether at least one referral was made in the visits sampled (generally about 20).

Because the authors were constrained in their choice of measures to information that was already available, there were limits on the extent to which the measures were specific to more conventional definitions of the primary care domains. Nevertheless, they were able to show that family physicians, general pediatricians, general internists, and general practitioners were much more oriented toward primary care than physicians in other specialties. General surgeons, nephrologists, and emergency medicine physicians also ranked relatively high on the measures, undoubtedly because data on continuity of care would favor physicians with a large proportion of patients under continuing care for a particular problem, because emergency medicine specialists would score high on the first-contact measure, and because general surgeons are known to have a wide range of diagnoses and therefore would score high on the Herfindahl index.

Based on their earlier work in evaluating care provided to individuals with chronic illness (see above), Safran. et al. (1998) developed an instrument to assess the view of adult state employees regarding their "regular personal doctor."

Known as the Primary Care Assessment Survey (PCAS), it has 11 scales of which 7 include more than one item that evaluates care. (The other four either have only one item and/or consist of reports of experiences.) The 7 scales are as follows:

1. Financial access: Two items assess the amount of money paid for visits and prescribed treatments.
2. Organizational access: Six items assess availability by phone, ease of getting appointments when sick, obtaining information and appointments by phone, office location and office hours.
3. Contextual knowledge of patients: Five items concern physician's knowledge of patient's medical history; responsibilities at work, home, or school; principal health concerns; and values and beliefs.
4. Communication: Six items deal with thoroughness of physician's questions about symptoms, attention to what the patient says, clarity of explanations, and advice and help in making decisions about care.
5. Interpersonal treatment: Five items evaluate physician's patience, friendliness, caring, respect, and time spent with patient.
6. Trust: Eight items evaluate physician's integrity, competence, and role as patient's agent.
7. Integration: Six items evaluate the physician's role in coordinating and synthesizing care received from specialists and/or while patient was hospitalized.

In addition, there are three items in two scales concerning "continuity": duration of relationship with physician (longitudinal continuity) and whether patient goes to that physician for check-ups and for sick care (visit-based continuity). Seven items report on prevention counseling: the physician's discussion of smoking, alcohol use, seat belt use, diet, exercise, stress, and safe sex. One additional component consists of an item that inquires as to thoroughness of physical examinations.

All scales had acceptable levels of reliability by standard psychometric testing.

The similarity of these scales to the four cardinal primary care domains is evident and is strengthened by analysis of the extent to which several of them are intercorrelated. Contextual knowledge, communication, interpersonal treatment, and trust all address aspects of interpersonal longitudinality (as discussed in Chapter 8), and all are highly intercorrelated. Preventive counseling, which represents aspects of the comprehensiveness of services provided, is separately identifiable, as are financial access, longitudinal continuity, and visit-based continuity. Organizational access is moderately correlated with most other scales; the Integration scale (which represents coordination) has moderate correlations with the interpersonal longitudinality scales. Thus there is evidence that the key domains of primary care can be assessed, at least in this sample of insured, employed adults.

Grumbach et al. (unpublished manuscript, 1998), in their study of differences between family physicians and general internists, constructed a score for accessibility that was derived from responses to four questions, to which respondents answered on a scale from "strongly agree" to "strongly disagree." The questions were

If I have a medical question during the day, I can usually reach my doctor for help
   without any problem.
I have easy access to specialists.
I am able to get care whenever I need it.
If I get very sick I can usually see my personal physician the same day.

The reader will note that the second of these questions does not pertain to
access to primary care but, rather, the extent to which the primary care services
facilitates access to specialists.

The scales for comprehensiveness consisted of four items asking individuals
whether they would make an appointment with their personal physician for a new
problem such as a sprained ankle or the flu, for flare-up of an ongoing problem
such as asthma or diabetes, for a check-up or physician examination, for a new
personal problem such as depression, a family crisis, or problems at work. It should
be noted that this series of questions does not specifically address services available
or provided by the primary care physician because responses could represent the
intent to seek first-contact care for advice about the best place to go for such
problems.

Three others scales in the instrument are related to comprehensiveness. The first
consists of four items concerning prevention services, including flu shots, check of
cholesterol level, breast examination, and routine pelvic (vaginal) examination. The
second concerns promotion of health life styles and inquires as to whether the
physician had talked with the individual about smoking, diet, use of alcohol, and
exercise. The third relates to health promotion and inquires as to whether the physician talked with the individual about emotional and psychological health, relationships with family members, violence in the home against women, sexuality and
sexual relationships, and how to prevent human immunodeficiency virus infection
and aquired immunodeficiency syndrome.

Coordination is addressed by asking whether the personal physician knows
about other health professionals that the person is seeing.

Stewart and colleagues (1997) developed a primary care assessment instrument
consisting of four domains that could be combined to develop a score for optimal
primary care. It was tested by means of a telephone survey of a random sample of
households in 41 randomly selected urban communities in California. The first
domain consists of five features of availability, including 1 day or less of average
waiting time for an appointment when sick; 20 minutes or less of average waiting
time in the office; after-hours telephone access; telephone access during weekdays;
and less than 20 minutes travel time. Temporal longitudinality is addressed by a
one-item "continuity" measure eliciting the years coming to the regular place.
Interpersonal longitudinality is addresses by a three-item "communication" scale
consisting of responses to how consistently doctors at the place take time to listen
and to explain and whether there is any trouble talking to the doctor or receiving
care because of a language problem. Comprehensiveness is a count of three items
inquiring whether the person would go to the place for a new problem such as a
sprained ankle or flu; for care of a flare-up of an ongoing health problem such as

asthma or diabetes; and for a check-up or vaccination or (for women) for a Pap test.

Primary care is considered "optimal" if the highest score is received on availability, comprehensiveness, and communication and with a score of 12 months or more on temporal longitudinality.

It should be noted that, except for the study using the National Ambulatory Medical Care Survey, all of the approaches described above concern only adults; the care of children is not included in any.

In contrast, Flocke and colleagues (1997) developed an instrument in the course of a collaborative study involving 4,454 patient visits to 138 family physicians participating in a research network in Ohio. Seven scales were initially developed to address the various postulated domains of primary care. The first three consisted of one item each: first-contact care ("If I am sick, I would always contact a doctor in this office first"); comprehensiveness of care ("I go to this doctor for almost all of my medical care"); and temporal longitudinality ("How many years have you been a patient of this physician?"). Interpersonal longitudinality was addressed by three scales, as follows

Accumulated knowledge

This doctor does not know my medical history well
This doctor knows a lot about my family
This doctor clearly understands my health needs
This doctor and I have been through a lot together

Interpersonal communication

I can easily talk about personal things with this doctor
I don't always feel comfortable asking questions of this doctor
This doctor always explains things to my satisfaction
Sometimes this doctor does not listen to me

Continuity belief

My medical care improves when I see the same doctor I have seen before
It is very important to me to see my regular doctor
I rarely see the same doctor when I go for medical care

The coordination scale consist of the following five items

This doctor does not always know about care I have received at other places
This doctor communicates with the other health care providers I see
This doctor knows about the results of my visits to other doctors

This doctor always follows up on a problem I've had, either at the next visit or by
phone
I want one doctor to coordinate all of the health care I receive

Psychometric testing revealed that the items in these scales collapsed to four
domains, which were relatively highly correlated with each other. The four were
patient preference for a regular physician (consisting of six items from continuity
belief items, coordination preference, first contact, and comprehensive care); interpersonal communication (four items); accumulated knowledge of patient (consisting of three knowledge items, the longitudinality item, and the item on "been
through a lot"); and coordination of care (four items).

The scores on this instrument were tested against patient satisfaction with the
visit, overall global satisfaction, and whether the patient's expectations were met.
It should be noted that, because testing took place on patients seen consecutively,
the findings cannot be generalized to patient populations or even to a random
sample of users of the facility because selection by visits proves an over-
representation of frequent users who might be expected to be both more ill and
more satisfied with care from that doctor or facility.

None of the instruments described in this section are oriented toward a full age
spectrum of individuals in communities. The primary care assessment tool (PCAT)
is an instrument intended for use in communities, among patients in facilities, and
(through a counterpart survey) for practitioners in health facilities. Although developed and tested for children and youth only, it is being adapted for adults
because the domains and subdomains of primary care the same for both.

The PCAT is a new tool designed specifically to evaluate the attainment of the
features of primary care as described in this book, from both a practice and a
population perspective. It is composed of the four primary care domains, each with
its two subdomains representing the capacity of the system and the performance
characteristics that represent the domain. In addition, it elicits information about
the three derivative domains of family-centeredness, community orientation, and
cultural competence. There are parallel forms for administration to people in community samples or those being seen in health care settings and for administration
to physicians or administrative personnel in health care facilities. Thus, it is possible
to examine the concordance between people and their health care practitioners on
primary care achievement. The instrument has been tested for reliability and validity (Cassady et al., 1998). When used in a comparison of primary care provided
by managed care and nonmanaged care settings, it showed that managed care settings achieved better performance of some but not all aspects of primary care,
whether judged by consumers or by their practitioners. Notable in this regard were
the significantly and consistently higher scores for first contact (access subdomain)
and comprehensiveness (services provided subdomain) of the managed care settings
(Starfield et al., 1998). Because the study was conducted in only one geographic
area, the specific findings might not be applicable in other areas. The contents of
the child versions of these instruments are in the Appendix to this book. The
content of the adult versions is identical, except where health needs of adults differ
from those of children (primarily in the comprehensive domain).

Evaluating the Impact of Primary Care on Health Status
from a Population Perspective

When the focus is on measures of health status, whether viewed generically or with a focus on particular disease, the challenge of measurement is demanding because of the difficulty in determining what aspects of health ought to be a responsibility of health services (as distinguished from other societal services) and of primary care services specifically. As Figure 2.1 showed, biological phenomena, genetic substrate, and prior health status provide a potential for good health that is influenced, positively or negatively, by a vast array of environmental characteristics all of which must be taken into account in assessing the impact of health services on health. This is particularly the case when different areas are compared, as similar services may have different impacts if the other influential factors are different.

The following approaches provide examples of the variety of measures that could be used to assess the impact of primary care services on health status; they range from the biomedical (including diseases as well as laboratory representations of them) to the much broader focus on ability to function adequately within the context of the social milieu.

For the most part, nations or other political subdivisions do not make the attempt to correlate the indicators of health of their populations with structural changes in the health system or modes of delivery of health services so that explanations for poor or good achievement or changes in the indicators are not available to inform subsequent decision-making. That is, they are used simply as trends in health status rather than as targeted outcomes for health services evaluation and planning. It is possible, however, to relate changes in these measures, or trends over time, to specific changes in health systems organization or delivery. For example, improvements in immunization rates can be tied directly to governmental efforts to facilitate vaccine availability and financing of their provisions (Blendon et al., 1990); improvements in infant mortality can be linked in time with improved access to abortion services; and improved postneonatal mortality was coincident in time to greatly expanded access to services as a result of the Medicaid program (Starfield, 1985). Thus, when applied at successive time periods, these methods provide a way to assess the extent to which health services are meeting selected important population needs.

For these assessments, the information may come from a variety of sources, including population surveys or population-based health statistics. Surveys in populations may include random samples or samples stratified to ensure the inclusion of populations of special interest. The U.S. National Health Interview Survey is the prototype of a source of data on population health at the national level. This survey, under the aegis of the National Center for Health Statistics, has been in operation continuously since 1957 and provides a wealth of information on reported health status and use of services and, because of its continuous nature, in trends in these characteristics over time. Information is available for broad regions in the United States, and there are also plans to collect data that would be more useful at the state level, at least for some states. There is a planned linkage of this survey with the more recent series of national medical care use and expenditures surveys conducted by the Agency for Health Care Policy and Research; these surveys are panel surveys in that they contact households several times over a period of a year and thus provide information on changes in health and utilization over a period of time. They also contact the sources of care (practitioners and facilities, including hospitals) for a sample of people in the household survey. This linkage provides a much richer understanding of health characteristics that can be related to particular sources of care. A further linkage with practitioner-based surveys such as the National Ambulatory Care Survey (see Chapter 16) would provide even more information about the relationship of patterns of practice on use of services and health status outcomes.

Guidance in the selection of measures to evaluate the impact of primary care at the population level comes from four compendia, each resulting from extensive work by panels of national experts in the United States.

The Year 2000 National Objectives (National Center for Health Statistics, 1997) provide a basis for selecting specific measures of the population's health in 22 priority areas, as listed in Table 13.5 (Sondik, 1996). These objectives cover a wide variety of clinical conditions and problems in their 319 objectives and an equal number of subobjectives for specific population groups. Two of the priority areas (environmental health and data; and surveillance systems) deal primarily with system structures rather than health services impact. Possible data sources include vital

Table 13.5. Year 2000 National (U.S.)
Objectives: Priority Areas

Physical activity and fitness
Nutrition
Tobacco use
Substance abuse: alcohol and drugs
Family planning
Mental health and mental disorders
Violent and abusive behavior
Educational and community-based programs
Unintentional injuries
Occupational safety and health
Environmental health
Food and drug safety
Oral health
Maternal and infant health
Heart disease and stroke
Cancer
Diabetes and chronic disabling conditions
Human immunodeficiency virus infection
Sexually transmitted disease
Immunization and infectious diseases
Clinical and preventive services
Surveillance and data systems

Source: Sondik (1996).

statistics, household surveys, surveillance systems, and, eventually, clinical data systems when they become standardized. Because the objectives are for the health system as a whole rather than for primary care in specific, it is not possible to use them to evaluate the performance of primary care systems without taking into account the relationship of that system to the larger health services system. However, the objectives do provide a basis for communities and health systems in general to set goals for themselves that take into account the likely contributions of primary care toward their achievement.

Of the 319 specific objectives, about 30% relate to structures, including the passage of necessary implementing legislation and developing programs to meet needs. Another 20% represent process, including the conduct of activities by health-related professionals that are designed to improve services to meet needs. About 50% relate to the achievement of outcomes directly, as measured by improvements in various aspects of health status or health behaviors known to be directly related to improved health status.

A subset of these 319 indicators was chosen by the U.S. Centers for Communicable Diseases for use by federal, state, and local health agencies with the aim to have them implemented in at least 40 states (Sutocky et al., 1996). The list of these "consensus" indicators includes nine mortality indicators, four disease incidence indicators, and five health risk factor indicators.

Two other reports, one in 1996 and one in 1997, proposed their own indicators, many (although not all) of them taken from the Healthy People 2000 objectives. The first of these reports was intended as a set of performance measures for public health agencies (Perrin and Koshel, 1997). There are 47 indicators, 26 of which concern physical health and 21 concern mental health. The 30 physical health indicators and the 17 mental health indicators are in 10 and 4 categories, respectively; most deal with outcomes (O), processes of health care (P), or processes known to be related to outcomes (P-O), as follows, with the number of individual indicators indicated in parentheses:

Smoking (4)	O
Weight/diet (2)	O
Physical activity (1)	O
Preventive care (5)	P-O
Diabetes care (3)	P-O
Sexually transmitted diseases/tuberculosis (2)	O
Sex behaviors (4)	P-O
Intravenous drug use (2)	P-O
Immunizations (3)	P-O
Disability (4)	O
Satisfaction with mental health services (1)	P
Decreased mental health distress and problems (6)	O
Substance abuse (9)	O
Sexual abuse (1)	O

The second report was intended as a set of indicators for community health to be used by both public health agencies and clinical medicine facilities and health plans as a basis for joint action (Durch et al., 1997). Five indicators reflect health status: infant mortality by race and ethnicity; age-adjusted number of deaths from motor vehicle crashes, work-related injuries, suicide, homicide, lung cancer, breast cancer, cardiovascular diseases, and all-cause by race and gender as appropriate); reported incidence of AIDS, measles, tuberculosis, primary and secondary syphilis, by age race and gender as appropriate; births to females aged 10–17 years as a proportion of total births; and number and rate of confirmed abuse and neglect cases among children.

Six indicators reflect health risk factors: proportion of 2 year olds completely immunized; proportion of individuals aged 65 and older who have ever received pneumococcal vaccine and influenza vaccine within the past 12 months; proportion of the population who smoke by age, gender, and race as appropriate; proportion of individuals aged 18 and older who are obese; number and type of U.S. Environmental Protection Agency air quality standards not met; proportion of assessed rivers, lakes, and estuaries that support beneficial uses (swimming and fishing).

Two indicators reflect functional status: proportion of adults reporting their health as good or excellent; and average days for which adults report their physical or mental health was not good in the past 30 days.

Two indicators reflect overall quality of life: proportion of adults satisfied with the health care system in their community; and proportion of persons satisfied with the quality of life in their community.

Although the limitations of many of these measures are evident, that is, no consideration of social class differences, paucity of indicators for children, inappropriate denominators (proportion of assessed rather than total rivers, lakes, and estuaries), and proportion rather than rates of teenage births, the breadth of the list and the implication that the indicators are obtainable is a considerable leap forward in evaluation of the impact of health systems.

In addition, an agency of the U.S. Congress tested the predictiveness of a set of indicators chosen both from the objectives for the nation and from an additional set of 17 indicators developed by a private organization. The effort was to determine if cross-state differences could be explained by a parsimonious set of indicators rather than the more extensive lists noted above. Analyses indicated that one indicator alone—years of life lost due to mortality from preventable causes before age 65—was by far the best in representing cross-state variability in health status (U.S. Congress, 1996).

Of the indicators proposed in the four compendia, no more than nine were proposed in all four, and nine were proposed in three of the compendia. These 18 indicators are listed in Table 13.6.

"Health of the nation" targets have been developed by many countries. Targets for the United Kingdom were developed in 1992 in six categories: coronary heart disease, stroke, cancer, mental illness, human immunodeficiency virus, and aquired immunodeficiency syndrome, and accidents. A survey of general practitioners in two large regions revealed considerable skepticism about the attainability of some of the 15 specific targets in these categories and variable implementation of strategies to meet them, largely as a result of excessive practice workload, unrealistic

Table 13.6. Indicators Common to Most U.S. National Compendia

Percentage of the adult population who smoke
Percentage of adults who are overweight
Appropriate immunization status in childhood and over age 65 years
Total mortality rates
Rate of mortality from cardiovascular disease
Rate of mortality from lung cancer
Rate of mortality from breast cancer
Rate of mortality from motor vehicle accidents
Rate of mortality from suicide
Rate of mortality from homicides
Infant mortality rate
Aquired immunodeficiency syndrome incidence
Syphilis incidence
Tuberculosis incidence
Measles incidence
Percentage of the population living in counties not meeting standards for good air quality
Percentage of deliveries with no prenatal care in the first trimester
Percentage of births to teenagers

Sources: Perrin and Koshel (1997); U.S. Congress (1996); Durch et al. (1997); National Center for Health Statistics (1997).

time scales, and unavailability of non-physician team members needed to address them adequately. However, half of the 257 respondents had practice-based strategies for meeting the targets (Cheung et al., 1997). Revised objectives (1998) contained 12 goals in 4 areas: heart disease and stroke, cancer, accidents, and mental illness.

A particularly primary care–focused compendium was proposed by the Bureau of Primary Health Care in the U.S. Department of Health and Human Services, which considered a variety of mechanisms for evaluating primary care in the many facilities under its jurisdiction. One approach focuses on comparisons of rates of hospitalization for ambulatory care–sensitive conditions. Also under consideration are evaluations of variations across area and explanations for them, reductions of gaps in health between deprived and nondeprived populations, and penetration of services in different areas. For the most part, however, the focus is on capacity, performance, and outcomes of clinical conditions in individual facilities, using techniques of medical record review, encounter data, visit surveys, and user surveys rather than on community statistic and health information systems (Bureau of Primary Health Care, 1995). A particular challenge to population-based evaluations of the impact of primary care is the absence of common data systems that would enable comparisons across different local practices or groups and link their respective performance to outcomes of the specific populations served by each of them.

Some indicators are less useful in reflecting the contributions of primary care, mainly because improvements in their occurrence rest not only on primary care but also on services provided by other levels of the health care system. For example, achievement of disease-oriented prevention goals such as breast cancer screening, Pap smears, cholesterol screening, and screening for hypertension may be as much a contribution of the specialty system as the primary care system if health policies dictate that services for them be provided by specialists (as is the case for Pap smears and mammography in some countries, e.g., Spain). Rates of handicap may be a result not only of the success of primary care physicians at prevention but also the success of physiotherapists in reducing handicap from disabilities and impairments. Indicators such as life expectancy at different ages, particularly at older ages, reflects a contribution of specialists who are successful in averting mortality from conditions that benefit from the application of complex technology for conditions of aging. For example, life expectancy at age 80 in the United States is better than that in almost all other countries, despite the poor primary care infrastructure in that country and due, in large measure, to the high use of death-delaying interventions.

Years of healthy life lost (HEALYs), quality-adjusted life years (QALYs), and disability-adjusted life years (DALYs) are other approaches that have been used to assess and monitor health needs (Morrow and Bryant, 1995). HEALYS are a measure based on the number of years of life in which the population suffers from specified diseases; the total disease burden is computed by summing the years of healthy life lost per 1,000 population resulting from disability and premature death attributable to these diseases with onset in a defined period of time. It has been used mainly in developing countries. Thus, from the viewpoint of the health system, reductions in equity across communities should be a measure of the success of the policy toward strengthening primary care.

QALYs, on the other hand, is a method developed for use in industrialized countries and generally takes into account the preferences of individuals for different outcomes that might result from a different intervention. Both observed disability (loss of function or mobility) and subjective distress (pain and anguish) are taken into account. One such system identifies eight levels of disability and four of distress, with a combined total number of 29 different combinations, each of which is given a value for each subject. Since preventable premature death is less of a pressing concern in developed countries, a method that focuses on disability and discomfort is more applicable than HEALYS. Although the system is oriented around making decisions about alternative interventions for individual patients, the individual QALYS might be aggregated for community use. No norms could be developed, however, because different populations could be expected to differ in their QALYS as a result of different priorities for different outcomes.

DALYS were developed to compare burdens of morbidity among different diseases, each of which has an associated DALY. Because of the difficulty in specifying disability and in attributing it to specific illnesses, this method of monitoring health needs has found less acceptance than the alternative methods.

Thus, achievement of many health status goals requires not only the contribution of primary care but also the contributions of specialists working in the variety of types of settings characteristic of health delivery systems. Because primary care is only one level of the health care system, the specific contributions that it makes to health status of populations and patients should be assessed with indicators that reflect its own contribution within the health care system. The unique contributions of primary care would be expected to be in those indicators that reflect care of people over time rather than care of specific conditions that afflict people and that, from time to time, may require health services other than primary care.

Recognizing that most outcomes require excellence not only of primary care services but also other levels of care, the Canadian plan for evaluating community-based health services (CBHSs) developed a compendium of CBHS-sensitive indicators to accompany the more encompassing set of population health goals. Notable among these are the indicators listed in Table 13.7.

Table 13.8, which derives from a series of informal focus groups held with presumed "experts" in the United States and elsewhere and on the basis of the European atlas of avoidable deaths (Holland, 1991), lists those outcomes that should be particularly related to the adequacy of primary care services.

Most but not all of the indicators in Table 13.8 are included in at least one of

Table 13.7. Examples of Indicators Particularly Amenable to Community-Based Health Systems (CBHS) in Canada

Improvement in personal health practices and behaviors	Smoking, alcohol consumption, nutrition, physical activity, illicit drug use
Physical/social environment	Actions to identify physical and social threats to health and percentage resolved through CBHS; demonstrated compliance with environmental health controls and resolution of social situations under the mandate of CBHS organizations; percentages of public policies and practices attributable to CBHS
Individual/community capacity	Consumer rating of increased ability to cope with health problems; improvement in health knowledge and attitudes and demonstrated acquisition of health skills
Relevancy	Responding to and collaborating with the community to address health incidents and issues; public perception of CBHS timeliness in responding to community concerns
Satisfaction	Consumer satisfaction with service outcomes; reported increase in health and well being attributed to CBHS by consumers
Costs	Absence of unnecessary service duplication and administrative inefficiencies (excessive paperwork)
De-institutionalization	Inappropriate hospitalizations and avoidable institutionalizations
Universality	Percentage of population covered, absence of exclusionary policies
Targeted services	Proportion of services delivered to vulnerable population groups, waiting time for assessment based on level of health need; waiting time for treatment by level of need
Community empowerment	Public satisfaction regarding process of policy development, perceived level of control in decision-making
Range of services	Number and type of core services provided: communicable disease control; community supports; dental health; basic emergency needs; environmental health; health promotion; healthy child development; home care, including palliative; mental health; nutrition; prenatal and obstetric care; prevention and treatment of common diseases and injuries, rehabilitation; sexual health/family planning; psychosocial services (non-justice system issues)

Source: Wanke et al. (1996).

Table 13.8. Indicators for Evaluating Primary Care at Population Levels

---

Accomplishments in prevention not related to specific diseases: immunization status; personal health
 behaviors (breastfeeding, not smoking, use of seat belts, use of smoke detectors, physical activity,
 good diet)
Unwanted pregnancies
Low incidence of vaccine-preventable diseases
Early detection of risk for child abuse
Low incidence of attempted suicide
Low incidence of accidental poisoning
Improved quality of life, including decreased disability from
 Asthma
 Osteoarthritis
 Postmyocardial infarct
Shortened duration of symptoms associated with peptic ulcers
Reduced use of unnecessary resources, including
 Laboratory test and procedures
 Unjustified medications (such as antibiotics for influenza, growth hormone treatment for short chil-
 dren
Low incidence of adverse effects of medications
Reduced frequency of conditions related to prevention: stroke, amputations resulting from diabetes
 complications, surgery for preventable eye conditions, incidence of sexually transmitted diseases and
 aquired immunodeficiency syndrome
Low postneonatal mortality rates
Improved quality of dying/terminal care
Rates of death due to
 Asthma
 Hypertensive and cerebrovascular disease
Hospitalizations for ambulatory care–sensitive conditions
For all health indicators—reductions in disparities across population subgroups.

---

the compendia mentioned above. Among the ones previously not included are hospitalizations for ambulatory-sensitive conditions, unwanted pregnancies, low incidence of adverse effects of medications, and low postneonatal mortality. The justification for including rates of hospitalizations for ambulatory-sensitive conditions
rests with the evidence from the several studies in the United States, Canada, and
Spain that suggest that good primary care services are associated with lower rates
than is the case in areas with poorer primary care resources. The justification for
unwanted pregnancies is that a good, long-term relationship with a primary care
source should provide the basis for more successful efforts at preventing births that
themselves are associated with higher rates of mortality and morbidity. The indicator concerning adverse effects of medications rests on the finding that such effects
may account for a larger proportion of morbidity than any other single condition
in the population, on the high level of predictability and hence preventability of
the many that are prescribed inappropriately, and from the likelihood that better
coordination of care associated with good primary care should reduce the likelihood
of inappropriate use. Postneonatal mortality, as distinguished from total infant mortality, is particularly amenable to minimization with good access to primary care
(Starfield, 1985).

In interpreting information on incidence and prevalence of these problems in the population, it is important to remember that primary care should not be expected to eliminate the effects of social and environmental determinants of ill health but, rather, to reduce the likelihood that external factors will cause adverse impact. Communities that vary in rates of occurrence of the problems listed in Table 13.8 are very likely to vary in social and environmental conditions that cause them. That is, comparing the adequacy of primary care in ameliorating these conditions in different communities has to take into account initial differences in the rates of these conditions. Rates may still be high even when primary care facilities are performing well, as manifested by progress toward reducing them. Thus, from the viewpoint of the health system, reductions in equity across communities should be a measure of the success of the policy toward strengthening primary care.

Finally, health services (including primary care services) can be evaluated according to overall principles concerning patients' rights. These "rights" are increasingly being incorporated into state laws and into the codes of professional organizations. For example, an association of health plans in the United States encouraged all of its members to adopt the following policies: patients should have the right to care, at the right time, in the right setting; all health care professionals should be held accountable for the quality of services they provide; patients should have choice within their plans of physicians who meet high standards of professional training and experience; physicians should be encouraged to share information with their patients on their health status, medical conditions, and treatment options; and working with people to keep them healthy is as important as making them well. Also, patients should be provided, on request, with clear information about how physicians are paid; procedures for control of utilization and the basis for specific decisions, whether a specific prescription drug is included in the formulary (and, presumably, the reason for exclusions), and how the health plan decides when a treatment is experimental and therefore not included in the services provided (American Association of Health Plans, 1997). A Consumer Bill of Rights was promulgated by a commission appointed by the President of the United States. The Advisory Commission on Consumer Protection and Quality in the Health Care Industry proposed eight areas of rights and responsibilities including information disclosure, choice of providers and plans, access to emergency services, participation in treatment decisions, respect and nondiscrimination, confidentiality of health information, complaints and appeals, and consumer responsibilities. (Advisory Commission on Consumer Protection and Quality in the Health Care Industry, 1997) In the future, it should be possible to assess the extent to which these criteria are met and the extent to which different types of health systems differ in their achievement.

References

Advisory Commission on Consumer Protection and Quality in the Health Care Industry. Report to the President of the United States. Consumer Bill of Rights. Washington, D.C., 1997

American Association of Health Plans. Report in Alpha Center. State Initiative in Health Care Reform, No. 21:5. Washington, DC: American Association of Health Plans. 1997.

Black C. Population-Based Measurement of Primary Care to Study Variations in Care Received by the Elderly. Dissertation. Baltimore: Johns Hopkins University, 1990.

Blendon R, Leitman R, Morrison I, Donelan K. Satisfaction with health systems in ten nations. Health Aff 1990; 9:185–92.

Bureau of Primary Health Care. Consensus Conference of Health Status Gaps of Low Income and Minority Populations: A Synopsis. Washington, DC: USDHHS, HRSA, December 1995.

Consumer Assessment of Health Plans. AHCPR Pub. No. 97-0001. Rockville, MD: Agency for Health Care Policy and Research, USDHHS, 1997.

Cassady, C., Starfield, B., Berk, R., Nanda, J., Friedenberg, L., Hurtado, M. Assessing consumer experience with their primary care. Unpublished manuscript, 1998.

Cheung P, Hungin A, Verrill J, Russell A, Smith H. Are the health of the nation's targets attainable? Postal survey of general practitioner's views. BMJ 1997; 314:1250–1.

Durch J, Bailey L, Stofo M (eds). Improving Health in the Community: A Role for Performance Monitoring. Washington, DC: National Academy Press, 1997.

Flocke S. Measuring attributes of primary care: Development of a new instrument. J Fam Pract 1997; 45:6474.

Franks P, Clancy C, Nutting P. Defining primary care: Empirical analyses of the national ambulatory medical survey. Med Care 1997; 34:655–68.

Grumbach K, Selby J, Schmittdiel J, Quesenberry C. Quality of primary care practice in a large HMO according to physician specialty (unpublished manuscript, 1998).

Holland WW. European Community Atlas of "Avoidable Death." Commission of the European Communities Health Services Research. Series No.6, 9, Vols. 1, 2. 2nd Ed., Oxford: Oxford University Press; 1991, 1993.

Institute of Medicine. Primary Care: America's Health in a New Era. Washington, DC: National Academy Press, 1997.

Larizgoitia I, Starfield B. Reform of primary health care: The case of Spain. Health Policy 1997; 41:121–37.

Morrow R, Bryant J. Health policy approaches to measuring and valuing human life: Conceptual and ethical issues. Am J Public Health 1995; 85; 1356–60.

National Center for Health Statistics. Healthy People 2000 Review, 1997. Hyattsville, MD: Public Health Service, 1997.

Noble J, Friedman RR, Starfield B, Ash A, Black C. Career differences between primary care and traditional trainees in internal medicine and pediatrics. Ann Intern Med 1992; 116(6):482–7.

Perrin E, Koshel J. National Research Council (U.S.) Panel on Performance Measures and Data for Public Health Performance Partnership Grants. Assessment of Performance Measures for Public Health, Substance Abuse and Mental Health. Washington, DC: National Academy Press, 1997.

Safran DG, Kosinki M, Tarlov AR, Rogers W, Taira DA, Lieberman N, Ware JE. The primary care assessment survey: tests of data quality and measurement performance. Med Care 1998; 36(5):728–739.

Safran D, Tarlov A, Rogers W. Primary care performance in fee-for-service and prepaid health care systems: results from the medical outcomes study. JAMA 1994; 271:1579–86.

Salenas-Jiménez J, Smith P. Data envelope analysis applied to quality in primary health care. Ann Oper Res 1996; 67:141–61.

Sondik E. Healthy people 2000: Meshing national and local health objectives. Public Health Rep 1996; 111:518–20.

Starfield B. Effectiveness of Medical Care: Validating Clinical Wisdom. Baltimore, MD: The Johns Hopkins University Press, 1985.

Starfield B, Cassady C, Nanda J, Forrest C, Berk R. Consumer experiences and provider perceptions of the quality of primary care: Implications for managed care. J Fam Pract 1998; 46:216–226.

Stewart A, Grumbach K, Osmond D, Vranizan K, Komaromy M, Bindman A. Primary care and patient perceptions of access to care. J Fam Pract 1997; 44:177–85.

Sutocky J, Dumbauld S, Abbott G. Year 2000 health status indicators: A profile of California. Public Health Rep 1996; 111:521–6.

U.S. Congress, General Accounting Office. Public Health: A Health Status Indicator for Targeting Federal Aid to States. GAO/HEHS 97–13. Washington, DC: General Accounting Office, 1996.

U.S. Department of Health and Human Services. Core Data Elements. Washington, DC: CDC, NCHS, 1996.

Wanke M, Saunders LD, Pong R, Church WJ. Building a Stronger Foundation: A Framework for Planning and Evaluating Community-Based Health Services in Canada 1995. Health Promotion and Program Branch, Health Canada. Ottawa: Canadian Dept of Supply and Services, 1996.

Weiner J, Kassel L, Baker T, Lane B. The Baltimore City primary care study: The role of the office based physician in a metropolitan area. MD State Med J 1982; 31:48–52.

Zapka J, Palmer H, Hargraves L, Nerenz D, Frazier H, Warner C. Relationships of patient satisfaction with experience of system performance and health status. J Ambulatory Care Manage 1995; 18, 73–83.

— 14 —

Public Health and
Community-Oriented Primary Care

In this chapter, we come full circle back to the concepts of primary care as expressed in the Declaration of Alma-Ata (see Chapter 1). In the paragraph defining primary care, the word *community* was used three times: "at a cost the community can afford to maintain," "an integral part of . . . the overall social and economic development of the community," and "the first level of contact of individuals, the family and community with the national health system. . . ." The declaration recognized the distinction between primary care as delivered to individuals or families and as delivered to the community; it required attention to both.

There is little doubt that access to effective medical care services improves health. Deprivation of access, as by withdrawal of previously provided services, has been followed in a relatively short period of time by declines in health (Fihn and Wicher, 1988; Lurie et al., 1986). Despite the clear importance of environmental and social conditions, including nutrition and housing, better access to health services makes a difference, particularly for those who have been relatively deprived of them. Improvements in access to care by virtue of the passage of legislation to provide funding and/or services for care of socially deprived individuals are followed by improvements in health. Examples include lower neonatal mortality rates through interventions that reduce work stress in pregnant women (Luke et al., 1995) and regionalized perinatal care (Starfield, 1985). Documented improvements in health also include lower postneonatal mortality rates, better survival from bacterial meningitis, and lower hospitalization rates from complications of diabetes when health services are improved. Easier access to abortions and family planning has been associated with lowered teenage pregnancy rates, and nationally funded programs to provide available immunization have been followed by greatly increased immunization rates (Starfield, 1985). Bunker et al. (1994) have calculated the substantial gains in life expectancy as a result of medical care interventions that are both preventive (early detection) and, even more salient, a result of greater availability of effective treatments. Gains have also been made in alleviating discomfort and disability, although quantitative estimation of the total effect of medical care is hampered by the absence of standard methods for assessing outcomes other than mortality (Bunker et al., 1994). These gains in health accrue either through targeted interventions imposed by national health policy (as in the case of national immunization programs) or through the application of technological development, which generally takes place according to professional prerogatives rather than through policy decisions. In the latter case, the benefits of medical progress often accrue inequitably and not according to decisions made on the basis of reducing disparities in health across different communities or population subgroups. The imperative of community-oriented care is to ensure that resources flow to areas where they are most needed, thus decreasing inequities within the populations.

Primary care, through its community orientation, shares responsibility with public health for maximizing the extent to which health services can overcome social disadvantage and its adverse health effects.

Primary Care From a Population Vantage

The presentation of the four characteristics of primary care in Chapters 7–11 explicitly distinguished the population vantage from the clinical vantage. However, most of the discussion and evidence of the usefulness of these characteristics was drawn from experiences in clinical settings. The reason for this is straightforward: Little has been done to explore the usefulness or benefits of community-oriented primary care in improving levels of health and reducing inequalities in health within and across different communities.

Conventional primary care, that is, care from the perspective of the clinician who has been exposed exclusively to patients appearing for care, has evident limitations. Such care cannot take into consideration the distribution of health problems in the community because many of those problems may never come to the clinician's attention and, even if they do, the relative frequencies of problems may not reflect their relative frequencies in the community. In addition, conventional primary care cannot be aware of the way problems initially are manifested because patients often wait for problems to progress or change before they seek care. Furthermore, traditional clinically oriented primary care practitioners have difficulty in understanding the relative impact of environmental, social, and behavioral factors in disease etiology and progression because they are often unfamiliar with the milieu in which patients live and work. Finally, monitoring the impact of health services is difficult in conventional primary care because follow up or feedback requires that the patients contact or re-visit the practitioner.

There are several reasons why a population-based focus to clinical care is a desirable goal. The first is that knowledge about the distribution of health problems cannot be derived from experiences in medical centers or in individual practitioners' practices. Analyses conducted by White et al. (1961) conclusively demonstrated that most experiences with an illness do not result in a visit to a physician; a maximum of one-third result in seeking help. Therefore, information about the nature and distribution of health problems cannot and should not be based on the experiences of practitioners in medical centers or offices. The second reason is that knowledge of how disease presents is not obtainable without a population-based focus. Evidence on this point derives from studies such as one in which physicians were asked to indicate how people with several genetic metabolic diseases usually describe their problem when they first seek care. The physicians generally cited the classic signs of disease as described in standard textbooks, which in fact are seldom the problems for which attention is sought (Holtzman, 1978).

The third reason for a population-based focus is that physicians overestimate their roles in providing care. In health systems in which individuals may seek care from any practitioner and there is no repository of information on visits made by individuals, there is no way for any individual practitioner to achieve any of the features of primary care. Physicians can report that most of their patients are "regular" even when a substantial minority of patient-initiated visits are made elsewhere (Dutton, 1981; Starfield et al., 1976). Better coordination with social services has much to offer in the ongoing care of the elderly, chronically ill, and mentally handicapped.

The fourth reason concerns the importance of feedback for the continuing education of the practitioner. When patients fail to return to the practitioner for follow up, either because they were not satisfied with the care or because they were not happy with the results, the practitioner loses information critical in learning from experience. A community focus would enable practitioners to develop information systems that could monitor the loss of patients to their care and to assess reasons for it.

The final reason for a population-based focus for clinical care derives from the imperative to add new knowledge about diseases, their natural course in the absence of treatment, and how that course can be modified by various interventions. Most of what is known about illness and especially its management results from experiences with patients in medical research centers. Although community interview surveys obtain information concerning people's perceptions of their problems, and population examination surveys provide additional information about aspects of health that can be detected by examinations and laboratory tests, neither approach can link medical care interventions with health status because clinical data generally are not available or linkable with survey data. Researchers in medical centers usually focus their attention on particular diseases. However, professional knowledge about disease does not necessarily reflect the illness experiences of people. As medical care becomes more and more effective in reducing mortality from specific causes, people will survive and thus be at risk of multiple diseases that may interact in unknown ways and may be differentially responsive to various interventions. The disease-focus approach, which characterizes most of clinical research, will increasingly have to be supplemented by a person-focused one, and such a focus can only be achieved by viewing the individual in a community context as well as in the clinical facility.

What Is Community-Oriented Primary Care?

Community-oriented primary care (COPC) has been defined in many different ways. Common to all of them is the idea that it is an approach to primary care that uses epidemiological and clinical skills in a complementary fashion to tailor programs to meet the particular health needs of a defined population. It gives explicit recognition to the interactions in the diagram of the determinants of health as presented in Chapter 1; these include the overlap of the health services system and the social and physical environment as well as the overlap of the health services system and individual behaviors that influence health.

A community-oriented approach applies the methods of clinical medicine, epidemiology, social sciences, and health services research and evaluation to the following tasks (Nutting and Connor, 1986):

• Defining and characterizing the community
• Identifying community health problems
• Modifying programs to address these problems
• Monitoring the effectiveness of the program modifications

The application of epidemiological methods in which data are more representative than those derived from clinical practices should especially improve certain aspects of care. Diagnosis and management would be more appropriate because of better recognition of etiological factors, many of which arise from social and environmental exposures. Improved "problem recognition" also should result, as more complete data will provide information on the characteristics of early stages of illness; more complete data will also facilitate the recognition of new types of disorders and of clusters of unusual symptomatology. Definitions of *normal* health also can be refined with more complete descriptions of the characteristics of those individuals who rarely appear for care.

The application of social sciences techniques should improve the recognition of existing problems through understanding of the impact of social and economic factors on health, including those of poverty, unemployment, and other stressful states.

Application of health services research techniques would provide a better understanding of the impact of various aspects of medical care and of the relationships between components of the structure, process, and outcomes of health services.

In approaches to measuring the attainment of primary care, community orientation is considered a "derivative" feature in the sense that it would "derive" from a high level of attainment of the unique features of primary care. In the process of optimally achieving a high degree of longitudinality of care, a program would have defined the population eligible for care and, in addition would have made sure that the population knew that the program assumed responsibility for its health services. The program would have thus achieved the first functional step of COPC, that of defining and characterizing the community in such a way that nonusers of services are not systematically excluded.

The second step in achieving comprehensiveness through COPC involves identifying the health needs of the enrolled population, including those individuals or groups who rarely appear for care.

The third and fourth steps, modifying the health care program and monitoring the effectiveness of the modification, would follow from the two derivative steps involving longitudinality and comprehensiveness.

The conceptual basis for COPC dates back to the writings of Will Pickles (1938) in Great Britain; Sidney Kark (1974, 1981) further developed the concept first in South Africa and then later in Israel. Several models have been evolving in the United States, although not as a formal movement toward COPC. In 1982, the Institute of Medicine of the National Academy of Sciences sponsored a conference and a study of COPC as it existed at that time in the United States.

To describe the degree to which COPC has been attained, the Academy specified the stages of achievement of each of the four aspects of COPC. Tables 14.1–14.4 describe the staging. Table 14.1 contains the stages in defining the community. At the lowest level, no effort has been made. At the highest level, there are systematic efforts that ensure a current and complete enumeration of all individuals in the community, including pertinent demographic and socioeconomic data.

Table 14.2 lists the stages in identifying community health problems. At the lowest level no systematic efforts are made to understand the health status or health needs of the community; the results from studies of the patient population are assumed to reflect the health problems in the community as a whole. At the highest level there are formal mechanisms to identify and set priorities among a broad range of potential health problems in the community, to determine their correlates and determinants, and to characterize the existing patterns of health care related to the problems.

Table 14.3 presents the stages in modifying the health care program and extends from no modifications made in response to the needs of the community (Stage 0) to Stage IV, in which modifications in the program involve both primary care and community or public health components and are targeted to specific high-risk groups with active efforts to reach these groups.

Table 14.4, which lists the stages in monitoring the effectiveness of modifications in the primary care program, has five levels. At the lowest level, examination of program effectiveness is limited to the impact on the active users of health services. In the highest stage, the effectiveness of the program is determined by techniques that are specific to program objectives, which account for differential impact among risk groups and which provide information on positive and negative impacts of the programs. Intermediate stages of achievement of these four functions describe progress toward attaining the highest level of the function.

Achieving Community-Oriented Primary Care

In the Institute of Medicine study, seven facilities seeking to provide COPC were identified and characterized. Although none of the programs had achieved a high level of COPC, several had attained relatively high levels of performance on some of the four functions (Nutting and Connor, 1984).

A notable attempt to achieve COPC in clinical practice was made by Dr. Julian

Table 14.1. Staging Criteria for COPC Function—Defining and Characterizing the Community

Stage 0	No effort has been made to define or characterize a community beyond the active users of the practice
Stage I	There is no enumeration of the individuals who comprise the community. The community is characterized by extrapolation from large area census data
Stage II	There is no enumeration of the community; it is characterized through the use of secondary data that correspond closely to the community for which the practice has accepted responsiblity
Stage III	The community can be enumerated and is actively characterized through the use of a database that includes all members of the community and that contains information to describe its demography and socioeconomic status. (Often such a data system is constructed over time from the active users of services, but approximates the community closely, e.g., at or above 90% coverage of the community.)
Stage IV	Systematic efforts ensure a current and complete enumeration of all individuals in the community, including pertinent demographic and socioeconomic data. For each individual, information exists that facilitates targeted outreach (e.g., address, telephone number)

Source: IOM (1984).

Tudor Hart in Great Britain. Dr. Hart, whose practice was located in a Welsh mining town, took responsibility for both community and clinical functions. In his concept, the "community general practitioner is a new type of physician who is engaged in local participatory democracy in the pursuit of the maximization of health" (Hart, 1983).

Mant and Anderson (1985) proposed that general practitioners accept responsibility for auditing the state of health of their patients and for publicizing the results, monitoring and controlling environmentally determined disease, auditing the effectiveness of preventive programs, and evaluating the effects of medical

Table 14.2. Staging Criteria for COPC Functions—Identifying Community Health Problems

Stage 0	No systematic efforts have been made to understand the health status or health needs of the community; the results from studies of the patient population are assumed to reflect the health problems in the community as a whole
Stage I	Community health problems are identified through general consensus of the providers and/or community groups
Stage II	Community health problems are identified by extrapolation from systematic review of secondary data, such as vital statistics, census data, large area epidemiological data, and so forth
Stage III	Community health problems are examined through the use of datasets specific to the community, but perhaps focusing on single health problems or health care issues
Stage IV	Formal mechanisms (usually but not always epidemiological techniques) are used to identify the set priorities among a broad range of potential health problems in the community, identify their correlates and determinants, and characterize the existing patterns of health care related to the problem

Source: IOM (1984).

Table 14.3. Staging Criteria for COPC Functions—Modifying the Health Care Program

Stage 0	No modifications are made in the primary care program in specific response to health needs of the large community
Stage I	Modifications address health problems believed to exist in the community, but are made more in response to a national or organization-wide initiative than in response to a particular problem specifically identified within the community
Stage II	Modifications address important community health problems, but are chosen largely due to the availability of special resources to address the particular problem and closely follow guidelines that may not be tailored to the community needs
Stage III	Modifications in the health care program are tailored to the unique needs of the community and involve (where appropriate) both the primary care and the community/public health components of the program
Stage IV	Modifications in the program involve both primary care and community/public health components and are targeted to specific high-risk or priority groups, with active efforts (e.g., outreach) made to reach specific high-risk or priority groups within the community

Source: IOM (1984).

intervention. In Great Britain, responsibility for community functions was, until recently, vested in a cadre of community medicine specialists. Mant and Anderson proposed that the functions be assumed by the primary care practitioners, with transfer of resources from the current community medicine structure to the primary care practices; such a transfer has been occurring since the early 1990s.

Some clinical organizations have found ways to link with the community in novel ways. For example, the Group Health Cooperative of Puget Sound in the state of Washington has been active in community organizations to develop automated vaccine registries and has supplied free vaccines to underserved communities. It also participates in activities to encourage the state legislature to pass laws to require greater safety in consumer product use. Its strategy to increase the use of bicycle helmet use depended on a community education cam-

Table 14.4. Staging Criteria for COPC Functions—Monitoring the Effectiveness of Program Modifications

Stage 0	Examination of program effectiveness is limited to the impact on the active users of health services
Stage I	Program effectiveness is viewed in terms of impact on the community as a whole, but is based on subjective impressions of the practitioners and/or community groups
Stage II	Program effectiveness is estimated by extrapolation from large area data or vital statistics
Stage III	Program effectiveness is determined by systematic examination of a dataset that is specific to the community
Stage IV	Program effectiveness is determined by techniques that are specific to the program objectives, account for differential impact among risk groups, and provide information on the positive and negative impacts of the program

Source: IOM (1984).

paign, the distribution of discount coupons, and the institution of a low-cost helmet campaign by the health plan (Thompson et al., 1995). Thus, its focus on
prevention was not limited to individual clinical interventions but, rather, it
adopted a community-based approach that reached far more people than an approach that depended for its success on changing the behavior of separate individuals.

In general, medical schools throughout the world have not yet recognized the
desirability of population-based approaches to the provision of health services. A
notable exception is McMaster University in the province of Ontario, Canada,
which has attempted, since its inception, to integrate the skills of population medicine with those of clinical practice. The Rockefeller Foundation in the United
States has used this model to encourage the development of programs in many
medical schools throughout the world.

In some European countries (Sweden, Finland) and in rural areas of many other
industrialized countries, physicians are actively involved in community and public
health activities. Several Latin American countries are actively pursuing an agenda
for COPC. In Cuba, an intensive effort to train family physicians has been underway since the mid-1980s. These new physicians live and work with an associated
nurse in the community they serve, which is intended to be about 600–700 people.
The family doctors spend half their time providing services in community organizations such as schools, day-care centers, and factories and in collecting information on community health needs. These physicians are expected to document
the frequency of health problems in their practices and to plan their clinical work
to address population needs (UNICEF, 1991). In Mexico, Costa Rica, Nicaragua,
and several other countries, medical education is directed at training physicians
with a community orientation; in some schools, work in the community is part of
the curriculum during each year of training in medical school (Braveman and Mora,
1987).

Several trends, in both the United States and elsewhere, may facilitate increasing community orientation of primary care practice. First, organizations such as
integrated health systems are now assuming responsibility for the care of populations. Many of these, particularly in health systems that historically organized their
health services by geographic area, may increasingly assume responsibility for community-oriented services. Second, the physician will no longer be the sole "captain
of the ship." As patients survive longer and the burdens of morbidity increase in
community settings, other health personnel will become increasingly central to the
avoidance of morbidity and the maintenance of well being. Third, there will be
heightened attention to making training programs for practitioners more relevant
to the changing population needs. Fourth, realization of the need for more effective
and more efficient health care will draw attention to COPC. COPC can help communities organize more efficiently to prevent disease and promote health and to
encourage more discriminating use of medical technologies. Finally, the advent of
increasingly better information processing resulting from highly efficient and high-
capacity computers will greatly facilitate the management of data from a variety
of sources and linkages of data from diverse sources.

Identifying and Monitoring Community Health Needs

Community health needs are notoriously difficult to specify with precision and completeness. Part of the difficulty derives from the difficulties in defining *needs,* and part is due to difficulties in ascertainment.

What is meant by a *need*? Are needs to be defined primarily by the occurrence of conditions that result in premature death, or is prevalence of the condition itself a sufficient cause for concern? Or should the disability associated with health problems determine the priorities? Or the extent to which conditions result in absence from work or school? Or, alternatively, are *needs* to be defined by failures to implement preventive strategies so that health in the community is jeopardized?

The definition of *need* will vary from time to time and from place to place depending on society's values and on the availability of data. In large measure, the definition is a matter of values: who values what for whom. Because some needs are easier to measure than others, the definition will also depend on what can be assessed at any given time or place.

In most industrialized countries, vital statistics systems provide basic information about the causes of death and about various routinely ascertained health problems, such as low birth weight or reportable diseases. Vital statistics have been used for many years as a starting point for assessment of community health needs and continue to be useful. For example, when infant mortality rates are greater in one city than in another, an investigation into the reasons for the differences is often launched. Needs are therefore defined empirically, that is, by comparison of one area with others. A "normative" approach sets specific standards or targets that are thought to be justifiable based on current knowledge of prevention and treatment.

One technique of measuring needs normatively involves a list of *sentinel* conditions, that is, those that should occur only rarely in the presence of adequate care. The method is a systematic application of differences observed from vital statistics (Rutstein et al., 1976). The list contains over 100 conditions or diagnoses. For most of the conditions on the list, death is preventable with early and appropriate medical care. For others, either preventive or treatment strategies will prevent premature death from the condition. Death statistics or, in some cases, case registries or hospitalization statistics provide the means for identifying these sentinel conditions. The occurrence of a condition on the list should signal an investigation to determine if it occurred because of inadequate or inappropriate health services in the community.

This sentinel conditions list was the basis for developing an atlas of preventable mortality that provided detail for each local region in several European countries and allowed for an empirical study of differences across areas (Holland, 1991, 1993). Notable differences in mortality were found both within and among countries. Although no effort was made to determine if the indicators could be related specifically to primary care performance rather than general health systems performance, a review of the data in this atlas provides evidence that countries with stronger primary care had lower mortality from infectious diseases (such as tuber-

culosis and intestinal infections) and lower maternal and perinatal mortality. However, conditions for which preventive interventions might be delivered in specialist
care rather than in primary care, such as breast cancer and uterine cancer, were
lower in specialty-oriented health systems. For other conditions (such as deaths
from other types of cancer, cardiovascular diseases, or asthma), which are likely
to be heavily influenced by factors other than medical care (such as climate, diet,
or living styles), there were no consistent differences across the countries.

The suggestion that the benefits of primary care would accrue more from the
way in which it manages problems and needs than from disease-oriented preventive
care is consistent with evidence that disease-oriented specialists may be better at
dispensing preventive care within their area of expertise than is the case for primary
care physicians. Thus, the benefits of prevention in primary care might be greater
for those that are generic rather than for those that are condition or organ-system
related. Although there is some evidence that this may be the case (see Chapter
8), there has been little exploration of this subject.

A *normative* approach to the assessment of health needs is *goal-setting*. This
method gained currency in the early 1980s with the publication of the U.S. Surgeon
General's "Goals and Objectives for the Nation" (U.S. Department of Health and
Human Services, 1980). These goals derived from committees of experts that selected important health problems they believed to be sensitive to change. Each
community could adopt all or some of the goals and could target resources to meet
them where the baseline frequencies suggested that a treatable problem was present.
Many goals for the year 1990 were met on the national level. The degree of variability in attainment of the goals across local areas or even states has not been
ascertained, although it is likely that many local communities modified the
goals.

Goals for the United States for the year 2000 were published in 1990 (U.S.
Department of Health and Human Services, 1990). The objectives were divided
into four main types: health promotion, health protection, preventive services, and
surveillance. They are adaptable for use at the community or state level. In small
communities, where the frequency of events is low or where estimates of frequency
may be unstable, data may have to be aggregated over several years to be useful.

Goals have also been set for each nation in the European region. The Regional
Office of the World Health Organization (1994) provided the framework with the
setting of 37 objections, as noted in Table 14.5. A comparison of the U.S. and
European goals suggests a much greater focus on the health system for achieving
health goals in Europe. In particular, primary care is identified as a priority in
Europe but is mentioned in the U.S. compendium only in the context of coordinating preventive and episodic care and reaching clinical preventive medicine goals
such as screening tests and immunizations.

The empirical approach to defining health needs, in which the goals are to
reduce disparities among different areas and population subgroups, has also undergone refinement. Computerization of health records and standardized reporting
of diagnoses from hospitalizations makes possible the detection of differences in
rates of illness in local communities. Known as the *small area variation* approach,
this method provides information that suggests the existence of systematic differ-

Table 14.5. Health for All by the Year 2000:
Areas in the WHO European Region Where
Specific Goals Were Specified*

Equity in Health
  Adding life to years
  Better opportunities for the disabled
  Reducing disease and disability

Elimination of Specific Diseases
  Life expectancy at birth
  Infant mortality
  Maternal mortality
  Mortality from diseases of the circulation
  Cancer mortality
  Deaths from accidents
  Suicides

Health Public Policy
  Social support systems
  Knowledge and motivation for healthy behavior
  Positive health behavior
  Reduction in health-damaging behavior

Environmental health policies
  Monitoring and control mechanisms
  Control of water pollution
  Control of air pollution
  Food safety
  Control of hazardous wastes
  Human settlements and housing
  Working environment

A System Based on Primary Health Care
  Resources for and content of care (2)
  Care providers and community resources (2)
  Quality of services (2)

Research Strategies
  Policies for health for all
  Planning and resource allocation
  Health information systems
  Human resource development (2)

*Figures in parentheses indicate number of specific
goals within the category.

Source: World Health Organization (1994).

ences in health needs among different communities. Small area variations can occur for several reasons, including true differences in morbidity because of different environmental exposures or because of variations in medical practice that result in different propensities to hospitalize for the same condition. Systematic differences in hospitalizations for conditions thought to be amenable to prevention, or believed to be treatable in an early stage so as to avoid hospitalization, suggest the existence of health needs that are not being adequately met in some communities. Billings

et al. (1989) pioneered this method in a study of hospitalizations in various metropolitan areas.

They examined rates of hospitalization for conditions where good primary care
should avoid progression of illnesses to the stage where they require hospitalization.
The first study, in New York City, found rates of such admissions to be three times
higher in low-income areas than in high-income areas (Billings et al., 1993). In a
similar study in Washington, DC, patients with a single practitioner in charge of
their care or treatment were half as likely to be hospitalized for such a condition
as those without such a practitioner in both low- and high-income patients (Billings
and Teicholz, 1990). Similar studies by the same group of investigators in 15
different urban areas across the United States confirmed the existence of disparities
in these hospitalization rates across income groups but failed to find them in three
cities in Ontario, Canada, where access to care is universal and people of low
income have similar access to primary care services as more advantaged people
(Billings et al., 1996). A parallel study in one area in Spain, a country with universal access to good primary care services, also found no differences in rates of
childhood hospitalizations across income groups (Casanova and Starfield, 1995). A
study in three areas in the northeast United States supported the importance of a
source of primary care by showing that children hospitalized with acute illnesses
had more severe illnesses if their linkage with a source of primary care was poor.
Furthermore, the adequacies of both first-contact care and coordination, as manifested by whether the patient was seen by the primary care practitioner before
hospitalization, whether the practitioner made the referral to the hospital, and
whether the practitioner followed the patient in the hospital, varied by area and by
type of health plan. The only findings that were consistent across the three areas
were the high rates of coordination of services by physicians in community-based
private practice or in staff model health maintenance organizations (Perrin et al.,
1996). The linkage between primary care services and lower rates of hospitalization
for these ambulatory-sensitive conditions was further strengthened by a study in
the entire state of Pennsylvania. Only the number of family physicians per population was significantly associated with lower rates of hospitalization for these conditions in both adults and children, even 'after controlling for the income of each
of the 27 areas in the state. Neither the supply of pediatricians nor of general
internists showed the same association (Parchman and Culler, 1994).

Many other studies have shown that rates of hospitalization, in general and for
ambulatory care–sensitive conditions in particular, are higher in areas where access
to care is poorer, as measured by changes when financial access is withdrawn
(Roemer et al., 1975), by community surveys (Bindman et al., 1995), or by absence
of insurance (Weissman et al., 1992). A variant of the studies on small area variation used national data from the Child Health Supplement of the National Health
Interview Survey of 1988 linked to county level data from the Area Resource File
of the Department of Health and Human Services. The study demonstrated that
children residing in counties where the supply of primary care physicians was in
the top quintile had half the odds of having an emergency department facility as
their source of primary care as children in low quintiles (Halfon et al., 1996). Thus,
differences in use of emergency department facilities, particularly when the need

for care is not urgent, can serve as a measure of adequacy of the organization and delivery of services to meet population needs.

Any community with higher than expected rates of hospitalization for ambulatory-sensitive conditions should examine its ambulatory services to determine if they are adequate in providing needed care in the community. For example, would additional social services or visiting nurses help to keep individuals under care at home when the severity of their illness alone does not require hospitalization? Are health services located so that needy individuals can reach them? Are the economic incentives for providing certain services perverse? Are the physicians' services of poor quality? Is the excess hospitalization just a result of idiosyncratic differences in the propensity of local physicians to hospitalize patients because of particular characteristics of those patients?

Responding to Community Health Priorities

Many experts working in the area of local health services throughout the world, particularly in developing countries, believe that community orientation requires attention not only to community health needs but also to empowerment of communities to play the major role in identifying the determinants of these needs and devising solutions to meet them. Such approaches are uncommon in industrialized countries, but, where they exist, they can serve as models for others.

Experience in both developed and developing countries indicates that sustainable behavior change is best promoted by family and community participation rather than the usual approach that encourages dependency by telling people what is in their best interests (Taylor, 1995).

In some areas of Canada, the need for community-based health services is well recognized. Community-based health services (CBHSs) imply a focus on a comprehensive range of noninstitutional health and related services that are generally synonymous with primary care services. Because the idea of CBHS developed from experience with a variety of different types of facilities in different provinces (including community health centers and the Centres Locaux des Services Communautaires [CLSC] in Quebec, as well as networks of primary care organizations and public health agencies), there is no one organizational model. CBHSs share common goals, however, including service effectiveness, economic efficiency, equity, consumer and community empowerment, and quality of worklife for those working in the system. Although there is little experience anywhere that enables specification of organizational characteristics to achieve these goals, there are a few fundamental principles that guide the activities, including greater attention to identifying consumer preferences for participation in health services decision-making (see Chapter 9); integration of services with multiservice and interdisciplinary approaches (see Chapter 5); the use of population-based funding with adjustments for different levels of health to achieve greater services equity; and a clear definition of the service catchment area (although it is recognized that the optimal catchment size is unknown).

The community orientation of the Canadian effort is evident from the goals for the structural elements of a local health system. Table 14.6 indicates the goals for defining the population, the resources that are needed to provide the services and the skills of the personnel, the funding mechanisms, governance structure, organizational structure, and information system. The emphasis on involving the community at all levels of decision-making is evident. No specific goals for CBHS performance or outcomes are prescribed, as it is recognized that communities differ and that needs change from place to place and time to time. However, a template for developing community plans and evaluation based on structure, process, and outcome components guides the activities of the different communities.

Individual primary care practices can also engage in activities that identify and respond to community health needs. One such effort, the Patient Advisory Council, has been used successfully in a fee-for-service family practice in Minnesota. The practice defined its patient population and invited all members to join the council and attend the four meetings held during each year. In addition, ongoing activities of the Council are directed at improving various aspects of the services. Decision-making in the practice is shared with the Council. One committee of the Council

Table 14.6. Community-Based Health Services: Structural Goals

---

Population Served

CBHS organizations serve an identifiable community defined by either geographic territory or common need

CBHSs are readily accessible to the population served and subgroups targeted

Resources

CBHS organizations use and support the most cost-effective service providers

Provider Skills

CBHS providers possess the skills necessary for their assigned functions

Organizational Regulation

The legislation under which CBHS providers operate enables cost-effective human resources management

Funding

Funding mechanisms for CBHS organizations and providers facilitate cost-effective and creative use of available health services dollars

Governance

The governance structure ensures adequate representation and involvement by the community served in the formation, implementation, and evaluation of CBHS policy

The mandate of CBHS governance boards, as expressed in provincial or territorial legislation, is clear

CBHS board members understand their legal mandate and possess the necessary skills to effectively govern the organization

Organizational Structure

CBHSs are structured to facilitate cost-effective and consumer-oriented service delivery approaches

Information Systems

Information systems that facilitate the planning, delivery, monitoring, and evaluation of CBHS are present and used

---

Source: Wanke et al. (1996).

(Services Improvement Committee) has helped the practice to better understand the needs of the community. As a result, the practice has lower malpractice premiums than others in the area. In addition, epidemiological data show that the practice identifies psychosocial problems in the population at rates comparable with those ascertained from community studies, whereas the rates in other practices are much lower (Seifert and Seifert, 1982).

As the capacity to collect data from an increasing number and variety of sources increases, new possibilities for identifying different types of community health needs will arise. A standardized dataset for ambulatory care that routinely reports all problems and diagnoses made in office- and center-based practice will illuminate the existence of problems not generally causing death or hospitalization. New systems for eliciting and categorizing different types of disability, limitation of activity, and interference with social roles as a result of health problems will make possible the use of these types of information to assess community health needs in ways other than by traditional morbidity and mortality statistics. Better and less expensive approaches to surveying populations outside of health facilities will provide yet another avenue to identify new types of health needs and will, in addition, provide a more complete picture of health needs than that obtained from data on individuals who have already received services.

The development of technology for collecting and processing information will certainly facilitate achievement of the initial steps in COPC. Improved medical technology will expand the definition of *health needs*; as existing problems are solved, new challenges at another level of need will emerge. Community-oriented care may not be achieved everywhere and to the same degree in all places. However, it is a concept that is now appropriate for consideration as the challenges of the 21st century approach.

Community-Oriented Primary Care and Public Health

The advent of managed care, wherein clinical medicine practices take responsibility for all care of a defined population, is likely to blur the boundaries between conventional public health and clinical medicine. Table 14.7 outlines the different types of interventions within the health services systems. The rows of the tables designate the type of population for which the intervention is designed, moving vertically down from aggregated populations (in which the intervention is targeted at the population as a whole rather than at individuals), at whole populations but targeted at individuals within those populations, at individuals within those populations who are selected according to the presence of some known or suspected risk factor, or at individuals because they have some individual characteristic. The columns of the table are divided according to the type of function ranging from primary (wherein the intervention is designed to avert the occurrence of a problem), to secondary (in which pathology is detected before it becomes overt), to tertiary (which involves avoidance of progression of pathology, its reversal, or remediation of its effects). Table 14.8 identifies the locus of responsibility for the intervention by its type. It is unlikely that clinical medicine services would assume primary

Table 14.7. Examples of Interventions by Type of Function and Target Group

Target	Type of Function		
	Primary	Secondary	Tertiary
Generalized populations	Environmental planning	Environmental monitoring and product control	Public advocacy, community mobilization (legal and social remedy)
individuals	Health education campaigns, immunizations	Phenylketonuria screening, breast cancer screening	Information systems†: data standardization, collection, analysis, and dissemination
Selective	Genetic engineering‡	Blood lead screening	Outreach/access, e.g., home visiting
Indicated	Communicable disease control, prophylactic antibiotics, practice guidelines	Frequent follow up for disease recurrence	Address problems: quality assessment of clinical services

* Type of function: Primary: intervention to prevent a problem from occurring; secondary: intervention at a stage before problem is manifested; tertiary: remediation to reverse manifestations of problem.

† Activities involve monitoring health statistics and surveying health status, access, and people's experiences with services.

‡ Should such an effort ever be considered ethical or practical.

responsibility for all or most activities in the top row of the table involving activities concerning environmental planning, monitoring, or regulation; product monitoring or regulation; or social and legal remedies to address threats to health of the population. On the other hand, interventions in all nine of the other cells could theoretically or actually fall within the realm of responsibility of either the public health or the clinical medicine sector, particularly if public health is defined as "organized community efforts aimed at the prevention of disease and promotion of health" (Holland et al., 1991).

Table 14.8. Locus of Responsibility for Interventions by Type of Function and Target Group

Target	Type of Function		
	Primary	Secondary	Tertiary
Generalized			
Populations	PH	PH	PH
Individuals	PH/CM	PH/CM	PH/CM
Selective	?	PH/CM	PH/CM
Indicated	PH/CM	PH/CM	PH/CM

PH, public health; CM, clinical medical care.

Source: Starfield (1996).

The potential for collaboration between clinical medicine and public health was documented by a review of over 500 initiatives existing in the United States in the mid-1990s (Lasker, 1997). Six types of "synergies" were identified:

- Improving services by coordinating care for individuals
- Improving access to care by establishing frameworks to provide services for the uninsured
- Improving the quality and cost effectiveness of services by applying a population perspective to medical practice
- Using clinical practice to identify and address community health problems
- Strengthening health promotion and health protection by mobilizing community campaigns
- Shaping the future direction of the health system by collaborating around policy, training, and research

Thus, it appears likely that the field of community-oriented primary care may, over time, merge with that of public health with many different models of teamwork merging in different areas depending on choices made by the localities themselves. The role of central and regional governments will be to set the framework for needs assessments and the general principles for evaluation of impact. The general lack of success worldwide in achieving a strong community orientation of any primary care system, other than local models such as described earlier in this chapter, may well be due to the fluidity of the boundaries between the two population-oriented fields and especially to the absence of clear goals and mandates to focus the attention and energies of communities.

References

Billings J, Zeitel L, Lukomnik J, Carey TS, Blank AE, Newman L. Impact of socioeconomic status on hospital use in New York City. Health Aff 1993 12(1):162–73.

Billings J, Hasselblad V. Use of Small Area Analysis to Assess the Performance of the Outpatient Delivery System in New York City. Lyme, NH: The Codman Research Group, Inc., 1989.

Billings J, Anderson G, Newman L. Recent findings on preventable hospitalizations. Health Aff 1996; 15:239–49.

Billings J, Teicholz N. Uninsured patients in District of Columbia hospitals. Health Aff 1990; 9:158–65.

Bindman AB, Grumbach K, Osmond D, Komaromy M, Vranizan K, Lurie N, Billings J, Stewart A. Preventable hospitalization rates and access to health care. JAMA. 1995; 274:305–11.

Braveman P, Mora F. Training physicians for community-oriented primary care in Latin America: Model programs in Mexico, Nicaragua, and Costa Rica. Am J Public Health 1987; 77:485–90.

Bunker J, Frazier H, Mosteller F. Improving health: measuring the effects of medical care. Milbank Q 1994; 72:225–58.

Casanova C, Starfield B. Hospitalizations of children and access to primary care: A cross-national comparison. Int J Health Serv 1995; 25(2):283–94.

Dutton D. Children's Health Care: The Myth of Equal Access. In: Select Panel for the

Promotion of Child Health, Better Health for Our Children: A National Strategy. U.S. Department of Health and Human Services, PHS Pub. No. 79-55071. Washington, DC: US-GPO, Vol 4, 1981, pp 357–440.

Fihn S, Wicher J. Withdrawing routine outpatient medical services: Effects on access and health. J Gen Intern Med 1988; 3:356–62.

Hart JT. A new type of general practitioner. Lancet 1983; ii:2729.

Halfon N, Newacheck PW, Wood DL. St Peter RF. Routine emergency department use for sick care by children in the United States. Pediatrics 1996; 98(1):28–34.

Holland WW. European Community Atlas of "Avoidable Death." Commission of the European Communities health services research. Series No.6, 9. Vols. 1, 2. 2nd Ed., Oxford: Oxford University Press, 1993.

Holland WW, Detels R, Knox G (eds). Oxford Textbook of Public Health. Vol. 1, 2nd Ed. Influences of Public Health. Oxford: Oxford University Press, 1991.

Holtzman N. Rare diseases, common problems: recognition and management. Pediatrics 1978; 62:1056–60.

Institute of Medicine (IOM). Community Oriented Primary Care: A Practical Assessment. Vol I. Washington, D.C. : National Academy Press, 1984.

Kark SL. Community Oriented Primary Health Care. New York: Appleton-Century-Crofts, 1981.

Kark SL. From medicine in the community to community medicine. JAMA 1974; 228: 1585–6.

Lasker R, and the Committee on Medicine and Public Health. Medicine and Public Health: The Power of Collaboration. New York: New York Academy of Medicine; 1997.

Luke B, Mamelle N, Keith L, Munoz F, Minogue J, Papiernik E, Johnson TR. The association between occupational factors and preterm birth: A United States nurses' study. Research Committee of the Association of Women's Health, Obstetric, and Neonatal Nurses. Am J Obstet Gynecol 1995; 173(3 pt 1):849–62.

Lurie N, Ward N, Shapiro M, Gallego C, Vahaiwalla R, Brook R. Termination of Medi-Cal benefits. A follow-up study one year later. N Engl J Med 1986; 314:1266–8.

Mant D, Anderson P. Community general practitioner. Lancet 1985; ii:1114–17.

Nutting P, Connor E. Community Oriented Primary Care. A Practical Assessment. Vol. II, Case Studies. Washington, DC: National Academy Press, 1984.

Nutting P, Connor E. Community-oriented primary care: an integrated model for practice, research, and education. Am J Prev Med 1986; 2:140–7.

Parchman M, Culler S. Primary care physicians and avoidable hospitalizations. J Fam Pract 1994; 39(2):123–8.

Perrin JM, Greenspan P, Bloom SR, Finkelstein D, Yazdgerdi S, Leventhal JM, Rodewald L, Szilagyi P, Homer CH. Primary care involvement among hospitalized children. Arch Pediatr Adolesc Med. 1996; 150:479–86.

Pickles WN. Epidemiology in Clinical Practice. Bristol: John Wright and Sons, 1938.

Roemer M, Hopkins C, Carr L, Gartside F. Copayments for ambulatory care: Penny-wise and pound-foolish. Med Care 1975; 13:457–66.

Rutstein D, Berenberg W, Chalmers T, Child C, Fishman A, Perrin E. Measuring the quality of medical care: A clinical method. N Engl J Med 1976; 296:582–8.

Seifert M, Seifert M Jr. The patient advisory council concept. In Connor E, Mullan F (eds): Community Oriented Primary Care. Conference Proceedings. Institute of Medicine. Washington, DC: National Academy Press, 1982. pp 307–312.

Starfield B, Simborg D, Horn S, Yourtee S. Continuity and coordination in primary care: Their achievement and utility. Med Care 1976; 14(7):625–36.

Starfield, B. Effectiveness of Medical Care: Validating Clinical Wisdom. Baltimore: Johns Hopkins University Press, 1985.

Starfield B. Public health and primary care: A framework for proposed linkages. Am J Public Health 1996, 86(10):1365–9.

Taylor C. E.H. Christopherson Lecture: Lessons for the United States from the Worldwide Child Survival Revolution. Pediatrics 1995; 96:342–6.

Thompson RS, Taplin SH, McAfee TA, Mandelson MT, Smith AE. Primary and secondary prevention services in clinical practice. Twenty years' experience in development, implementation, and evaluation. JAMA 1995; 273(14):1130–5.

UNICEF/UNFPA/OPS/OMS/MINSAP. Cuba's Family Doctor Programme (monograph). Distributed at the 3rd International Seminar on Primary Care. Havana, Cuba, March 12–16, 1991.

U.S. Department of Health and Human Services. Public Health Service. Promoting Health/Preventing Disease. Year 2000 Objectives for the Nation. Washington, DC: U.S. Department of Health and Human Services, 1980.

U.S. Department of Health and Human Services. Public Health Service. Promoting Health/Preventing Disease: Year 2000 Objectives for the Nation. DHHS Pub. No. (PHS)90-50212. Washington, DC: U.S. Department of Health and Human Services, 1990.

Wanke M, Saunders LD, Pong RW, Church WJB. Building a Stronger Foundation: A Framework for Planning and Evaluating Community-Based Health Services in Canada 1995. Health Promotion and Program Branch, Health Canada. Ottawa: Canadian Dept of Supply and Services, 1996.

Weissman J, Gatsonis C, Epstein A. Rates of avoidable hospitalization by insurance status in Massachusetts and Maryland. JAMA 1992; 268:2388–94.

White KL, Williams TF, Greenberg BG. The ecology of medical care. N Engl J Med 1961; 265:885–92.

World Health Organization. Implementation of the Global Strategy for Health for All by the Year 2000. 2nd evaluation. Vol. 5, European Region. Copenhagen: Regional Office for Europe, 1994.

— V —
Health Policy
and Primary Care

— 15 —

Primary Care Systems in Western Industrialized Nations

Chapter 1 contains a description of the relationship between the characteristics of primary care in 11 different western industrialized nations and their relationship with health levels and costs of health services. That study used information concerning the late 1980s. Since that time, the health systems of many countries have undergone reforms in financing and organization. Most of the reforms, which are still ongoing, were designed to reduce the inexorable rise in the costs of health care worldwide, as a result of new and expensive technologies, ageing of the population, and changing morbidity patterns. The extent to which the reforms have changed the practice of primary care is not well known; only some of them were specifically designed to do so. Although the philosophical underpinnings of most national health systems may not have been affected, this might not be the case for specific health policies related to the achievement of primary care objectives. For example, the imposition of co-payments might affect access to primary care physicians and achievement of first contact care, particularly if the reforms are not accompanied by ''gatekeeper'' requirements. Reorientation of primary care services from individual physicians to groups might interfere with longitudinality if it interferes with maintenance of strong interpersonal relationships between patients and their practitioners. Better planning and organization of services consequent to the formation of formal groups or health systems that integrate primary care services with consultative (secondary) and referral (tertiary) services might alter the comprehensiveness of services provided by primary care practitioners and change the nature of coordination of care in unpredicted ways.

This chapter presents data on the characteristics of national health systems that are conducive to a primary care orientation (policy priorities at the national level) as well as information on practice characteristics that reflect good primary care. Only industrialized nations are included in the comparison to minimize the possible confounding effects of widely disparate historical, cultural, and philosophical characteristics of eastern and western countries and the impact of national wealth on

335

health system characteristics and functions. Only countries with populations of 5 million or more are presented, although comparable information is available on several smaller countries (see, for example, Grant., et al. [1997] concerning New Zealand). Other countries that fulfill these criteria were omitted because comparable current data are not available.

Policy characteristics include the extent to which the system regulates the distribution of resources throughout the country; the modal type of primary care practitioner; the mode of financing of primary care services; the percentage of active physicians involved in primary care rather than other specialty care; the ratio of average professional earnings of primary care physicians compared with other specialists; the most common site of primary care services; the requirement for patient lists to identify the community served by practices; 24-hour access arrangements; the requirement for cost sharing by patients; the mode of reimbursing primary care physicians and other specialists; the role of primary care physicians in providing in-hospital care to their patients; whether or not specialists have practices in the community outside of hospitals; and the strength of academic departments of primary care of general practice.

The practice characteristics include first-contact care; longitudinality; comprehensiveness; coordination; family-centeredness; community orientation; and the frequency of home visiting.

The following section describes the countries and their characteristics.* To rate the primary care orientation of each country, each characteristic was assigned a score from 0 (connoting the absence or poor development of the characteristic) to 2 (connoting a high level of development of the characteristic). A score of 1 was assigned if there was moderate development of the characteristic. Table 15.1 describes the criteria for scoring the health system and practice characteristics. The unweighted scores for each country were averaged to derive a "primary care score."

The scores for each country reflect the characteristics of the most common form of services only and not other systems that may provide more adequate primary care to certain segments of the population.

In the following country descriptions, the rating for each of the characteristics that were scored is indicated in parentheses.

---

*Major sources of information are Organization for Economic Cooperation and Development Health Policy Studies No.7 (1995); Fry and Horder (1994); Boerma et al. (1994) (reprint from 1993 publication); Statistics Netherlands (1996); and official documents (such as the WHO-EURO country profiles). I am particularly indebted to John Horder, who led me to many published sources of information and provided me with the benefit of his great wisdom. Other individuals (and organizations) who were of great help include Juan Gérvas (Madrid); Wienke Boerma at NIVEL; Ellie Tragakes and Janet Leifelt (WHO-EURO); Stephen Buetow, Martin Roland, Francois Mennerat (St. Eienne); Simone Sandier (Paris); Jande Maeseneer (Ghent); Ruut de Melker (Utrecht); Margo Rowan and the staff of the Canadian Medical Association (Ottawa); Robert Reid (Canada); Bronnie Veale (Flinders, Australia); Anne Staehr Johansen (Copenhagen); Esko Kalimo, Ilkka Vohlonen, and Pertti Kekki (Helsinki); Lennart Carlsson and Lars Linder (Stockholm); Alexandra Prados (Granada); Jon Orueta (Bilbao); Sebastian Juncosa (Barcelona); and Javier Elola (Madrid).

Country Characteristics Regarding Primary Care

Australia

Type of system: Partially unregulated primary care: incentives for practice in rural areas; billing numbers to be rationed by area (1)

Financing: National health insurance, universal, tax based (2)

Type of primary care practitioner: Family/general practitioner (2)

Percent active physicians who are specialists: More generalists than specialists (2)

Professional earnings of primary care physicians relative to specialists: Approximately 1:2 (0)

Cost sharing for primary care: 80% of general practitioners bulk-bill (patients pay nothing). Otherwise, low co-pay. (2)

Patient list: No (0)

Requirements for 24-hour coverage: Part of vocational registration obligation (deputizing services) (0)

Strength of academic departments of family medicine: Moderate (1)

Most common site of primary care practice: Solo practice

Reimbursement of primary care physicians: Fee for service, extra billing allowed (20% of general practitioners do so)

Reimbursement of specialists: Fee for service (in office-based practice)

General practitioners care for patients in hospital: No, except rural areas

Specialists restricted to hospital: No

Primary care organized by defined geographic area: No

First Contact: Yes; access to specialists by referral from primary care (2)

Longitudinality: Variable (1)

Comprehensiveness: Extensive range (2)

Coordination: Poor between general practitioners and specialists (0)

Family-Centeredness: Yes (2)

Community orientation: Moderate to poor (0)

Belgium

Type of system: Unregulated primary care (0)

Financing: Virtually universal (98%); over half (52%) by employer–employee contributions (1)

Type of primary care practitioner: Family (general) practitioner (2)

Percent active physicians who are specialists: 46% (1)

Professional earnings of primary care physicians relative to specialists: Not available

Cost sharing for primary care: High (25%), except 10% for ''vulnerable'' groups (0)

Patient list: No (0)

Requirements for 24-hour coverage: No (0)

Strength of academic departments of family medicine: Fair (1)

Table 15.1. Criteria for Rating of Health System and Practice Characteristics Related to
Primary Care

Health System Characteristics

Type of system. Regulated primary care or public health centers are considered to have the highest
commitment to primary care. Regulated primary care implies that national policies influence the
location of physician practice so that they are distributed throughout the population rather than
concentrated in certain geographic areas. Public health centers are also assumed to represent the
equitable distribution of physician resources. Intermediate scores connote systems where incentives
for equitable distribution are present and moderately effective

Financing. Tax-based systems are given the highest score because they are generally more
progressive in financing than other forms of financing. Social security–based systems are given an
intermediate score because the percentage for employee contributions are not generally tied to
level of income. Financing primarily through private insurance agencies is given the lowest
score

Type of primary care practitioner. Generalists (family or general practitioners) are the prototypical
primary care physicians because the nature of their training is exclusively devoted to primary care
practice. General pediatricians and general internists are considered "intermediate" primary care
practitioners because their training has a major subspecialty focus. Other specialists are not
considered primary care physicians because their training is focused on subspecialty issues

Percent active physicians who are specialists. A value equal to or below 50% is considered
indicative of an orientation toward primary care. Values of 51%–69% are considered intermediate,
and values above 70% are considered to indicate a specialty-oriented system

Professional earnings of primary care physicians relative to specialists. A high ratio (0.9:1 or above)
of average salary of primary care physicians to specialty physicians is considered an incentive
toward primary care. A low ratio (0.8:1 or less) is considered an incentive toward a specialty-
oriented system. Ratios between 0.8 and 0.9 are considered intermediate

Cost sharing for primary care services. The highest score is assigned where there are none or very
low requirements for co-payments. Intermediate scores are assigned where required co-payments
are low and/or where there are ceilings on the level of payments. Low scores are assigned where
co-payments are substantial and/or where there is no ceiling

Patient lists. Highest scores are assigned where there are system requirements for personal lists.
Intermediate scores are assigned where there are group lists and/or where the existence of such
lists is de facto rather than required. The lowest score is assigned where neither is present

Requirements for 24-hour coverage. Where either personal or delegated 24 hour coverage exists by
legal obligation, the maximum score is assigned. Where there is a social rather than a legal
obligation, an intermediate score is assigned. The lowest score reflects the absence of either

Strength of academic departments of family medicine. Highest scores are given when these are as
strong as departments of other specialities. Intermediate scores are given where strength is not
uniform across the country, and low scores are given where family medicine is accorded low
priority or prestige in medical education and training

System characteristics not scored for primary care are where care is provided (because there is no
evidence that one type of site is better than another), the type of reimbursement of generalists and
of specialists (because the impact of type of reimbursement on incentives for primary care practice

Most common site of primary care practice: Solo general practitioner offices
Reimbursement of primary care physicians: Fee for service, direct from patient,
partially reimbursed, except low income exempt from pay. Negotiated fee, phy-
sician not bound by it (extra billing allowed)
Reimbursement of specialists: Fee for service
General practitioners care for patients in hospital: No
Specialists restricted to hospital: No
Primary care organized by defined geographic area: No

Table 15.1. —Continued

is unknown), whether or not generalists care for patients in hospitals (because there is little evidence on the impact of this feature of a health services system), whether or not specialists are restricted to hospitals (because consultations with primary care physicians might be enhanced by limited specialty practice in the community), team work, and extent of home visiting because the contributions of these to primary care functions is unknown. Even though the assignment of primary care services to a defined geographic area is considered conducive to community orientation and hence potentially pursuant to a high level of primary care, no points are assigned because community orientation is assessed directly

Rating Practice Characteristics

First contact. First contact implies that decisions about the need for specialty services are made after consulting the primary care physician. Requirements for access to specialists via referral from primary care are considered most consistent with the first-contact aspect of primary care. The ability of patient to self-refer to specialists is considered conducive to a specialty-oriented health system. Where there are incentives to reduce direct access to specialists but no requirement for a referral, an intermediate score is assigned

Longitudinality. Longitudinality connotes the extent of relationship with a practitioner or facility over time that is not based on the presence of specific types of diagnoses or health problems. Highest ratings are given where the relationship is based on enrollment or registration (patient lists) with a particular practitioner. Lowest rates are given where there is not an implicit or explicit relationship over time, and intermediate scores are assigned where this relationship exists by default rather than intent

Comprehensiveness. The extent to which a full range of services is either directly provided by the primary care physician or specifically arranged for elsewhere is the measure of comprehensiveness. Highest ratings are given to arrangements for the universal provision of extensive and uniform benefits and for care of children, elderly, and women as well as other adults, routine obstetric care provided by primary care practitioners, consideration of mental health needs in primary care practice, performance of minor surgery, and various aspects of preventive care. Highest scores are assigned when most of these services are performed in primary care practice. Intermediate scores are assigned when fewer than a majority are provided or when less than a majority provide most, but it is routine. Lowest scores are assigned when the provision of most of these services is not usually characteristic of primary care practice

Coordination. Care is considered coordinated where there are formal guidelines for the transfer of information between primary care physicians and specialists. Where this is present for only certain aspects of care (such as long-term care), intermediate ratings are given. Low ratings reflect the general absence of guidelines for the transfer of information about patients

Family-centeredness. High ratings are given to explicit assumption of responsibility for family-centered care

Community orientation. High ratings are given where practitioners use community data in planning for services or for the identification of problems. Intermediate values are assigned where clinical data derived from analysis of data from the practice are used to identify priorities for care. Low ratings are assigned when there is little or no attempt to use data to plan or organize services

---

First contact: No (0)

Longitudinality: No (0)

Comprehensiveness: Poor. Preventive care done mainly by public health, including pregnancy-related care, outpatient mental health, school health, occupational health, under age 5 preventive care (0)

Coordination: Poor (0)

Family-centeredness: Poor (0)

Community orientation: Poor (0)

Canada

Type of system: Partially regulated (incentive). In Quebec, regulated, but poor distribution of family practitioners overall (1)
Financing: Universal coverage; tax based (2)
Type of primary care practitioner: General practitioners and pediatricians (1.5)
Percent active physicians who are specialists: 49% (2)
Professional earnings of primary care physicians relative to specialists: approximately 2:3 (higher in rural areas) (0)
Cost sharing for primary care: No (2)
Patient list: No. Some proposals to introduce registration (0)
Requirements for 24-hour coverage: Moderate (by social obligation) (1)
Strength of Academic departments of family medicine: Strong (2)

Most common site of primary care practice: Group practices (67%)
Reimbursement of primary care physicians: Fee for service (negotiated), but fee for procedures is low. Some provinces set global cap
Reimbursement of specialists: Fee for service (negotiated)
General practitioners care for patients in hospital: In rural areas primarily
Specialists restricted to hospital: No
Primary care organized by defined geographic area: No

First contact: Yes, through incentives (specialists paid less if patient self-referred) (1)
Longitudinality: Variable (1)
Comprehensiveness: Good. Preventive care good in primary care; in rural areas, general practitioners do half of all normal deliveries and 20% of cesarean sections (2)
Coordination: Moderate. Professional policy but not often followed (0.5)
Family-centeredness: Generally good (1)
Community orientation: Variable (0.5)

Denmark

Type of system: Regulated primary care (2)
Financing: Virtually universal; tax based (2)
Type of primary care practitioner: Family (general) practitioners (2)
Percent active physicians who are specialists: 75% , including community-based specialists with direct access (0)
Professional earnings of primary care physicians relative to specialists: 1:1 (2)
Cost sharing for primary care: Low (2)
Patient list: Yes (2)
Requirements for 24-hour coverage: Yes, legal obligation (2)
Strength of academic departments of family medicine: Strong (2)

Most common site of primary care practice: Solo/group practice (33%/49%)
Reimbursement of primary care physicians: About 1/4 capitation, 3/4 fee for ser-

vice including minor surgery, some diagnostic tests, pregnancy-related care, certificates, but *not* for preventive care

Reimbursement of specialists: Fee for service in community; salary in hospital

General practitioners care for patients in hospital: No

Specialists restricted to hospital: Yes, except ophthalmologists and ENT as well as "Midi" specialists who do day surgery, angiography

Primary care organized by defined geographic area: Yes (radius 10 Km)

First contact: Yes, but direct access to otolaryngologists and ophthalmologists (2)

Longitudinality: Yes, but must change if move out of doctor's area (2)

Comprehensiveness: High. Preventive services strongly developed; excellent relationships with community nurses, mental health (2)

Coordination: Moderate. General practitioners receive feedback from outpatient specialists and nurses, but poor communication with hospital specialists (1)

Family-centeredness: High. Children assigned to same general practitioner as parent (2)

Community orientation: Moderate (1)

Finland

Type of system: Public, center based (regulated primary care) with substantial private sector (2)

Financing: 100% ; tax based (2)

Type of primary care practitioner: Family (general) practitioners (2)

Percent active physicians who are specialists: 63%–68% (1)

Professional earnings of primary care physicians relative to specialists: 1:1 (2)

Cost sharing for primary care: Substantial ($17–$20 or 50 marks for first three visits in a year, except children and elderly) (1)

Patient list: Only one-third of general practitioners have lists (1)

Requirements for 24-hour coverage: Yes, by doctors in health centers (2)

Strength of academic departments of family medicine: Strong (2)

Most common site of primary care practice: Health centers (55% of all visits)

Reimbursement of primary care physicians: Salary and fee for service for overtime for 60%; capitation and fee for services for overtime (40%)

Reimbursement of specialists: Salary, but substantial private sector with fee for service with direct billing to patients; 40% of private visits are referred by public sector

General practitioners care for patients in hospital: No, but most health centers have chronic care/nursing home beds

Specialists restricted to hospital: Yes in public sector (about 70%), no in private sector (about 30%). Hospital specialists often work after hours in private sector

Primary care organized by defined geographic area: Yes

First contact: Yes, in public sector. Effectively, only about 25% of people have first-contact care. Any patient can go to a private doctor and ask for a hospital referral (1)

Longitudinality: Moderate. Choice of physician is limited but possible. Overall, poor during 1990–95, but getting better because use of list is increasing (36%) (1)

Comprehensiveness: Extensive range; excellent range of services (2)

Coordination: No formal guidelines; poor coordination with specialists, good with long-term care (1)

Family-centeredness: Poor (0)

Community orientation: High (2)

France

Type of system: Unregulated (0)

Financing: 100%; employer–employee social insurance (65%) (1)

Type of primary care practitioner: Family (general practitioners) and specialists (gynecologists for many women and pediatricians for child preventive care) (1)

Percent active physicians who are specialists: 50% (2)

Professional earnings of primary care physicians relative to specialists: 1:2 (0)

Cost sharing for primary care: High: 30% of agreed fee schedule and over-billing common, but co-payments are zero for vulnerable groups and long-term illness. Patients pay and are reimbursed by social insurance or private insurance if they have it (0)

Patient list: No. Some proposals to institute registration (0)

Requirements for 24-hour coverage: Moderate (social obligation) (1)

Strength of academic departments of family medicine: Poor (0)

Most common site of primary care practice: Solo practice (80%).

Reimbursement of primary care physicians: Fee for service (according to fee schedule with overall cap on expenditures for general practitioner services); there is a list of over 4,000 services that are reimbursable); one-third of general practitioners are hospital based and thus salaried; 15% work in health centers (salaried)

Reimbursement of specialists: Fee for service except in hospital (salaried)

General practitioners care for patients in hospital: No

Specialists restricted to hospital: No

Primary care organized by defined geographic area: No

First contact: No (0)

Longitudinality: Although most patients can name their general practitioner, they often go elsewhere (0)

Comprehensiveness: Poor; preventive care not generally integrated in general practice (0)

Coordination: Poor. No exchange of information between generalists and specialists. Starting in 1997 patients are supposed to bring carte sante (record of visits and procedures), but fewer than 50% do (0)

Family-centeredness: Poor (0)

Community orientation: Poor (0)

Germany

Type of system: Unregulated* (0)

Financing: Over 1,000 separate funds cover over 90% of population (employer–employee contributions) (1)

Type of primary care practitioner: General practitioners (although other specialists may provide "primary care" (1)

Percent active physicians who are specialists: 81% (0)

Professional earnings of primary care physicians relative to specialists: 1:1.4 in ambulatory sector; much greater disparity in system as whole (0)

Cost sharing for primary care: Only certain services; low income exempt (2)

Patient list: No. Chip card links patient and physician for 3 month periods (0)

Requirements for 24-hour coverage: Doctors in local areas share coverage (1)

Strength of academic departments of family medicine: A few are strong (1)

Primary care organized by defined geographic area: No
Most common site of primary care practice: Solo practice
Reimbursement of primary care physicians: Fee for service
Reimbursement of specialists: Fee for service (salary in hospital)
General practitioners care for patients in hospital: No
Specialists restricted to hospital: No

First contact: No* (0)
Longitudinality: Poor (0)
Comprehensiveness: Poor* (0)
Coordination: Poor (0)
Family-centeredness: Poor (0)
Community orientation: Poor (0)

Netherlands

Type of system: Regulated (2)

Financing: 70% of population in "public" system (employer–employee social insurance system); 30% private insurance; 100% in catastrophic coverage scheme (tax based) (plans to convert entire system to tax based) (1)

---

*In 1993, the Health Care Structure Law changed some policies regarding health services in the ambulatory structure. For the first time, there is a clear separation of general practitioners and specialists in the ambulatory sector, with mandatory training in general practice and required consultations with a general practitioner before consulting a specialist. Certain general practitioner services (especially preventive) will receive higher fees, although broad scope of practice including diagnostic procedures will remain discouraged.

Legislation to establish fixed physician to population ratios for each geographic area, with a ratio of 1 general practitioner to 2,000 population and with almost 60% of all areas closed to new practices (and fewer open areas for general practitioners than for specialists), is opposed by doctors and is expected to be fought in court.

Type of primary care practitioner: Family (general) practitioners; independent community nurses; independent midwives; independent physiotherapists (2)

Percent active physicians who are specialists: 67% (1)

Professional earnings of primary care physicians relative to specialists: 2:3 (0)

Cost sharing for primary care: None for "public" patients (70%) (0)

Patient list: Yes. Average list size 2,350 patients. In groups, list may be group list (2)

Requirements for 24-hour coverage: Yes (legal obligation) (2)

Strength of academic departments of family medicine: Strong (2)

Most common site of primary care practice: Solo office practice (54%) or small groups

Reimbursement of primary care physicians: Capitation for "public" patients (2/3); 1/3 fee for service

Reimbursement of specialists: Salary as of 1995

General practitioners care for patients in hospital: No

Specialists restricted to hospital: Yes

Primary care organized by defined geographic area: Yes

First contact: Yes, both public and private sectors (2)

Longitudinality: Yes (2)

Comprehensiveness: Prevention separate from general practice, that is, primary care is comprehensive although not necessarily through general practitioner. Teamwork extensive (2)

Coordination: Poor. Letters between general practitioners and specialists are required, but often not done (1)

Family-centeredness: Yes (2)

Community orientation: Poor except for relationships with visiting nurses, physiotherapists. (1)

Spain

Type of system: Regulated (2)

Financing: 99%; mostly tax based (2)

Type of primary care practitioner: Family (general) practitioner and pediatricians (1.5)

Percent active physicians who are specialists: 63% (1)

Professional earnings of primary care physicians relative to specialists: Approximately equivalent (2)

Cost sharing for primary care: No (2)

Patient list: Yes (2)

Requirements for 24-hour coverage: In rural areas. Deputizing service in urban areas (high emergency department use) (0)

Strength of academic departments of family medicine: Weak (0)

Most common site of primary care practice: Health centers (in reformed areas)

Reimbursement of primary care physicians: Salary (some experimentation with capitation)

Reimbursement of specialists: Salary (in hospital); salary in ambulatory sector (part of hospital job)

General practitioners care for patients in hospital: No

Specialists restricted to hospital: No

Primary care organized by defined geographic area: Yes, health centers serve 5,000–25,000 population

First contact: Yes, but free access to pediatricians and ophthalmologists (2)

Longitudinality: Strong affiliation with individual primary care doctor (2)

Comprehensiveness: Moderate. Little gynecology or minor surgery (1)

Coordination: Poor quality of communication (0)

Family-centeredness: Good. List size includes family members (2)

Community orientation: Poor to good (depends on health center) (1)

Sweden

Type of system: Regulated (health centers), although shortage of general practitioners in some urban and rural areas (2)

Financing: 100%; tax based (2)

Type of primary care practitioner: Family (general) practitioners (2)

Percent active physicians who are specialists: 90% (0)

Professional earnings of primary care physicians relative to specialists: Greater than 1 (2)

Cost sharing for primary care: Yes, with maximum for the year; free care for children and adolescents (1)

Patient list: No, although experiments and plans to change system to list with about 2,000 patients (0)

Requirements for 24-hour coverage: No (0)

Strength of academic departments of family medicine: Fair (1)

Most common site of primary care practice: Health centers, although increasing number of independent general practitioners paid for through social security system and county councils

Reimbursement of primary care physicians: Salary

Reimbursement of specialists: Salary

General practitioners care for patients in hospital: No

Specialists restricted to hospital: No. Some work in health centers

Primary care organized by defined geographic area: Yes

First contact: No. Many people go directly to hospital outpatient department. There are attempts to introduce gatekeeping (0)

Longitudinality: No (0)

Comprehensiveness: Range of services diminishing due to demands for high productivity (1)

Coordination: Poor (0)

Family-centeredness: High (2)

Community orientation: Primary care centers responsible for many aspects of public health. Good community data on morbidity (1)

United Kingdom

Type of system: Regulated (2)
Financing: 100%; tax based (2)
Type of primary care practitioner: Family (general) practitioners (2)
Percent active physicians who are specialists: 40% (2)
Professional earnings of primary care physicians relative to specialists: 1:1 (2)
Cost sharing for primary care: No (2)
Patient list: Yes (2)
Requirements for 24-hour coverage: Yes, legal obligation (2)
Strength of Academic departments of family medicine: Strong (2)

Most common site of primary care practice: Groups (75% of general practitioners work in practices of 3 or more)
Reimbursement of primary care physicians: Capitation plus fees for minor surgery, immunizations, home visits at night, contraception services, maternity care, Pap smear, child health surveillance, management of chronic diseases, plus practice allowances
Reimbursement of specialists: Salary
General practitioners care for patients in hospital: No
Specialists restricted to hospital: Yes
Primary care organized by defined geographic area: Yes

First contact: Yes, except for sexually transmitted diseases (2)
Longitudinality: Yes (2)
Comprehensiveness: Wide variety of types of services provided (2)
Coordination: Poor with specialists/inpatient, although improving rapidly (1)
Family-centeredness: Yes (explicit assumption of responsibility for families) (2)
Community orientation: High, with reporting of data and growing recognition of need to study communities (2)

United States

Type of system: Unregulated; about 20% health maintenance organizations (HMOs), 50% other managed care; 30% other (0)
Financing: 16% uncovered, probably twice as many at some time during the year (0)
Type of primary care practitioner: Family (general) practitioners, general internists, pediatricians (1)
Percent active physicians who are specialists: 61% (if general internal medicine and pediatrics are counted as primary care; over 80% if not) (1)
Professional earnings of primary care physicians relative to specialists: 0.6–0.7 (0)
Cost sharing for primary care: High (20% in excess of deductible, generally lower if HMO) (0)

Patient list: Yes in HMOs, sometimes in other managed care; No in other (0–1)

Requirements for 24-hour coverage: Yes in HMO; no in other (0–1)

Strength of academic departments of family medicine: A few excellent ones (1)

Most common site of primary care practice: Generally groups (single specialty and multispeciality)

Reimbursement of primary care physicians: Variable. Most still fee for service

Reimbursement of specialists: Majority fee for service (salary and bonuses in academic settings)

General practitioners care for patients in hospital: Variable

Specialists restricted to hospital: No

Primary care organized by defined geographic area: No

First contact: Yes in HMOs; variable in other managed care; no in other (0–2)

Longitudinality: Variable, probably decreasing over time (0)

Comprehensiveness: Variable. Preventive care increasing (HMOs); overall coverage probably decreasing with new exclusions from financial coverage (0)

Coordination: Variable, depends on setting and aegis. Probably poor overall (0)

Family-centeredness: Good for family physicians; poor for others (overall poor) (0–1)

Community orientation: Poor (0)

The distribution of scores for the "modal" form of organization (Table 15.2) indicates two general types of systems. In the first group are Belgium, the United States, France, and Germany, all with scores below 0.5. All of these countries are characterized by an absence of one key characteristic—regulation of the distribution of resources—although Germany may be moving toward more regulation. The second group contains the other seven countries, all of which have scores of 0.9

Table 15.2. Primary Care Scores*

Country	Score
Belgium	0.4
France	0.3
Germany	0.4
United States	0.4
Australia	1.1
Canada	1.2
Sweden	0.9
Denmark	1.7
Finland	1.5
Netherlands	1.5
Spain	1.4
United Kingdom	1.9

*Countries arranged in three groupings according to strength of primary care. The higher the score, the stronger the primary care.

and above and, at least to some extent, regulate the distribution of resources. Three
of these countries have an intermediate primary care score (0.9–1.2), whereas the
other five are 1.4 or greater.

One characteristic of primary care emerged from these updated comparisons
that was not noticed in the earlier comparison (Starfield, 1992). That is, the strength
of the primary care system is not synonymous with the primary care orientation of
primary care physicians themselves. Some countries have strong primary care but
not because of practice characteristics of primary care physicians. For example, in
Figure 1.5, the Netherlands was found to have the highest ranking for system
characteristics conducive to primary care but only the sixth ranking for practice
characteristics. Sweden tied for fourth (with Spain) for system characteristics but
ranked eighth for practice characteristics. This is because both of these countries
organize their primary care so that personnel other than physicians, often working
for separate nonprofit organizations (as in the Netherlands) or the county councils
(in the case of Sweden), undertake many of the functions of primary care, especially
regarding aspects of its comprehensiveness. In the United Kingdom, this is also
the case, but because these personnel are usually attached to practices, the practices
themselves are rated high on the characteristics. Thus, conclusions about the
strength of primary care as a level of the health system must be distinguished from
the strength of primary care as represented by the characteristics of individual
clinical practices. Historical and cultural considerations will determine the best way
of achieving the functions of primary care in each country.

As compared with the earlier findings (Starfield, 1992) there is a rather striking
similarity of ratings for the individual characteristics and for the rankings of the
different countries despite the fact that the sources of information were completely
different. Furthermore, health care reform efforts oriented primarily at cost containment have not altered each country's orientation. Countries that were poorly
oriented to primary care a decade ago still are; countries strong in primary care
before reforms started remain strongly oriented to primary care.

The ranking of the countries as obtained in this survey of data and experts is
confirmed by studies done by others using similar but not identical methods. Wen-
sing and colleagues (unpublished) surveyed a sample of patients attending at least
12 general practices in 8 European countries to determine their expectations of
general practice. They independently characterized the strength of primary care in
the countries using data from the European Study of referrals, from the Organization for Economic Cooperation and Development, and from the literature. Using
the 11 criteria presented by Starfield (1992) as described in Chapter 1, the rankings
(for those countries included in this chapter) were as follows (from highest to
lowest): Denmark; United Kingdom and the Netherlands (tied for second); Sweden;
Germany. Roland and Sibbald (unpublished) surveyed a knowledgeable individual
in 24 European countries. Data are available for five of the nine European countries
described in this chapter. Their rankings for strength of primary care were (from
best to worst): United Kingdom, Sweden, Finland, Belgium, France. The scores
and the rankings were the same regardless of whether only the primary care characteristics as described in this chapter were used or whether an enlarged set in-

cluding several additional items* were used. Thus, it appears that the ratings and rankings as presented in this chapter are relatively robust and likely to be adequately describing the state of primary care in the different countries.

Satisfaction of Population with Its Health Systems

Although comparable telephone surveys were conducted in many of the countries in the late 1980s (Blendon et al., 1990, 1991) these have not been repeated. However, satisfaction ratings are available for 1996 from face-to-face interviews in the 15 members of the European Union (Mossialos, 1997). The survey obtained information on two aspects of satisfaction: general satisfaction and needed changes. Three groups of countries could be distinguished based on the combined data on these two aspects, as follows:

- Countries with high population satisfaction: Denmark, Finland, Austria
- Countries with intermediate population satisfaction: Belgium, Germany, the Netherlands, Sweden, France
- Countries with low population satisfaction: Spain, United Kingdom, Italy, Greece, Portugal, Ireland

Although the methods of the earlier telephone survey and the more recent household survey are different, the nature of the questions (which referred to the health system as a whole rather than to primary care in specific) was relatively similar so that it is possible to draw tentative conclusions about changes over time. In the earlier study, the ranking for satisfaction was (from highest to lowest) Canada, the Netherlands, France, West Germany, Australia, Sweden, Japan, United Kingdom, Italy, Spain, United States, thus suggesting consistency at least for countries in both comparisons.

Interpretation of satisfaction responses cross-nationally are necessarily tenuous because cultural differences may be responsible for different expectations and hence different evaluations. It seems more plausible that perceived satisfaction is a response not only to characteristics of the system but also to the stability of the system. In the earlier surveys, two countries in particular (the United Kingdom and Spain) had already started major reforms; populations of both countries reported low satisfaction. The populations of these countries are still among the most dissatisfied, perhaps because their reforms are still incomplete or inadequate. In the case of the United Kingdom, they are being reversed to some extent. Unfortunately, the highest ranking countries (Denmark and Finland) were not included in the prior surveys so that it is not possible to judge the nature of trends in these countries or across countries.

---

*Training of primary care physicians in primary care setting; comprehensive patient medical histories held by primary care physicians; primary care physicians practice in multidisciplinary teams including community-based nurses; people of all incomes have approximately equal access to primary care; existence of government-organized welfare schemes for disadvantaged populations.

Health Indicators in 12 Countries

Sixteen indicators were available for the 12 countries. Four pertained to indicators in infancy (Tables 15.3 and 15.4), 10 pertained to life expectancy at ages 1, 15, 40, 65, and 80 for males and females separately. (Table 15.5), and two (male and female) pertained to total years of potential life lost before age 70 from preventable conditions. (Table 15.6) In addition, years of life lost from suicide and external causes is available separately for both females and males. Some of the tables contain additional information on health indicators not included in the final tabulations of the rankings of the countries.

Table 15.7 contains information on the percentage of women and men who smoke and alcoholic beverage intake in liters per capita at ages 15 and older.

Cost of care

Table 15.8 shows the cost per capita (in U.S. dollars). They are expressed in purchasing power parities, which express the conversion of the different currencies to a standard value that purchases the same set of goods and services in the different countries. The data in Tables 15.2 and 15.8 show that those countries that are more primary care-oriented have lower overall costs for their health services.

Table 15.3. Percentage of Infants Who Are of Low Birth Weight (less than 2,500 g) of Infants Delivered in Hospitals, Early to Mid-1990s

Country	Percentage
Belgium[d]	6.5
France[a]	6.2
Germany[a]	6.1
United States[c]	7.2
Australia[c]	6.3
Canada[b]	6.0
Sweden[a]	4.4
Denmark[b]	5.2
Finland[a]	4.1
Netherlands[d]*	4.9
Spain[c]	5.4
United Kingdom[b]	7.0

[a] 1995; [b] 1994; [c] 1993; [d] 1992.

* Because almost one-third of infants are born out of hospital in the Netherlands, and these are less likely to be of low birth weight, the figure for all births in the Netherlands is likely to be somewhat lower

Source: Organization for Economic Cooperation and Development data tapes (1997).

Table 15.4. Neonata, Postneonatal, and Total Infant Mortality Rates, 1993 and 1996*

	Neonatal Mortality Rate (1993)	Postneonatal Mortality Rate (1993)	Infant Mortality Rate (1993)	Infant Mortality Rate (1996)
Belgium	4.2	4.0	8.2	7.0
France	3.3	3.5	6.8	5.0
Germany	3.1	2.7	5.8	5.3
United States†	5.3	3.1	8.4	8.0
Australia	3.9	2.2	6.1	5.7
Canada	4.2	2.2	6.3	6.0
Sweden	3.1	1.7	4.8	4.0
Denmark	3.6	1.8	5.4	5.5
Finland	3.0	1.4	4.4	4.0
Netherlands	4.5	1.8	6.3	5.2
Spain	4.6	2.6	7.2	5.5
United Kingdom‡	4.1	2.1	6.2	6.0

*Except for Belgium and France (1992) and Spain (1991) in the case of neonatal and postneonatal rates.

† The relatively high mortality rates for the United States as a whole are also found among the white (majority) population only, with a neonatal mortality rate of 4.3, a postneonatal mortality rate of 2.5, and a total infant mortality rate of 6.8.

‡ England and Wales only. Rates for Northern Ireland are 4.94, 2.13, and 7.07, respectively.

Source: NCHS, 1997, p. 105; and Organization for Economic Cooperation and Development data tapes (1997).

Overall performance

Table 15.9 is a summary table that provides the primary care score, the primary care rank (with the best considered as No. 1), and the ranks for the health indicators considered core indicators for a country's health.

Comparisons of these data with data from the late 1980s (Starfield, 1992) reveal general consistency in the ranking for the individual countries. However, there are two countries for which ranks have changed substantially for several indicators. The Netherlands has relatively lower ranks than was previously the case for neonatal and postneonatal mortality rate, life expectancies at age 1, during adolescence, at age 65, and at age 80, and years of potential life lost. In contrast, Australia has improved its relative ranks for life expectancy at age 1 and in adolescence and for years of potential life lost.

The extent to which these changes are consequent to change in the orientation to primary care deserves further study. However, it is worthy of note that Australia has improved its primary care system in many regards, including strengthening the academic base for training in family practice. Although its primary care score does not reflect this improvement, this may be because the new ratings of primary care contain four additional items, on which Australia rated relatively low. Using only the original 11 indicators, the score for Australia improved from 1.1 to 1.3.

There is a general relationship between the extent of primary care orientation of countries and their ranking on the health indicators such that countries with a

Table 15.5. Life Expectancy

	At Age 1 Year		At Age 15 Years		At 40 Years		At 65 Years		At 80 Years	
	Females	Males	Females	Males	Females	Males	Females	Males	Females	Males
Belgium[n,a,d]	na	na	na	na	41.2	35.3	18.3	14.0	8.1	6.3
France[d,e]	81.5	73.3	67.7	59.6	43.2	36.3	20.6	16.1	9.0	7.1
Germany[c,c]	79.0	72.5	65.2	58.7	40.7	35.0	18.3	14.6	7.9	6.4
United States[e,c]	78.8	72.0	65.1	58.3	40.7	35.5	19.0	15.5	9.0	7.2
Australia[d,b]	80.5	74.6	66.7	60.9	42.1	37.2	19.7	15.7	8.9	7
Canada[d,b]	80.4	74.3	66.6	60.5	42.5	37.5	20.1	16.2	9.5	7.5
Sweden[d,b]	80.2	74.9	66.4	61.1	42.4	37.6	19.2	15.6	8.7	6.9
Denmark[d,c]	77.3	72.2	63.5	58.4	39.0	34.6	17.6	14.1	8.1	6.4
Finland[c,b]	79.6	72.2	65.7	58.4	41.3	34.8	18.6	14.5	7.9	6.4
Netherlands[c,b]	79.8	74.0	65.9	60.3	41	35.7	18.7	14.4	8.1	6.2
Spain[e,a]	80.6	73.3	66.9	59.6	42.9	36.7	19.8	15.8	8.5	7
United Kingdom[c,c]	78.9	73.6	65.1	59.8	40.6	35.9	18.4	14.7	8.6	6.7

[a] 1996; [b] 1995; [c] 1994 [d] 1993; [e] 1992 [na] not available (first letter[s] refer to birth, age 1, age 15; second letter refers to age 40, 65, 90)

For age-standardized death rates: 1994 except Australia, Canada, France, Sweden, 1993; and United States, Denmark, Spain, 1992.

Source: Birth, age 1, age 15: WHO (1993, 1994, 1995); age 40, 65, 80: Office of Economic Cooperation and Development data tapes (1997).

Table 15.6. Potential Years of Life Lost per 100,000 (Under Age 70)

	All, Except Suicide		Suicides		All, Except External Causes	
	Female	Male	Female	Male	Female	Male
Belgium[e]	3,952.8	7,020.4	221.3	588.0	3,157.8	4,986.4
France[b]	3,296.5	7,212.7	231.8	703.5	2,557.7	5,031.4
Germany[a]	3,494.3	6,671.4	141.3	477.9	2,994.3	5,101.0
United States[c]	4,656.1	8,503.9	121.5	523.5	3,861.8	5,976.0
Australia[b]	3,201.6	5,485.1	119.3	535.9	2,683.2	3,799.2
Canada[c]	3,413.0	5,789.1	157.3	601.2	2,811.9	3,988.7
Sweden[b]	2,875.5	4,739.3	223.9	488.3	2,315.1	3,392.4
Denmark[b]	4,167.3	6,373.4	244.7	594.4	3,488.9	4,728.7
Finland[a]	2,930.1	6,228.8	298.2	1208	2,157.4	3,350.9
Netherlands[b]	3,406.5	5,501.8	151.5	324.3	3,035.7	4,538.4
Spain[d]	3,333.2	7,450.5	56.2	216.6	2,837.1	5,604.1
United Kingdom[c]	3,762.3	5,941.1	83.1	346.8	3,359.2	4,710.8

[a] 1994; [b] 1993; [c] 1992; [d] 1991; [e] 1989.

Source: Office of Economic Cooperation and Development data tapes (1997).

Table 15.7. Percentage of Individuals Who Smoke and Alcoholic Beverage Intake Liters per Capita at Ages 15 and Older—1991

	Smoke*		Alcoholic Beverage Intake†
	Female	Male	
Belgium	24.0	33.0	11.8
France	19.2	37.8	15.7
Germany	21.5	35.6	14.2
United States	23.5	28.1	9.6
Australia	26.6	29.9	10.0
Canada	26.0	26.0	8.8
Sweden	24.4	25.7	6.3
Denmark	40.6	47.3	11.6
Finland	22.0	33.0	9.2
Netherlands	32.7	44.3	9.9
Spain	24.5	43.5	13.6
United Kingdom	29.0	31.0	8.9

*1991 except Australia, 1989; Germany, 1995; France, 1990; Spain, 1995; United Kingdom, 1994.

†1991 except the Netherlands and Spain, 1990; and United States, 1987.

Sources: Office of Economic Cooperation and Development data tapes (1997); Schieber et al. (1994).

Table 15.8. Cost of Care per Capita (in U.S. Dollars)*

Belgium	1693
France	1978
Germany	2222
United States	3708
Australia	1776
Canada	2002
Sweden	1405
Denmark	1430
Finland	1389
Netherlands	1756
Spain	1131
United Kingdom	1304

*In purchasing power parities

Source: Anderson, 1997

Table 15.9. Primary Care Score and Rank, and Ranks* on 18 Health Indictators

	Primary Care Rank	Infancy† (4)	Childhood‡ (2)	Young Adult** (4)	YPLL†† (2)	Older** Adults (4)
Belgium	10	11	11.5	10.5	9	12
France	12	5.5	5	4	5	2
Germany	10	4	9	9	9	9
United States	10	12	11.5	10.5	12	3.5
Australia	7	7	2	2	3	3.5
Canada	6	8	4	1	4	1
Sweden	8	2	3	5	2	11
Denmark	2	3	10	12	11	10
Finland	3.5	1	6	8	1	7
Netherlands	3.5	5.5	7	6	6	8
Spain	5	9	1	3	9	5
United Kingdom	1	10	8	7	7	6

*To obtain the rank, the ranks for each of the groups of indicators (which often included decimal places) were re-ranked according to their order. Components of composite indicators were equally weighted.

† Neonatal mortality, postneonatal mortality, infant mortality, low birth weight ratio.

‡ Consists of life expectancy at age 1. While not exclusively a childhood indicator, it excludes the substantial impact on life expectancy of infant mortality.

** Life expectancy at ages 15 and 40 (not available for Belgium) and at ages 65 and 80, respectively.

†† Under age 70, all but external causes. Average of male and female rankings. When all causes are included the country rankings are (best to worst) Sweden (1), Australia (2), Netherlands (3), Finland (4), Canada (5), United Kingdom (6), Spain (7), Germany (8), France (9), Denmark (10), Belgium (11), United States (12).

354

better primary care orientation tend to have better rankings on these health indicators than countries with a poor primary care orientation. However, once primary care ratings reach an average level there does not appear to be further improvement in health status. In particular, Denmark, Finland, and the United Kingdom do not rank as highly for health indicators as might be expected given their very high primary care scores. In Denmark, the less favorable improvement in life expectancy and mortality than in other countries has been analyzed and attributed to an increase in female work force participation in the absence of lack of improved social supports, an increase in unemployment, high rates of smoking and heavy alcohol drinking, and an increase in social inequality (Ministry of Health, 1994). In at least some parts of Finland, diets are high in saturated fat. In the United Kingdom, the poor health levels may reflect many years of poor funding of the health system so that even though the primary care infrastructure is strong, it may not have been well enough supported financially.

On average, however, it is clear that the four countries with low primary care orientation (Belgium, France, Germany, United States) also have worse performances for all groups of health indicators. In all countries, building a primary care focus appears to first require a national policy commitment and appropriate practice organization. Once such an infrastructure is in place, attention shifts to the adequacy of primary care services in meeting population needs—an imperative for *all* countries.

Unfortunately, the indicators that are available to assess the state of health of the countries are not the ones most appropriate to assessing the impact of primary care because many of them reflect the adequacy of services provided by physicians other than primary care physicians. Monitoring of the indicators suggested in Chapter 13, should they become available, may provide more of an opportunity to assess the special contributions of primary care to health both within as well as across countries.

References

Anderson GF. In search of value: an international comparison of cost, access, and outcomes. Health Affairs 1997; 16: 163–71.

Baggesen O. The Danish Health Care System. 5th ed. Organization of General Practitioners in Denmark, August 1994.

Battista R, Banta HD, Johnson E, Hodge M, Gelband H. Lessons from the eight countries. Health Policy 1994; 30:397–421.

Blendon R, Donelan K, Jovell A, Pellisé L, Lombardía E. Spain's citizens assess their health care system. Health Aff 1991; 10(3):216–28.

Blendon R, Leitman R, Morrison I, Donelan K. Satisfaction with health systems in ten nations. Health Aff 1990; 9(2):185–92.

Boerma W, de Jong F, Mulder P. Health Care and General Practice Across Europe. Utrecht: Nivel/Dutch College of General Practitioners, 1994.

Boerma W, van der Zee J, Fleming D. Service profiles of general practitioners in Europe. Br J Gen Pract 1997; 47:481–6.

Buetow S. What do general practitioners and their patients want from general practice and are they receiving it? A framework. Soc Sci Med 1995; 40:213–21.

Buetow S, Arias L, Peterson C. Defining the core content of general practice in Australia. Aust Fam Physician 1995; 24:1495–9.

Canadian Medical Association. Cost-effectiveness of primary health care providers: A systematic review. Working Paper (95–04). Ottawa: Canadian Medical Association, April 25, 1995.

Fry J, Horder J. Primary Health Care in an International Context. London: The Nuffield Provincial Hospital Trusts, 1994.

Gérvas J, Pastor Sánchez R, López Miras A, Pérez Fernández M. La Organización y la práctica de la medicina general/de familia en Europa. Rev Salud Publica 1997; 5:33–48.

Gérvas J, Pérez Fernández M, Starfield B. Primary care financing and gatekeeping in western Europe. Fam Pract 1994; 11:307–17.

Grant C, Forrest C, Starfield B. Primary care and health reform in New Zealand. NZ Med J 1997; 110:35–9.

Harris M, Frith J. Continuity of care: In search of the Holy Grail. Med J Aust 1996; 164:456–7.

Ministry of Health. The Life Expectancy Committee. Lifetime in Denmark. Copenhagen, Denmark. Ministry of Health, 1994.

Mossialos E. Citizens' views on health care systems in the 15 member states of the European Union. Health Economics 1997; 6:109–16.

National Center for Health Statistics (NCHS), Health, United States 1996–7 and Injury Chartbook. Hyattsville, MD: DHHS Pub. No. (PWS) 97–1232, 1997.

Organization for Economic Cooperation and Development. The Reform of Health Care. A Comparative Analysis of Seven OECD Countries. Health Policy Studies, No. 2. Paris; Organization for Economic Cooperation and Development, 1992.

Organization for Economic Cooperation and Development. New Directions in Health Care Policy. Health Policy Studies No. 7. Paris, 1995.

Ortún V, Gérvas J. Fundamentos y eficiencia de la atención médica primaria. Med Clin (Barc) 1996; 106:97–102.

Schieber G, Poullier J-P, Greenwald L. Health System Performance in OECD Countries, 1980–1992. Health Affairs 1994; 13:100–112.

Starfield B. Primary Care: Concept, Evaluation, and Policy. New York: Oxford University Press, 1992, Chapter 15.

Statistics Netherlands. International Comparison of Health Care Data. Phase I: Intramural Health Care. Voorburg: Heerlen, 1996.

Swedish Institute for Health Services Development. Health Care in Sweden: The facts. Stockholm: Spri, 1996.

Vohlonen I, Pekurinen M, Saltman R. Reorganizing primary medical care in Finland: The personal doctor program. Health Policy 1989; 13:65–79.

Webster I. General practice—A rising phoenix. Med J Aust 1996; 164:709–10.

World Health Organization. General Practice Profiles. Copenhagen: World Health Organization, Regional Office for Europe. Germany, August 1995.

— 16 —

Information Systems
for Primary Care

The information you have is not what you want, the information you want is not
what you need, and the information you need does not exist.   An Irish wit

Medical records have always been important in the care of patients. Information
systems are an extension of medical records to serve not only individual patient
needs but also population needs for primary care services (as well as for other
levels of health care). This chapter first deals with the traditional uses of medical
records for clinical care and with the changes that have been made to make them
more useful. The discussion then turns to computerization and its potential for
enhancing not only clinical care but also planning, delivering services, evaluation
of services for populations, and the knowledge base on which progress in health
services delivery rests. Although the importance of medical records and information
systems transcends primary care, the focus of this chapter is on issues of special
relevance to primary care because primary care practitioners are the coordinators
of care and therefore the main repository of information about patients.

To a large degree, medical care depends on a transfer of information. For this
reason both medical systems and professionals must maintain and provide information, both general and specific, so that other systems as well as other professionals who provide care or who assess quality of care not only have access to
information but can find it in a form applicable to the practice of general medical
care and its associated aspects. In addition, information transfer is often required
for medicolegal purposes to document care provided.

A quite different type of information transfer involves the relationship between
patient and physician. This chapter discusses the former aspects, and Chapter 9
considered the latter ones.

Medical Records

Medical records and information systems serve four functions. First, they are important as an aid to the memory of practitioners in caring for patients and as an

epidemiological tool in the planning of care for populations. Second, medical records are important legal documents: What goes into records is considered to reflect the processes of care, and therefore provides evidence when these processes are called into question. Third, medical records influence the processes of care. Chapter 11, concerning coordination of care, documented how the contents of medical records affect what patients know about their care and how they respond to that knowledge. Fourth, medical records serve as a source of information about the quality of care and clues as to how to improve it.

Because primary care is long term rather than episodic (as in hospitalizations), the demands on the record differ from those in inpatient care. Records must facilitate review of the patient over a period of time rather than only at one point. As yet, information science has not perfected techniques optimally suited to this challenge. Most uses of medical records still focus on review of particular visits or, at best, episodes of illness. These uses are further limited by their focus primarily on only certain processes of care, most notably the processes of diagnosis and treatment within a visit or within an episode. As a result, records are of less help in examining the practitioners' recognition of patients' needs, their understanding, acceptance, and participation in the processes of care, or the process of reassessment that spirals the cycle of care into time.

There is little doubt of the importance of records in clinical care. Records are often better than physicians' recollections for some types of information. For example, when patients were followed to determine their health status 6 months after a hospitalization, the accuracy of a prediction about their prognosis made at the time of discharge depended on the basis for the prediction. When the prediction was based on information from the medical record, it was often more accurate than when it came from recollections of the physician who had cared for the patient (Linn et al., 1974). Even though there are systematic deficits of information in medical records (Thompson and Osborne, 1976; Zuckerman et al., 1975) they do accurately reflect many aspects of care. These include important problems that have been identified by physicians as requiring follow up, medications prescribed (although not necessarily all those that the patient is taking), and tests with abnormal results (Starfield et al., 1979). The patient's chief complaint, at least as interpreted by the practitioner, is usually recorded; information related to the history of the present illness is recorded about three-fourths of the time. Elements of the past medical history are recorded infrequently (Romm and Putnam, 1981), and certain types of information, such as social characteristics, are rarely present in the medical record (Chamberlin, 1971). Family history and family characteristics are also rare in medical records.

The conventional complete medical record is a handwritten document of the patient's visit and contains a summary of the patient's "chief complaint," a section of variable length containing the "past medical history," a section containing the history related to the complaint followed by a section labeled "physical examination" (which is often limited to describing the state of the part of the body most related to the chief complaint). There is also a section containing the "diagnoses" or "impressions," which can contain any number of items with no requirement that they be in any standard or codable form, and yet another section called a "plan" or "disposition." These practitioner notes are in one section of the record;

laboratory reports and consultation notes are in other sections. Records kept in this format are known as "source oriented" because each item is inserted into a record according to its source. One modification of the "source-oriented record" is the "structured" medical record. Use of forms structured to require the recording of information in specific categories results in higher levels of performance and better recording (Duggan et al., 1990; Holmes et al., 1978; Cheney and Ramsdell, 1987). However, when the structured form is merely a list of items requiring a check for completion, items may be recorded as done even if they were not (Duggan et al., 1990).

Another modification of source-oriented notes employs algorithms to guide and document care. In New York City such a system was implemented in several hospital-based primary care clinics. These guidelines improved documentation in medical records; they also improved adherence to guidelines in the management of several conditions for which the guidelines were developed; these included asthma, otitis media, and gastroenteritis (Cook and Heidt, 1988).

Time orientation is an alternative or, more usually, a supplement to source orientation. In a time-oriented chart, the information is entered by a particular item that is followed, over time, on a flow chart. This type of record is particularly suited to specialty care where there are a limited number of items that are followed over time. These types of records, because of their organization and dependence on recording over time, often depend on computer technology.

Problem orientation is a third format useful for primary care. A problem-oriented medical record (POMR) contains a problem list, usually in the front of the chart, consisting of a list of all currently active problems updated at each visit. Resolved problems are crossed off. In some cases, the problem may be a symptom or sign that has not yet, and may never be, resolved into a standard diagnosis. In a complete POMR, each record contains a database with a complete history, physical examination, and laboratory results at the initial visit. Each encounter is recorded in SOAP format. That is, for each problem listed on the problem list, there is recoding of *s*ubjective data (what the patient says about the problem), *o*bjective data (what the practitioner finds on examination or testing), *a*ssessment (the practitioner's account of the status of the problem), and *p*lan (what is to be done about the problem). Although the full impact of the SOAP format has not been documented, the problem list improves the recognition and follow-up of problems from one primary care visit to the next particularly if there is a different practitioner (Simborg et al., 1976). The list of problems, as well as therapies and follow-up appointments, readily lends itself to computerization; these computerized lists provide the same benefits as do the handwritten lists (Johns et al., 1977). One important advantage of this type of record is that it clearly specifies the patient's problems, thus making it possible to link the diagnosis and treatment to what is important to the patient and to outcomes assessments.

Information Systems

An older woman has a good relationship with her family physician but she was also seeing a number of specialists, was admitted to the hospital every so often, and was

taking six different medications. It was difficult for her to update each of her practitioners on the care the others were giving. Once her records were put on a computer, a printed summary of her illnesses, treatments, and responses was available
and updated regularly. Each practitioner knew exactly what medications and tests
she was receiving. With a written record of her care, the woman understood her
health better, felt more comfortable, and was able to communicate more effectively
with her providers   An account from Canada, 1996

Information systems are aggregations of individual records, or at least of certain
parts of those records. These systems may include individual identifiers (usually in
the form of a unique number) or may be anonymous. If the former, it is possible
to link information from the different times and places where individuals have
sought care. If the latter, linkage is possible only to the level of aggregation of the
data, usually geographic area. That is, relationships between different characteristics
can be studied on the aggregate level, which may not reflect relationships at the
individual level, i.e., the ecological fallacy. Figure 16.1 depicts the different types
of information that are often linked in information systems with the capacity to do
so (Roos et al., 1998). Information systems in primary care have three main purposes: administrative, clinical care at both the individual and population levels, and
knowledge generation.

Traditional administrative functions require that information be obtained and
transferred to keep track of the processes of health services delivery so that financing and reimbursement are appropriate and timely. With the advent of more
formal institutionalized evaluations of the quality of care, information systems are
increasingly being used for review of care by others than those who generate it,
that is, peer groups, managers, and external review organizations.

Clinical care involves the basic functions of transferring needed information
about individuals' health needs and health care in clinical management, follow up,

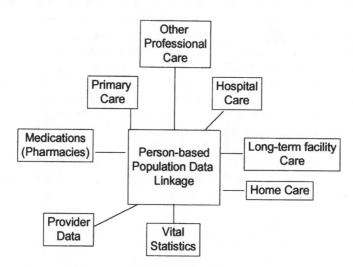

Figure 16.1. Types of information in information systems. Adapted from Roos et al. (1977).

and coordination of care that takes place at different times and in different places. Increasingly, information systems are serving an additional clinical function: quality assessment and assurance by individual practitioners and practice groups themselves so that they may engage in continuous quality improvement. The first systematic attempt to make physician records useful for research occurred in England by the Royal College of General Practitioners. Morbidity studies carried out in the mid-1950s by the College and the General Register Office of England and Wales showed that a substantial proportion of diagnoses in primary care could not be assigned disease codes and that almost half (45%) of conditions seen in general practice could not be classified by the International Classification of Diseases (ICD) because they were symptom complexes rather than diseases. Because they could not be coded, it was impossible to conduct studies of their natural history and of the impact of medical care on them. The College subsequently supported the development of a coding scheme useful for primary care and applied it to a method of indexing called the *E-book* (for Eimerl, its developer). The system consisted of a series of small sheets, one for each patient, inserted into a loose-leaf ledger divided into separate sections according to diagnosis. It included information about the patient and type of encounter and had several spaces to code items of special interest to the practitioner. The system could provide the number of episodes of illness and the number of visits per episode over a given time period. When combined with an age–sex register (a list of all patients in the practice, with their sex and age), E-book data were useful for epidemiological research as well as for clinical investigations (Last, 1965).

Information from clinical practice is used not only for individual patients but also for the entire population eligible to receive care in the primary care practice. Three types of information are required for this purpose: geographic distribution (area of residence) of enrolled patients, characteristics of that population (such as social class indicators) that influence the incidence and prevalence of different illnesses, and characteristics that should be taken into account in deciding on appropriate management strategies, age–sex distribution of that population, and prescribing data. Shanks and Crayford (1996) provided graphic examples of the utility of this information for comparing health practices in different areas and judging the extent to which they are taking local needs into account in monitoring health. For example, a review of age–sex data indicated that men of all ages are less likely than women to be receiving treatment for hypertension, despite the higher prevalence of hypertension in men. The practice then had to decide whether to devote more attention to persuading men in the community to have their blood pressure measured.

Yet another use of an information system is for research on effectiveness of services. As justification for interventions is increasingly based on evidence from systematic studies, information systems are increasingly in great demand as sources of data to evaluate the relative merits of different approaches to the diagnosis and management.

Computerized medical records and information systems are becoming essential as medical practice moves into an era of accountability and evidence-based medicine. Three imperatives are driving health care systems to better modes of information transfer: disappearance of the traditional boundaries between clinical medicine and population health; blurring of the distinction between administrative functions and clinical functions; and increasing coverage of vulnerable groups of patients in private health systems rather than in government-sponsored health programs. Integrated health systems serving large defined populations are taking on functions that were previously undertaken in the public sector. Information about population health and health care is as essential as information about individual patients. The blurring of administrative and clinical functions is occurring as a result of the need for accountability for the expenditures of funds; payers need information to ensure that their expenditures are justifiable according to the current state of clinical knowledge, and information about clinical care is an increasingly important component of payment for services. In countries (such as the United States) in which vulnerable populations that heretofore received their care in separate government-sponsored organizations are now being absorbed into private health systems, accountability for the quality of their care needs attention.

A model for the application of practice-based information for population-based purposes is provided by the Population Health Information System (POPULIS) in the province of Manitoba, Canada (Roos and Shapiro, 1995). This system uses a well-designed administrative database derived from claims records that can be linked to hospital information, vital statistics and census data, and survey data. Indicators of health are in six categories: demographic profile of the geographic area, low birth weight, indicators of the penetration of the health care system, mortality indicators, hospitalization data, and practice data. Claims data from physician visits contain diagnoses coded by the ICD—Clinical Modification.

A wide variety of questions of clinical and policy relevance have been addressed by this system, including correlates of variation in hospitalization, medical procedures, and surgery, and the relationship between these processes of care and costs as well as outcomes (both desired and adverse). Thus, data systems that are relatively common in industrialized countries using claims forms for reimbursement or encounter forms for monitoring services can be adapted to serve purposes far greater and equally as important as reimbursement for individual clinical services, that is, for knowledge generation and population health monitoring (Roos et al., 1995).

The Potential of the Office-Based Computer

The widespread availability of computers facilitates many aspects of information retrieval, storage, and transmission. Both medical record functions and information system functions can be achieved simultaneously. Legibility of handwriting is no longer a problem, and even security of information is technically easier to ensure because safeguards can be placed on the retrieval of electronic information more easily than is the case for paper records. Information for administrative purposes, quality monitoring, and research purposes no longer needs to be coded manually; software can take words, place them in appropriate categories, and convey them as needed.

Computerization of certain types of information facilitates some aspects of care even in the absence of a computerized medical record. For example, the use of microcomputer-generated reminders by primary care physicians increases the ordering of indicated mammograms (Chambers et al., 1989), as well as of other indicated preventive services such as tetanus immunization, Pap smears, breast examinations, and tests for occult stool blood (Turner et al., 1989).

However, the clear direction is toward the more widespread implementation of electronic medical records. These have been in use in many places for over 25 years. The best known and earliest of the clinical prototypes is the Computer-Stored Ambulatory Record (COSTAR), which has been used for many years in the Harvard Community Health Plan (now Harvard-Pilgrim). The system allows information transfer across the facilities so that the records of individuals who visit another facility are always available to the physician seeing them. This record replaces all handwritten or typewritten medical records; there is no medical record except for information that cannot be computerized, such as electrocardiograms and other graphic material, and full hospital discharge summaries. The computer receives input when the practitioner records information on a self-encoding form specifically designed for the needs of each specialty in the Health Plan. There may be free-text entries, either in writing or by dictation. Computer output is available in three forms: an encounter form containing data from individual encounters, a status report summarizing the current medical status of the patient, and flow charts showing the change in a given item over time. The system includes billing information, accounts receivable, electronic claims transfer, scheduling of personnel and resources, preventive services guidelines, reminders to physicians of needed vaccines (Barton and Schoenbaum, 1990), and medical information. Several hundred sites in the United States were using such systems as of 1993 (Barnett et al., 1993).

The potential of computerized patient records has been most exploited in the Netherlands, where more than one-fourth of the 6,400 general practitioners have instituted them in their offices; almost 40% of these clinicians actually did away with their paper medical records. As a result, over one-fourth of Dutch general practitioners rely completely on computerized medical records (van der Lei et al., 1993). The success of the electronic medical record in the Dutch system is a result of achievements in meeting four critical challenges: development of a standard clinical vocabulary, development of methods to facilitate direct physician interaction with the system, the support of key professional societies in developing standards and education programs (in particular, the Dutch College of General Practitioners and the Dutch Association of General Practitioners), and government contributions to the costs of development and use. The Dutch government, for example, reimburses 60% of the costs to the general practitioner for automating offices with computerized patient records.

The system uses free text as the basis of the clinical record; however, certain items require coding to use the full potential of the system. Diagnoses are coded by the International Classification of Primary Care, which was designed specifically for primary care but is compatible with the ICD maintained by the World Health Organization. Leadership by the professional societies in the Netherlands was key in adopting this system as the standard coding system for problems and diagnoses.

Drug names and dosages are required to link the computer system to pharmacy computers. Other data that are coded include laboratory tests, vital-sign measurements, referrals to other health care providers, and enrollment in research studies. (The system itself will identify the appropriate code for these items of information.)

A controlled and standard vocabulary is as crucial in the implementation of computerized patient records as standard vocabularies and codes are to coding systems used in claims forms, encounter forms, and other abstracts of records. It allows computers to search and sort quickly, summarize information, identify important clinical information, and retrieve selectively as instructed. Adjuncts to the record, such as drugs that should not be used simultaneously, and clinical guidelines for preventive care or care of particular conditions can easily be incorporated in the information system to automatically highlight contraindicated or indicated care for individual patients.

The Dutch success in achieving direct physician input is important in minimizing errors in transcription and providing the opportunity for direct feedback and reminders to the clinician as data are entered. The professional organizations led the way in developing the standard vocabulary and the standards for patient identification, record security, and electronic transmission of data. The Dutch National Board of Health has responsibility for providing the standards for electronic exchange of information (van der Lei et al., 1993). As is the case everywhere, decisions about the extent to which information for other than clinical use should be anonymous and the type and extent of use of unique patient identifiers that do not allow the linkage of number to name of person except for clinical purposes are subjects of intense discussions and policy consideration.

"Smart cards" are another technology with considerable utility in health care, including primary care. Developed over 20 years ago in France, they offer a mechanism of information transfer with excellent opportunities for confidentiality and security of information. The information on the cards is owned by the patient, who has the right and opportunity to decide what information should not be entered and the right to delete information already on the card. Entry of information is permitted only to authorized users and patients must enter their own personal identification number every time anyone seeks access to the information on the card. The card itself is owned by the issuer (generally the government or insurer); a copy is usually retained by the patient's primary care practitioner. Smart card technology creates a record of users so that there is a nonerasable trail of transactions. A particular utility, which is also shared by automated clinical records, is the facilitation of prescription writing and filling. Certain data fields can be protected and reserved for use only by certain practitioners. For example, information from psychiatric visits can be protected against entry by anyone designated by the patient or restricted to entry by only selected individuals. Because of these limitations, smart cards are primarily used for clinical care, particularly concerning coordination of care of individual patients, rather than for data analyses useful for documenting problems in populations, for use by practitioners to analyze their own practices, or to answer complex research questions, although there is potential for use in compiling statistics and for limited aspects of research.

Several models of the successful use of smart cards document their contributions to primary care practice. For example, the Exeter Care Card pilot included 13,000 patients, eight community pharmacists, two general medical practices, one general dental practice, a community hospital, and a general hospital, all within one district in the United Kingdom. Data could be entered into cards either directly or from an automated clinical record. Evaluation of the system showed that use of the system was associated with reduced cost of prescribing, reduced costs of laboratory investigations, reduction in risk of iatrogenic illness (especially in relation to dental care), reductions in time for communication of information, and ready access to needed patient care information. Patient acceptance of the card system was high (Neame, 1997).

The cards have also been in use in a town (Rimouski) in the province of Quebec, with 7,250 patients and 300 health professionals (including general practitioners and primary care teams). Five categories of information were included on the card: identification, emergency, vaccinations, medications, and ongoing care (history, consultations, follow-ups). The card was designed to reduce redundancy of tests, reduce the risk of drug interactions, and improve the quality, continuity, and integrity of care. As a result of this pilot test, Quebec was set to issue 7 million smart cards as of 1998.

The use of smart cards has considerable potential for care provided when patients travel. For that reason, the European Community is developing the standards, including privacy standards) for "Eurocards" (Tervo-Pellikka and Schaefer, 1995).

A considerable barrier both to the implementation of the computerized patient record and to the use of smart cards is the general absence of computer literacy among practitioners. Although most physicians in industrialized countries have computers in their offices, in fee-for-services systems they are often used only by administrative personnel for billing and other administrative transactions. The percentage of primary care doctors who use computers for clinical purposes varies considerably across countries (Wilson and Purves, 1996). The low end of the range is represented by Switzerland, the United States, and Austria, with the high end represented by Iceland, the United Kingdom, Canada, the Netherlands, and Sweden. Thus it appears that countries with a stronger orientation toward primary care (see Chapter 15) are more likely to have practitioners who use computers for clinical purposes. Although the data derive from a small survey of selected respondents and may not be precisely accurate, they do provide the relative magnitude of the challenge toward improving the potential of information use in different countries.

Codes and Coding Systems

The ICD, maintained by the World Health Organization, was originally developed to code causes of mortality. Over the years it has been modified and expanded, first to facilitate coding of hospital diagnoses and then coding of morbidity in outpatient practices. Subsequent revisions of the ICD included codes for symptoms so that it was at least theoretically possible to track illnesses from their initial presentation to their eventual diagnosis.

Despite this potential, the ICD has not been very useful in primary care because it is a compendium of all possible diagnoses, most of them uncommon and rarely if ever seen in primary care practice. Thus it is a cumbersome instrument not readily useful to primary care practitioners, at least for purposes other than those of assigning a diagnosis for billing purposes. In 1979, the World Organization of National Colleges Academies, and Academic Associations of General Practitioners/ Family Physicians developed a classification specifically for use in primary care (World Organization of National Colleges, 1979). This classification, known as the International Classification of Health Problems in Primary Care (ICHPPC-2), is compatible with the ICD but is much briefer and easier to use in clinical practice. Thus, since the 1980s, a practical mechanism for coding diagnoses in primary care has been available.

Although many researchers recognized the need for a better information base, it was the involvement of the government in financing and providing care directly that gave it widespread attention in the United States. If public programs were to be accountable to the taxpayers, there had to be a method of generating and using information. In the late 1960s, the U.S. National Center for Health Statistics sponsored a series of conferences, which led to the publication of three sets of "minimal data": a set for long-term care, a set for inpatient care, and a set for ambulatory care. Part of this effort led to the recognition of the importance of coding presenting problems as well as diagnoses. When presenting problems are elicited and recorded, it becomes possible to study and understand the natural history of evolution of problems and their responsiveness to different modes of intervention, thus facilitating both knowledge generation and better patient care. The pioneering work of the National Center stimulated an international collaborative project to devise and test a system of nomenclature for problems in primary care (Lamberts and Wood, 1987). The basis for the coding scheme, the International Classification of Primary Care (ICPC), is a bi-axial alpha numeric matrix in which there are "components" and "chapters." Each reason for visit is categorized as one of seven components:

- Symptom or complaint
- Diagnostic, screening, or preventive procedure
- Treatments, procedures, or medications
- Receipt of test results
- Administrative
- Diagnosis
- All others

Each reason is also assigned to 1 of 17 chapters indicated by letter, 15 of which are body systems, one is for problems that cross systems or are general in nature, and one is for social problems. Within the chapters are specific codes, organized in a similar way across the chapters according to the appropriate component. For example, the first 29 codes in each chapter refer to specific symptoms or complaints; codes 30–49 refer to specific diagnostic procedures; codes 50–59 are therapeutic modalities; codes 60 and 61 are, respectively, results of tests or procedures and results from other providers; code 62 is an administrative procedure; codes 63–69 are various other reasons (including the institution of a referral or an encounter initiated by someone other than the patient); and codes 70–99 are the most common specific diagnoses within the chapter. The coding system for the symptoms/complaints and diagnosis components is compatible with the ICD, ICHPPC-2, and the Classification of Diseases, Problems, and Procedures of the British Royal College of General Practitioners (1984). The second edition of the ICPC contains definitions for all rubrics, a classification of severity, and a tool to measure functional status (World Organization of National Colleges, 1998).

The availability of uniform systems to code presenting problems and reasons for visits will greatly facilitate both research and delivery of primary care services. It will lead to greater understanding of the distribution of health problems and the impact of various methods of managing them, and it also will focus attention on a most critical but relatively neglected aspect of care: recognition of the patients' problems by practitioners.

Challenges to Advances in Medical Record and Information Systems

Technological capacity is no longer the barrier to effective information systems. The state of the art in development of computer systems is such that there are essentially no barriers to the rapid and accurate transfer of information, with appropriate safeguards to maintain its confidentiality. The challenges result from the absence of a framework to decide what information should be included; how the information should be recorded, with what detail, and in what form; and mechanisms to ensure standardization so that the same information is interpreted in the same way regardless of its source. In 1996, the U.S. Congress enacted a law (PL 104–191) that required the Department of Health and Human Services to recommend standards for privacy of individually identifiable information for administrative transactions and for the clinical information that accompanies them. The imperatives that underlie this ''administrative simplification'' are that information

- Must be linkable across places so that it is possible to follow patients across different sites and levels of care
- Must be linkable across time so that it is possible to trace patients' problems from onset to resolution
- Is conducive to linking ''inputs'' to ''outputs,'' that is, to help determine whether clinical problems improve and the mechanism by which health services interventions do or do not contribute to that improvement.

Pursuant to the goal of standardizing the content of medical records, whether paper based or computer based, the U.S. National Committee on Vital and Health Statistics held hearings and conducted investigations on the items of information in major health services information systems throughout the country. Its deliberations resulted in a proposed ''core data'' set that contains 42 items of information in three categories: patient enrolment data, provider data, and encounter data (further categorized as inpatient, outpatient, and all types of encounters regardless of where they occur). Table 16.1 lists the items of information according to whether or not they are deemed ready for implementation because of long-standing expe-

Table 16.1. Core Health Data Elements Proposed for Standardization
Listed by Readiness for Implementation

Elements Ready for Implementation

2. Date of Birth
3. Gender
4. Race and Ethnicity
5. Residence
6. Marital Status
10. Years of Schooling
11. Patient's Relationship to Subscriber/Person Eligible for Entitlement
14. Admission Date (inpatient)
15. Discharge Date (inpatient)
16. Date of Encounter (outpatient and physician services)
20. Location of Address of Encounter (outpatient)
24. Principal Diagnosis (inpatient)
25. Primary Diagnosis (inpatient)
26. Other Diagnoses (inpatient)
27. Qualifier for Other Diagnoses (inpatient)
29. Diagnosis Chiefly Responsible for Services Provided (outpatient)
30. Other Diagnoses (outpatient)
31. External Cause of Injury
32. Birth Weight of Newborn
33. Principal Procedure (inpatient)
34. Other Procedures (inpatient)
35. Dates of Procedures (inpatient)
36. Procedures and Services (outpatient)
37. Medications Prescribed
39. Disposition (outpatient)
41. Injury Related to Employment

Elements Substantially Ready for Implementation, but Need Some Added Work

7. Living/Residential Arrangement
17. Facility Identification
18. Type of Facility/Place of Encounter
19. Health Care Practitioner Identification (outpatient)
21. Attending Physician Identification (inpatient)
22. Operating Clinician Identification (inpatient)
23. Health Care Practitioner Specialty
38. Disposition of Patient (inpatient)
40. Patient's Expected Sources of Payment
42. Total Billed Charges

Elements That Require a Substantial Amount of Study and Evaluation

1. Personal/Unique Identifier
8. Self-Reported Health Status
9. Functional Status
12. Current or Most Recent Occupational Industry
13. Type of Encounter
28. Patient's Stated Reason for Visit or Chief Complaint (outpatient)

Source: U.S. Department of Health and Human Services (1996)

rience and/or the availability of widely accepted approaches to categorizing the information. Definitions of each of the items that are ready for implementation are provided (U.S. Department of Health and Human Services, 1996).

There are additional challenges that require attention, especially for primary care. The most pressing of these is the certainty of the diagnosis. In primary care, patients are more likely than not to present initially with problems that cannot be assigned a diagnosis. As noted above, the ICPC provides a means of categorizing these problems in a standard way. However, in some countries there are powerful incentives for practitioners to assign a diagnosis code rather than a problem code, because systems of reimbursement are linked to the presence of a diagnosis (as is often the case where physicians are reimbursed by fee for service). Under such circumstances, medical records might record that a particular diagnosis is suspected, that is, is a "rule-out" (R/O) condition, but this is rarely the case. Health systems such as the Harvard Community Health Plan (now Harvard-Pilgrim) incorporated such modifiers long ago. They include "rule out," "status post," "in remission," and "partial remission" (K. Coltin, personal communication). Some of the facilities in the Kaiser Health Plan do similarly; typical modifiers are "rule out" (R/O) or "probable" (S. Cohn, personal communication, 1997). In the vast majority of instances in the United States, the administrative transaction records the diagnosis as if it were a firm diagnosis, thus making it impossible to track the course of problems from their first presentation to their resolution in computerized information systems. Furthermore, it complicates the task of understanding the diagnostic process, because diagnostic investigations cannot be linked to the nature of the patients' problems. As the unique needs of primary care practice are increasingly recognized, systems of classifying problems should become more widely acceptable and used. In some countries (such as the Netherlands), problems rather than diagnoses are coded if a firm diagnosis is not reached.

Another major challenge to coding of clinical information is the lack of standardization of methods to code diagnoses, diagnostic tests and their results, and therapeutic interventions. As noted above, the ICD, now in its tenth revision, is the mainstay of mortality and inpatient diagnoses throughout the world. Coding of problems in primary settings is most commonly done with the ICPC, but many countries, including most practices in the United States and the United Kingdom, do not use it. In the United Kingdom, the Read classification is the standard for coding of a variety of types of clinical and related information (National Health Service, 1995). These include:

Occupations
History and observations
Disorders
Investigations
Operations and procedures
Regimes and therapies
Prevention
Causes of injury and poisonings
Tumor morphology

Staging and scales
Administration
Drugs
Appliances and equipment
Units of measurement
Organisms
Anatomical site
Additional values
Context-dependent categories (certain qualifiers, such as "history of")
Attributes (such as onset)

Although there are still some limitations of the system, the national Department of Health in the United Kingdom purchased the system and is using it as the standard for all practices, maintaining it, and updating it as needed (Smith et al., 1995).

Various other coding systems are used throughout the world for various aspects of health services. Figure 16.2 indicates the number of countries using the major systems (Wilson and Purves, 1996). Each of these systems has its strengths and weaknesses, and none are widely accepted. Most have been developed for specific applications in particular institutions, and each has weaknesses and strengths (Cimino, 1996). As noted above, the Read classification system is promoted in the United Kingdom. In the Netherlands, the Elias system is in use in a majority of general practices and is based on the ICPC for coding diagnoses and reasons for visits in a computerized patient record context (Duisterhout et al., 1992). As electronic record keeping becomes more widely adopted, there may be convergence of the various systems into one that will support use of the information well beyond a particular clinical context or health system. The complexity of the challenge is evident from the large number of different attempts to devise a system with universal relevance, feasibility, and acceptability (Chute et al., 1998).

The Electronic Patient Record

Computerized patient records (CPR) are likely to become the routine method of storing information concerning health needs and health care in the near future, even replacing paper-based medical records. They will greatly facilitate the major objectives of health information systems: to support patient care and improve its coordination; to enhance the productivity of health care professionals and reduce administrative costs associated with a paper-based system; and to support clinical, epidemiological, and health services research.

There are no technical barriers to the entry of data and its maintenance in computerized form in countries in which computer use is widespread. However, there are impediments that may interfere with applications in health services.

When information is computerized, decisions must be made concerning the data to be entered and the detail that is included. At a very minimum, the elements

System

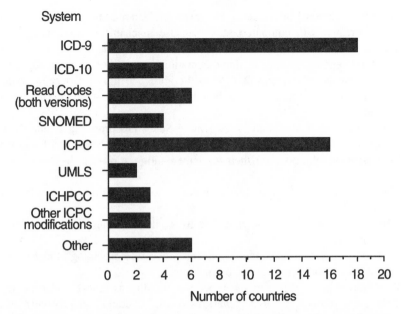

Figure 16.2. Number of countries using various primary care coding and nomenclature systems. ICD-9, International Classification of Diseases, 9th Revision; ICD-10, International Classification of Diseases, 10th Revision; SNOMED, Systematized Nomenclature of Human and Veterinary Medicine; ICPC, International Classification of Primary Care; UMLS, Unified Medical Language System; ICHPCC, International Classification of Health Problems in Primary Care (Wilson and Purves, 1996).

listed in the core dataset (see discussion earlier in this chapter) should be included to provide basic information in a standard way.

Threats to privacy are of no less a concern with computerized records than with patient records and may be greater because of the potential that many more people and agencies may have access to a system that is used for multiple purposes. Fulfilling the purposes of a CPR system requires that each individual in the population be assigned a unique identifier that is used for all health-related transactions. Although most countries assign such number to individuals in the population, some use numbers that are limited only to health-related information whereas others use a multipurpose unique identifier. In the latter instance, fears of loss of privacy are heightened because knowledge about health status and health care may be linkable with data from other systems such as the justice system and thus be used for purposes that threaten the rights of individuals. Limitation of the unique identifier to health-related purposes alone reduces but does not eliminate the potential for individual harm, particularly in health systems where the individual's access to health services and health insurance coverage may be compromised by the disclosure of their personal information. However, the potential for safeguarding privacy may be greater with computerization because mechanisms for making the data secure are easier than is the case with paper-based records.

A third potential barrier to implementation concerns networking capacity. Because one of the advantages of CPR is the ability to link a variety of sources of information about people and their health care, assurance of networking capability is essential.

The Institute of Medicine in the United States has proposed standards for the development and deployment of CPR systems (Dick and Steen, 1991; Dick et al., 1997). Several conditions for their implementation are proposed:

- The data must be entered by the individual who collects them in order to optimize accuracy
- The system must reliably include data from all sources and permit their retrieval when needed
- The record must be used actively in the process of providing clinical care, and all relevant information should be included
- The system is important in the process of quality assurance and generation of knowledge through research of various types, including that involving observations over time, in different places, and obtained through different mechanisms, including surveys, registers, and vital statistics
- Users must be proficient with the tools that are made possible by computerization, including bibliographic databases and clinical decision-support systems

For the potential of CPR to be realized, countries must develop standards for information components and the way in which they are entered into the computer, enact laws and regulations that protect patient privacy, and develop standards for ensuring confidentiality and procedures for maintaining the security of the system, with imposition of severe penalties for unauthorized use.

Fifteen recommendations in five categories of activities were made to maximize the security of CPR systems (National Research Council, 1997). Although the recommendations were specific to the United States, they can be generalized to apply to any national health system, as follows:

1. All organizations that handle patient-identifiable information—regardless of size—should adopt the set of technical and organizational policies, practices, and procedures set out below.
2. Governments and the health care industry should take action to create the infrastructure necessary to support the privacy and security of electronic health information.
3. There should be a publically accountable standing health information security standards committee to develop and update privacy and security standards for all users of health information. Membership should be drawn from organizations that represent the broad spectrum of users and subjects of health information.
4. Governments should provide initial funding for the establishment of an organ-

ization for the health care industry to promote greater sharing of information about security threats, incidents, and solutions to problems.

5. Governments should work with nongovernmental organizations to promote and encourage an informed public debate to determine an appropriate balance between the privacy concerns of patients and the information needs of various users of health information.

6. Organizations that collect, analyze, or disseminate health information should adopt a set of information practices that are consistent with privacy legislation.

7. National governments should work with area and local governmental units, health researchers, and the health care industry to establish a program to promote consumer awareness of health privacy issues and the value of health information for patient care, administration, and research. It should also conduct studies that will develop a set of recommendations for improving consumer awareness of health data flows and uses.

8. Professional and industry groups should continue and expand their leadership roles in educating members about privacy and security issues.

9. Governments should conduct studies to determine the extent to which, and the conditions under which, users of health information need data containing patient identifiers.

10. Governments should determine appropriate ways to provide consumers with a visible, centralized point of contact regarding privacy concerns.

11. Any effort to develop a universal individual identifier should weigh the presumed advantages of such an identifier against privacy concerns. Methods to identify individuals and link their records should be accompanied by an explicit policy framework that defines the nature and character of linkages that violate privacy and specifies legal or other sanctions for creating such linkages. They should facilitate the identification of parties that link records so that those who make improper linkages can be held responsible for their creation. They should be unidirectional to the degree that is technically feasible, facilitate the appropriate linking of health records given information about the person or provided by the person, but prevent a person's identity from being easily deduced.

12. Governments should take steps to improve information security technologies for health care applications.

13. Governments should establish formal liaisons with professional and nongovernmental groups to facilitate exchange of technical knowledge about information security.

14. Governments should support research on methods of identifying and linking records, on solving the problems of anonymous care and pseudonyms that necessarily would interfere with achieving quality of care for individual patients; concerning audit trails such that those who misuse CPR systems can be identified; and concerning tools for rights enforcement and management.

15. Governments should fund test sites to explore different approaches to controlling access to data that can be incorporated into existing operations.

In addition, it is recognized that each and every organization that collects, maintains, processes, or otherwise uses health care information must be constantly aware of threats to confidentiality and security of individually identifiable information and develop its own standards for maintaining confidentiality and identifying any breaches in policy designed to ensure it.

The use of computers in primary care practice does not necessarily facilitate the transfer of information between primary care and other types of care. A study in six Eurppean countries showed that practitioners in countries with stronger primary care systems (U.K., Denmark, The Netherlands) are more likely to use computers for keeping patient records, but the use of computers for transfer of information about patients is limited everywhere because of cultural and legal barriers (DeMaeseneer and Beolchi, 1995).

Each country will develop its own approaches, tailored to its own particular needs. National exchanges will be necessary to ensure relative compatibility because exchange of information across national boundaries concerning individual persons will be needed as a result of international commerce and travel.

Previous sections of this chapter indicate that many countries and groups of countries have already made impressive strides in addressing the challenges of computerized data and their translation into information. The potentials and possibilities for enhancing the effectiveness and equity of care that accrue from the new technologies are enormous and merit pursuit in the interests of improving health of patients and populations.

References

Barnett O, Jenders R, Chueh H. The computer-based clinical record—Where do we stand? BMJ 1993; 119:1046–8.

Barton M, Schoenbaum S. Improving influenza vaccination performance in an HMO setting: The use of computer-generated reminders and peer comparison feedback. Am J Public Health 1990; 80:534–6.

Chamberlin R. Social data in evaluation of the pediatric patient: Deficit in outpatient records. J Pediatr 1971; 78:111–6 .

Chambers C, Balaban D, Carlson B, Ungemack J, Grasberger D. Microcomputer-generated reminders, improving the compliance of primary care physicians with mammography screening guidelines. J Fam Pract 1989; 29:273–80.

Cheney C, Ramsdell J. Effect of medical records' checklists on implementation of periodic health measure. Am J Med 1987; 83:129–36.

Chute C, Cohn S, Campbell J. A framework for comprehensive health terminology systems in the United States: Development Guidelines, Criteria for Selection, and Public Policy Implications. J Am Med Informatics Assoc 1998 (In press).

Cimino J. Review paper: Coding systems in health care. Methods Inform Med 1996; 35: 273–84.

Cook CD, Heidt J. Assuring Quality Out-Patient Care for Children: Guidelines and a Management System. New York: Oxford University Press, 1988.

DeMaeseneer J, Beolchi L. Telematics in Primary Care in Europe, Amsterdam: IOS Press, 1995.

Dick R, Steen E (eds). The Computer-Based Patient Record: An Essential Technology for Health Care. Washington, DC: National Academy Press; 1991.

Dick R, Steen E, Detmer D (eds.). The Computer Based Patient Record: An Essential Technology for Health Care. Revised Edition. Washington D.C.: National Academy Press, 1997.

Duisterhout J, van der Meulen A, Boersma J, Gebel R, Kjoo K. Implementation of ICPC coding in information systems in primary care. In Lun K, Degoulet P, Piemme T, Reinhoff O (eds): MEDINFO 92. Amsterdam: North Holland, 1992, pp 1483–8.

Duggan A, Starfield B, DeAngelis C. Structured encounter form: The impact on provider performance and recording of well-child care. Pediatrics 1990; 85:104–13.

Holmes C, Kane R, Ford M, Fowler J. Toward the measurement of primary care. Milbank Q 1978;56:231–52.

Johns C, Simborg D, Blum B, Starfield B. A minirecord; an aid to continuity of care. Johns Hopkins Med J 1977; 140:277–84 .

Lamberts H, Wood M (eds). International Classification of Primary Care (ICPC). World Health Organization of National Colleges, Academics, and Academic Associations of General Practitioners/Family Physicians. Oxford: Oxford University Press, 1987.

Last J. Primary medical care. Record keeping. Milbank Q 1965; XLIII(2):266–76.

Linn B, Linn M, Greenwald S, Gurel L. Validity of impairment ratings made from medical records and from personal knowledge. Med Care 1974; 12:363–8.

National Health Service. The Read Codes Version 3. Centre for Coding and Classification, Loughborough, England: NHS Centre for Coding and Classification, 1995.

Neame R. Smart cards—The key to trustworthy health information systems. BMJ 1997; 314:573–7.

National Research Council. For the Record: Protecting Electronic Health Information. Washington, DC: National Academy Press, 1997.

Romm F, Putnam S. The validity of the medical record. Med Care 1981; 19:310–5.

Roos L, Romano P, Fergusson P. Administrative databases. In: Encyclopedia of Biostatistics. Colton T and Armitage P. (eds.). Chichester, England: John Wiley and Sons, 1998.

Roos N, Black C, Roos L, Tate R, Carriere K. A population-based approach to monitoring adverse outcomes of medical care. Med Care 1995; 33(12, suppl):s127–38.

Roos N, Shapiro E. Health and health care: Experience with a population-based health information system. Med Care 1995; 33(12, suppl), DS1–146.

Shanks J, Crayford T. Information for a primary care–led health service—Health needs assessment. In Littlejohns P, Victor C (eds): Making Sense of a Primary Care-Led Health Service. Oxford: Radcliffe Medical Press, 1996. pp 30–44.

Simborg D, Starfield B, Horn S, Yourtee S. Information factors affecting problem follow-up in ambulatory care. Med Care 1976 14:848–56.

Smith N, Wilson A, Weekes T. Use of Read codes in development of a standard data set. BMJ 1995; 311:313–5.

Starfield B, Steinwachs D, Morris I, Bause G, Siebert S, Westin C. Concordance between medical records and observations regarding information on coordination of care. Med Care 1979; 17:758–66.

Tervo-Pellikka R, Schaefer O. Eurocards. The AIM DGXIII concerted action on Patient Data Cards. Privacy Aspects. Committee on European Normalization-Technical Committee, Finland: Tervo-Pellikka and Schaefer, 1995.

Thompson H, Osborne C. Office records in the evaluation of quality of care. Med Care 1976; 14:294–314.

Turner B, Day S, Borenstein B. A controlled trail to improve delivery of preventive care: Physician or patient reminders? J Gen Intern Med 1989; 4:403–9.

U.S. Department of Health and Human Services. Report of the National Committee on Vital and Health Statistics. Core Data Elements. US-GPO No. 1996-722-677/83245. Centers for Disease Control. Washington, DC: National Center for Health Statistics, 1996.

van der Lei J, Duisterhout JS, Westerhof HP, van der Does E, Cromme PV, Boon WM, van Bemmel JH. The introduction of computer-based patient records in the Netherlands. Ann Intern Med 1993; 119(10):1036–41.

Wilson RG, Purves IN. Coding and nomenclatures: A snapshot from around the world. In Moving Toward International Standards in Primary Care Informatics: Clinical Vocabulary. AHCPR Pub. No. 96–0069. October 1996. Rockville, Maryland: US Department of Health and Human Services, Agency for Health Care Policy and Research, 1996.

World Organization of National Colleges, Academies, and Academic Associations of General Practitioners/Family Physicians.) ICPC-2 (International Classification of Primary Care. 2nd Ed.) Oxford: Oxford University Press, 1998.

World Organization of National Colleges, Academies, and Academic Associations of General Practitioners/Family Physicians. ICHPPC-2 (International Classification of Health Problems in Primary Care. 2nd Ed.) Oxford: Oxford University Press, 1979.

Zuckerman A, Starfield B, Hochreiter C, Kovasznay B. Validating the content of pediatric outpatient medical records by means of tape-recording of doctor–patient encounters. Pediatrics 1975; 56:407–11.

— 17 —

Primary Care
Research Needs

Research is to see what everybody has seen and to think what nobody else has
thought.   Albert-Szent-Gyorgyi

Continuous accrual of evidence-based knowledge is the basis for progress in every
field of endeavor. Primary care is no exception. The previous chapters of this book
have documented the current state of knowledge of the organization and delivery
of primary care services; the astute reader will recognize that there is still much to
learn! This chapter identifies those areas that are of high priority for research in
primary care in the hope that an increasing number of academicians and clinical
practitioners will become engaged in the exciting process of contributing knowledge to improve the effectiveness, efficacy, and equity of the basic level of all
health services systems.

Since Starfield's earlier book on primary care was written (1990), much has
been learned about primary care and its contributions to the work of health services systems. Many of the advantages of primary care have now been documented, largely by means of studies on the benefits of the separate components
of primary care. Most of the documentation concerning the advantages of primary care as a whole is based on a few studies that compared costs and outcomes in areas that differ in the strengths of their primary care as measured by
the number of primary care physicians or by the presence of health system characteristics that reflect strong primary care. As a result of the historical neglect of
primary care itself as a subject of scholarly interest, there still is a tremendous
backlog of questions that require answers. Most of the questions are the same as
they were in 1990, but research conducted in the most recent few years has at
least helped to sharpen their focus.

Two main types of research are needed to promote the effectiveness of primary
care: basic research and policy-related research. Basic research includes the methods that are important in measurement, and policy-related research contributes information that helps in decision-making. The latter concerns both clinical research
and research on modes of organizing, financing, and delivering services and on

primary care training. (A fourth type of research, health systems research and evaluation relevant to primary care, is considered in chapter 18.)

Basic Research

Many aspects of basic research would greatly facilitate the measurement of primary care. This section summarizes the issues that are of special importance in enhancing knowledge about primary care problems and primary care practice.

Measurement of health status

The ultimate justification for a health services intervention is its impact on health status. As noted in Chapter 2, health status has several components; any, either individually or in combination, may be influenced by health services. Although there are several techniques for assessing health status in adults (McDowell and Newell, 1996), much remains to be done, particularly in the development of measures that are clinically useful. The World Organization of National Colleges and Academies (WONCA) of general/family practice has developed a pictorial method for assessing health status in adults. The instrument (COOP/WONCA) is generally completed by patients themselves. The charts address physical fitness, feelings, daily activities, social activities, change in health, and overall health. An additional chart for pain and one for sleep are under development. The charts have been published in Chinese, Danish, Dutch, Finnish, French, German, Hebrew, Italian, Japanese, Korean, Norwegian, Portuguese, Spanish (Catalan, Castilian, and Gallego), Slovak, Swedish, and Urdu (WONCA, 1998). A prime area for research is the testing of this and other instruments for their usefulness in improving recognition and management of patients. Another prime area for developmental work concerns health status of children; the need is great for methods that are appropriate in the different age periods in childhood (Starfield, 1987).

Measurement of case mix and severity of illness

Comparisons of effectiveness of care, either over time or across facilities or health systems, should take into account initial differences in the extent or degree of illness of the different populations. Although there are several techniques for measuring this (Gold, 1988), none has been sufficiently well developed to gain widespread acceptance. WONCA (1998) has also developed and tested a measure of severity of illness for use in adult patients. Known as the DUSOI (Duke University Severity of Illness) system, it involves physician ratings of symptoms, complications, prognosis, and treatability for each problem dealt with in visit. Scores can be aggregated when there is more than one health problem. Tested in 22 volunteer practices in nine countries, it was thought (by the practitioners) to be most useful for research. Further testing for wider applicability and utility is indicated.

Primary care needs a case-mix measure that facilitates the categorization of individuals with more than one diagnosis or type of morbidity. Techniques have been developed (Starfield et al., 1991) and used for purposes of profiling the practices of individual clinicians and groups of health practitioners. Although developed in the United States using the International Classification of Diseases—Clinical Modification (ICD-CM), it has been modified for use with the International Classification of Primary Care (ICPC) in Europe. The developmental work of Juncosa and Bolibar and the organized application and testing of its use in collaborative practice-based research directed by Prados-Torres, Orueta, and colleagues in Spain are noteworthy in this regard. Wider application and testing in a greater variety of settings is indicated, however, to ascertain the method's contribution to understanding the epidemiology of problems in primary care, and how they inform the use of resources, for both primary care and the totality of care provided to populations (Starfield et al., 1991, 1994; Tucker et al., 1996; Weiner et al., 1996; Salem-Schatz et al., 1994). Finally, there is a need for measures of severity of illness that would make it possible to standardize or stratify populations that may differ in this aspect of illness (Iezzoni, 1997).

Procedures for assessing quality of care

Most assessments of the quality of care address only single diagnoses. Little is known about the extent to which judgements are consistent across diagnoses, and no techniques are available to assess this. Interventions to improve the quality of care depend on whether care is consistently poor or is poor in only a few areas; consistently inadequate care calls for a different type of intervention than does inadequate care for only one type or just a few types of specific health problems. There is a need for quality of care measures that do not depend on the presence of particular diagnoses. Such measures would be of considerable usefulness in primary care because many of its health problems never reach the stage of a diagnosis and, conversely, patients may have several co-existing and interacting health problems under care at any one time. Most research on quality of care has focused on identifying and understanding errors of omission. Studies have consistently shown that about 20% of care is inappropriate, but the vast majority of these studies have been conducted in inpatient settings. Moreover, while research on the causes and correlates of medical malfeasance (including medical malpractice) has documented the extent of errors of judgment, few if any have distinguished errors of omission from errors of commission and the relative impact of each on damage to patients. There is a compelling need to focus attention on errors in ambulatory settings as well, particularly concerning interventions (both pharmacological and nonpharmacological) that are unnecessary and potentially dangerous. Furthermore, it is important to determine what methods of ascertainment are best in sorting out the relative responsibilities of organizations and individuals in improving the quality of services because most evidence of poor quality is at least partly ascribable to the organizational setting in which the practitioner works.

The capacity to improve quality of care might be extended by developing new types of techniques. In particular, what might be gained by mechanisms that involve patients in designing and conducting quality enhancement activities? To what extent is satisfaction with care on the part of patients an adequate proxy for professional judgments about the quality of care? What particular components of satisfaction are most related to these other types of judgments about quality, and to what extent do they enhance knowledge about effective care above and beyond professional assessments?

Measurement of the need for referral and characteristics of referral care

What types of problems are always referred, which are rarely referred, and for which is there variability?* What is responsible for the variability? To what extent do the expectations of patients drive referrals, and what types of referrals can be attributed primarily to the requests or insistence of patients? To what extent does provider reimbursement policy influence decisions to refer? What types of problems require long-term involvement of specialists, and which are best managed by short-term consultation, repeated if necessary at various times in the course of illness, or by shared care? What are the most effective methods of communication with specialists, and do they vary with the nature of the relationship of the specialist with the patient? When tertiary care specialists must assume responsibility for long-term management, what is the appropriate role of the primary care practitioner, and what are the best methods for achieving coordination between them? To what extent can specialty care be streamlined so that patients who no longer need ongoing care from specialists are promptly returned to their primary care physician? Can methods be developed to distinguish consultant (short-term) care from referral (long-term) care so that specialists are appropriately trained for their respective roles, making the organization of referral care more rational? Another needed area of research concerns the development of guidelines to help practitioners decide when a referral to a consultant is desirable.

Development and adaptation of methods to manage presenting problems

Most assessments of the quality of diagnostic workups start with a study of the diagnosis and retrospectively examine the adequacy or appropriateness of the procedures used to reach it. With the exception of the algorithm approach to assessing quality of care, no techniques start with the presenting problem. Chapter 16, concerning medical records and information systems, summarizes a method of classifying the presentation of problems in primary care. Techniques to apply it would enable facilities of health systems to judge the adequacy and appropriateness of all problems presented by patients not only of those that resulted in particular diagnoses. Emphasis on presenting problems is even more important in primary care than in other types of care because of its first-contact feature and because evidence indicates that about half of all "diagnoses" in primary care visits do not resolve into codable diagnostic entities. Because of the high degree of uncertainty of diagnosis in primary care, better methods are needed to characterize it. When diag-

---

*The Agency for Health Care Policy and Research in the United States has identified referrals as a particularly important areas for research because of past neglect of the subject. A summary of some of the salient issues is given by Lanier and Clancy (1996).

noses are unclear, watchful waiting sometimes involves the prescription of a trial of therapy, yet little is known about the justifiability and impact of various strategies for intervention when diagnoses are still tentative. Many systems of reimbursement (particularly in the United States) depend on the designation of a diagnosis. Thus, information that derives from official records (such as claims forms) generally provides overestimates of the incidence and prevalence of specific diagnoses. Pioneering health systems such as the Harvard Community Health Plan (now Harvard-Pilgrim) in Boston recognized this challenge in the design of their computerized medical record, which uses qualifiers for diagnoses that specify the stage of the diagnostic process and that, therefore, provides the basis for a better understanding of the relationship between diagnostic problems and resources used to solve them.

What methods are best for examining how patients and practitioners negotiate their differences regarding the needs and opinions about the cause and management of health problems and determining how they arrive at a solution that leads to a mutually acceptable plan of approach?

Techniques to measure the effectiveness of care and assessment of patients' cooperation

This involves the degree to which patients understand, accept, and participate in the process of care as prescribed by health professionals. Comparisons of continuous versus episodic care and evaluation of patients' participation in their care require the development of methods to collect information about patients more accurately, conveniently, and confidentially. Among the potentially useful techniques are health diaries, medical records, and abstracts of personal medical records kept by patients themselves.

What types of communication styles are most suited to patients from particular cultural subgroups? To what extent can differences across cultural subgroups be categorized and used for teaching primary care trainees? Are communication styles that are optimum in primary care the same as those for specialty care, or does the challenge of long-term interpersonal and patient-focused relationships that characterizes primary care call for a different type of interaction than is the case in short-term consultative care?

Procedures for assessing the responsiveness of patients to medical recommendations

There is a need for determining the point at which nonresponsiveness suggests inappropriate diagnosis or inappropriate therapy.

Improving the accuracy and efficiency of data collection and record keeping

This will result in improved auditing, patient follow-up, and coordination of care. Possible approaches range from patient-carried records to electronic information networks in primary care. Another approach is directed at the development and testing of information systems that would enhance the usefulness of large databases deriving from claims records and other accounting procedures. Other techniques that might be explored include small areas surveys and repeated observations of patient cohorts to monitor care over time.

Development of a method to estimate the community served by a primary care practice

The estimation of this "population at risk" is needed as a denominator for calculating rates, thereby permitting comparisons of relative frequencies among different settings or between different primary care practices.

Development of methods to facilitate the use of community data in primary care practice

Many, if not most, local and state health departments collect data that can be related to characteristics of geographically defined populations. These data are important in identifying health problems that should be addressed in primary care practice. Many if not most communities contain one or more subpopulations that are at high risk of health problems and their sequelae. These populations include the elderly (particularly those living alone), high-risk pregnant women and their infants, minority populations, socioeconomically disadvantaged populations, migrant workers, individuals with disabilities, handicaps, or impairments, and individuals at particular risk of specific diseases such as aquired immunodeficiency syndrome, hypertension, occupational hazards, environmental exposures, or stress-related illnesses. Examples of study topics include design and development of coordinated information networks that will enable health departments, community health agencies, and primary care practitioners to collect, analyze, and interpret data on health needs. The network will also make possible the development of plans for dealing with current and emerging health problems.

Development and testing of ways to examine the effectiveness of primary care training, certification, and educational activities

Methods are needed to compare the various ways in which residency programs are structured, the differences and similarities in educational approaches of the various primary care specialties, and the variations in training of physician and nonphysician practitioners. Additional methods are needed to seek out individuals who are trained in various types of programs and to assess the impact of their training on the nature, extent, and adequacy of primary care practice. Such assessment would be useful in helping training programs to improve their direction and intensity, as well as in guiding their continuing education activities.

How do physicians deal with scientific information, particularly when it contradicts their current mode of practice? What characteristics determine whether physicians can alter their practices on the basis of their own reading of the evidence or whether they require more formal group mechanisms that are based on group processes or on the advice of respected mentors or colleagues?

Policy-Related Research

Policy-related research addresses issues that pertain to decisions about services either directly by providing answers to important questions or indirectly by providing information that helps to understand a problem so that alternative solutions can be posed. In primary care, there are three types of policy-related research: clinical research, health services research, and research related to primary care training. Policy-relevant clinical research (sometimes known as *clinical epidemiology*) concerns the processes of care directed at recognition of symptoms, signs, and syndromes in primary care practice, the diagnostic processes associated with them, and the treatment and reassessment strategies that follow from the diagnosis. Health services research concerns the myriad relationships between the various components of the structure, process, and outcomes of care as described in Chapter 2. Research related to primary care training concerns the characteristics and impact of the process to educate primary care practitioners and to maintain their competence in practice.

Clinical primary care research

Within this area are several aspects in need of further investigation:

- Descriptions of the practice of primary care in various organizational configurations, settings, and communities, including the incidence of problems encountered, patterns of diseases seen, services provided, and resources employed. Such information will provide the basis for understanding the reasons for variations in practice patterns across different facilities. How much of the variation is a result of differences in the patients and their illnesses, and how much is a result of differences in specific modes of organization, financing, and practice? How much of the variation in use of tests, procedures, and referrals can be explained by practitioners' discomfort with uncertainty, how much to differences in patients' desires and demands, and how much to the conditions of the practice itself?
- Evaluations of the effectiveness of the drugs, devices, and procedures common in primary care practice. What are the benefits and risks of technologies or interventions employed in practice compared with the result of testing under controlled conditions of research? What is the impact on effectiveness of various characteristics of patients, providers, and settings?
- Design and testing of protocols for screening, diagnosis, and treatment. Protocols seek to provide more systematic review of the quality and of the costs of care, to permit the identification and evaluation of alternative services or providers, and to identify problems in presenting symptoms, disease incidence, or management effectiveness. Limited studies of the use of protocols for common conditions in pediatric practice suggest that they may be of some benefit; does the use of

such protocols make it possible for non-physician providers to assume some of the burden of care in busy ambulatory facilities?

- Examining the relative frequency of adverse effects on patients, on medical liability suits, and on other documentation of physician performance occurring because of inappropriate, unnecessary, or facility interventions (errors of commission) rather than failure to intervene (errors of omission). Is the widespread perception of physicians that doing too much is preferable to doing too little confirmed by experiences with patient's outcomes?

- Evaluation of prevention, patient education, and self-care activities. Although prevention of disease and promotion of health involve activities that extend beyond the health services system, aspects requiring changes in health behaviors of individuals are largely within the province of primary care. The effectiveness of various approaches, especially those based on group rather than on individual efforts, needs to be tested. Evaluation of the role of support groups in the management of common conditions such as childhood asthma or low back pain in adults would contribute in a major way to understanding the potential usefulness of group procedures rather than the usefulness of individual strategies to manage illness and to prevent it. Although there is substantial evidence of poor attention to preventive and health promoting activities in primary care and evidence that these activities can be increased by a variety of practical interventions (Yanos et al., 1995), little is known about the applicability and utility of the various interventions for the variety of types of preventive care and the populations to which they are provided.

- Analyses of the process of medical decision-making, including both careful descriptions of how diagnostic and therapeutic choices are made and the development and testing of methods to improve the process. How do primary care practitioners with different types and levels of training identify indicators of illness and plan management and follow-up strategies? Which prescribed strategies for decision-making are best for improving the effectiveness and efficiency of these processes, and what are their limitations and risks? Studies of this type include analyses of the role of mathematical models in medical diagnosis and of the use of utility theory in estimating and comparing preferences of patients for alternative treatments and outcomes.

- Examinations of the interrelationships between the physical and psychosocial aspects of illnesses, particularly as they are seen in primary care. Primary care is directed toward the treatment of persons rather than of diseases; practitioners frequently must sort through a wide variety of complaints and problems and assign them the correct diagnostic labels and therapeutic strategies. The interplay of physical and psychosocial disorders in patients may result in serious distortions in signs, symptoms, and treatment responses, and there is therefore a great need for information about how these interrelationships can be more easily recognized and effectively managed. Studies of this type include examinations of the relationships between stress and common complaints; analyses of the ways tranquilizers are used in office practice; and comparisons of nonpharmacological and pharmacological approaches to alleviating health problems. Variation in the way in which practitioners record symptoms and complaints may play an important role in determining the ensuing process of diagnosis and management. What proportion of patients present multiple "chief complaints"? Where there are multiple complaints, it is not clear that the first-listed is the most salient, yet little is known about how practitioners go about describing and prioritizing them. What systems can be developed that would be of use in characterizing "symptom complexes" when multiple complaints are encountered, and what can be learned about their prognostic value, both for resource use and for outcomes of care?

Is there a role in primary care for primary care practitioners who subspecialize in particular types of clinical problems? To what extent, if any, does this specialization improve the quality of care without raising its costs? If subspecialization is useful, what practice size is required to justify it? In the special case of women's health, can subspecialization provide better attention to women's health needs and improve the responsiveness of primary care for them?

- Examinations of differences between users and nonusers of health services by comparing individuals, families, communities, or practices. Such factors as variations in economic status, education, cultural values, life style, family and community support systems, and practice outreach activities may underlie the differing perceptions of providers, patients, and the public concerning necessary, appropriate, and adequate primary care. Studies of this type include examination of the adequacy and acceptability of care provided in medically underserved areas and investigation of barriers to seeking care in various population subgroups.
- Descriptions of the natural history of illnesses commonly encountered and managed in primary care practices. More complete information is needed, for example, about the course of disorders such as otitis media, arthritis, asthma, depression, and low back pain—disorders that are characterized by cycles of remission and exacerbation. Particularly important is the extent of functional impairment over time, the effects of co-existing physical or mental disorders, and the effectiveness of efforts to prevent recurrence or exacerbation.
- Can good primary care reduce the likelihood of co-morbidity in certain individuals or in particular population subgroups? For example, socioeconomically disadvantaged populations are not only more likely to become ill, they also are more likely to become ill with a variety of different types of illness (Starfield et al., 1991). Is this a result of more vulnerability to illness or a result of less adequate primary care? Can access to primary care that achieves longitudinality, comprehensiveness, and coordination reduce this tendency to co-morbidity in these individuals and populations?

Health services research related to primary care

The second area of policy-related research concerns several issues related to achieving the important functions of primary care and their interrelationships, to organizing and financing of primary care, and to the challenges of increasing technology available in the office and home:

- Studies related to longitudinality of care. Relatively recent research provides the basis for postulating that a relationship between patients and a particular practitioner are more salutary than a relationship with a particular place alone. Little is known, however, about the conditions under which, or populations for which, a particular place might be as advantageous as a particular practitioner. If coordination of care within the different personnel in a facility is at a high level, might having a "particular place" rather than a "particular physician" be just as advantageous in achieving the benefits of longitudinality? To what extent can the benefits of identification with a particular provider be achieved by methods other than by continuity of practitioner, and what are the conditions under which such alternatives are useful? What are the specific situations in which the maintenance of a long-term relationship between patient and practitioner might be detrimental to care? What problems arise when patients prefer a degree of autonomy and a less personal relationship with a provider than that which ordinarily develops in a primary care practice and which might compromise the effectiveness of care by reducing the patient's participation? To what extent is the "free choice" of a primary care practitioner conducive to achieving the benefits of longitudinality, particularly when longitudinality is assessed by ascertaining the strength of the interpersonal relationship between practitioners and patients?

• Studies related to first-contact care. How can the benefits of the gatekeeper role be maintained despite incentives that may reduce access to needed specialty services? Why do some patients chose to by-pass primary care physicians and go directly to specialists? Are there cultural variations in the acceptability of the primary care role? Do these differences result in different patterns of care and in different outcomes of care? What might be the disadvantages of discouraging the practice of self-referral to specialists?

• Studies related to comprehensiveness. What problems are best managed solely within primary care? Conversely, what problems should routinely be referred to secondary consultants for advice or to tertiary care specialists for long-term management? What role does increased empowerment of patients play in the improved recognition of problems by practitioners? What can be done to maximize the involvement of primary care practitioners in community outreach, long-term care, and preventive activities?

• Studies related to coordination. What mechanisms can optimally facilitate the communication of information about patients between practitioners and between levels of care?

• Studies concerning the relationships among the essential features of primary care. Less than a handful of research studies have simultaneously evaluated the achievement of multiple primary care goals; those that have been conducted suggest that achieving one may be at the expense of achieving others (Yanos et al., 1995). At an ecological level, that is, using aggregated data about each characteristic, international comparisons show that greater achievement of first contact is not associated with greater achievement of comprehensiveness (Boerma et al., 1997), but whether this is the case at the level of individual practices is unknown. To what extent does the maintenance of a long-term practitioner–patient relationship facilitate first-contact care, comprehensiveness, and coordination? Does greater comprehensiveness of care foster greater coordination? Are physicians or organizations that perform well on one characteristic likely to perform well on others, or are they unrelated? What factors are responsible for good performance on these characteristics? Are they primarily educational, or are they largely a function of the setting in which the practitioner works? What are the best ways to improve performance simultaneously of first contact, longitudinality, comprehensiveness, and coordination?

Studies related to referral practices

To what extent are the observed variations in referral rates related to differences in needs of patients rather than to either random or systematic differences in the patterns of physician practices? Is there evidence that there are differences in rates of referral for short-term advice or interventions and for long-term ongoing disease management, and do these differences in referral practices influence the health status of patients? Variability in referral rates might be associated with differences in (1) case mix, (2) patient characteristics such as sex and age, (3) physician characteristics such as training or duration in practice, (4) availability of resources within a practice setting as well as external ones, (5) accessibility of specialty practices to patients, and (6) differences in patterns of practice possibly related either to psychological variables associated with tolerance of uncertainty or general norms in the community. These characteristics require consideration when one explores variations in referral rates, understanding their basis and devising ways to change them to achieve the best outcomes expressed in terms of the health of patients.

Studies related to modifying pattern of referral

Studies in Great Britain show that specialists treat patients in instances when the latter could be treated by their general practitioner and that general practitioners express dissatisfaction when patients are cross-referred to other specialists without their consent (Wilkin and Dornan, 1990). To what extent can consultants' review of their medical records remind them of the involvement of the primary care physician? What other mechanisms for involving consultants could reduce the frequency of referral? For example, can the need for referrals be reduced by phone conversations between the consultant and the primary care physician (Hartog, 1988) or by specialty consultation sessions within the primary care setting (Tyrer, 1984)? How are differences of opinion between primary care physicians and specialists resolved? To what extent are patients involved in decision-making in such instances? These issues are all appropriate subjects for research.

Studies concerning the roles of primary care physicians and those of specialists

In many countries, the tasks of primary , secondary, and tertiary care physicians are clearly delineated. Primary care physicians work largely outside of the hospital; consultant specialists work in community hospitals, and tertiary care physicians work primarily in regionalized teaching and medical centers. In some countries, secondary care physicians may work outside of hospitals as well as in them. To what extent does restriction of the practice site of primary care and non-primary care physicians influence the quality, effectiveness, and cost of care?

Studies related to teamwork in primary care

Many useful contributions to primary care are made by personnel other than physicians, although there are no standards for the different roles and relationships. As noted in Chapter 5, the delegated tasks may substitute for those ordinarily performed by physicians, supplement what the physician does, or complement physicians' conventional activities. The training of non-physician personnel for primary care would be greatly facilitated by information on what function is most appropriately assumed by whom. How widespread is the use of non-physician personnel in providing clinical aspects of care and how variable are their tasks in primary care? Are nurse practitioners more effective than physicians in ensuring the provision of needed preventive services, and, if so, are there barriers to their deployment for these purposes? How often are home visits done, for what purpose, and by whom? Under what conditions do patients relate to a nonphysician as their "regular source of care" or as the individual who coordinates the various aspects of care, and how well are the major attributes of primary care achieved when compared with care by physicians?

Studies related to the organization and financing of primary care services

What financing and organizational arrangements best facilitate problem recognition, adequacy of diagnostic and therapeutic procedures, and reassessment after the institution of therapy? To what extent and under what conditions can telephone management substitute for face-to-face visits? What forms of organization and financing facilitate the development of information systems to enhance knowledge of community health needs, the recognition of patients' problems, and the responsiveness to interventions? How can we maximize the incentives to develop such systems?

Studies related to the use of technology in primary care

As technology expands, more procedures will be done at the level of primary care, and some will even be suitable for use by patients themselves. The expansion of technology beyond the confines of hospitals and large medical centers raises a host of issues for research. How does the availability of technology alter the nature of primary care? Does the availability of home testing increase or decrease the use of health services, and does it influence patients to by-pass primary care physicians and seek care directly from specialists? Will new testing technologies directed at screening for early stages of disease deflect attention from the need for its prevention? Will the widespread availability of home testing impose greater burdens of coordination of services on primary care physicians? What information systems would be required to facilitate the efficient use of data from these home- and office-based technologies? Will increasing use of technology facilitate or hamper the expansion of organized and integrated primary care services?

To what extent can concerted efforts to deal with problems in a family context facilitate both the process of care and its outcome?

Do practitioners who use the family as an integral part of management achieve more rapid or more complete resolution of problems than primary care physicians who deal with the family context only as an adjunct to management?

Research on primary care training

The third type of policy-related research has three areas that especially need investigation:

How can knowledge about the distribution of disease be included in medical curricula?

By what mechanism can primary care physicians learn the principles of primary care, and how can its content be made more adequate?

What techniques shall be used in teaching physicians-in-training the limitations of their expertise as well as the proper time for appropriate consultation and referral? Because much of primary care requires dealing with uncertainty, physicians-in-training must be taught how to recognize when "watchful waiting" has reached its limits and subsequent action is required. The primary care trainee should also be taught techniques to minimize the anxiety that accompanies uncertainty. How do physicians involve patients in dealing with uncertainty? What information do they provide to patients about the likelihood of the various possibilities concerning their undifferentiated problems and the prognoses associated with them? How do these mechanisms differ by cultural background of the patient? What are the best mechanisms to teach the appropriate techniques in the educational setting?

How can approaches to quality assessment and quality improvement be incorporated into physician training? Primary care trainees should learn how to keep abreast of scientific advances in subjects related to primary care and how to use computers to search the literature for current knowledge when it is required in the care of patients. Is such training best accomplished in conjunction with clinical activities or as part of basic science training?

Mechanisms To Facilitate the Conduct of Research in Primary Care

A very small proportion of published research concerns topics of importance in primary care. With the exception of a few journals devoted entirely to topics in family medicine and general internal medicine and pediatrics, fewer than 10% and in most cases well under 5% of papers published in peer-reviewed journals have any relevance to problems encountered in primary care practice (Starfield, 1990).

Even journals that focus on primary care are heavily overbalanced with clinical topics rather than basic research or health services research of relevance to primary care. Furthermore, less than one-fourth of all articles in these journals report on studies that take place in ambulatory care settings (Starfield, 1996).

The most straightforward approach to encouraging the conduct of primary care research involves the provision of public or private funding for it. The U.S. Government provides some targeted funding for such research, largely through the Agency for Health Care Policy and Research. However, the amounts of such funding are only a tiny fraction (much less than 1%) of funding for research related to the provision of health services. In the United Kingdom, where a focus on primary care is policy for both major political parties and the government, a substantial percentage (14%) of governmental money spent on research and development will be earmarked for primary care research (Groves, 1997).

Additional mechanisms for stimulating research in primary care include support for the strengthening of academic units in primary care, particularly in prestigious medical schools and universities, and providing visibility for the results of primary care research in public and professional media. A major primary care journal, or perhaps more than one, might undertake to commission an annual review of recent primary care research studies and their findings. The review by Yanos et al. published in 1995 concerning research published from 1980 to 1994 provides an interesting example of the potential for such a proposal.

Levels of Research in Primary Care

To exploit the tremendous potential of research, it is useful to divide the possibilities into three levels:

- Research done at the level of the individual practitioner or practice group
- Research done through collaboration among professionals in many practices (or health centers) in an area or country (or even across countries)
- Research done for the purposes of developing policies about the organization and delivery of services in a political jurisdiction, which might be a municipality, province or state, or nation

All three levels of research are important in the development and support of a research agenda, and they complement each other.

Research at the level of the individual practitioner or practice

The aim of this type of research is to encourage a spirit of inquiry among practitioners. Many if not most physicians enter medical training with a spirit of intellectual curiosity that is often lost as a result of the didactic nature of their training. Given time and encouragement, this spirit often can be recovered. Because knowledge in medicine is always incomplete and sometimes based on inadequate information, assumptions about "right" and wrong" practices must continually be subjected to validation. Physicians should be given incentives to ask questions about their own practices. For the most part, physicians will be interested in clinical subjects such as how their own diagnostic and therapeutic procedures compare with those of their colleagues in the same practice, how the problems of their own patients compare with the problems seen by their colleagues, and about the effectiveness of alternative treatment choices on improvement of problems experienced by their patients. To carry out these kinds of studies, it is only necessary to have information systems that can identify a core set of information about each patient, the visits they make, and what occurs in each visit (presenting problem, diagnosis, treatment, and disposition). Investment in training physicians to use data in computerized form and provision of easy access to computerized data will greatly facilitate their interest in and conduct of research of this type. Keith Hodgkin (1963) and John Fry (1966) described the conditions they encountered in their practices over 30 years ago. Fry, a general practitioner in Great Britain for 45 years (Fry, 1993), regarded the potential for long-term research in practice as exciting and challenging and as indispensable in providing information to improve the understanding and management of primary care problems. As examples of his contributions, he cited the following "discoveries":

1. The syndrome of recurrent upper respiratory infection in early childhood is generally outgrown by age 7–8 years.
2. Disorders such as asthma, migraine, hay fever, and duodenal ulcer do not persist forever.
3. Although high blood pressure and ischemic heart disease are conditions of aging, not all require long-term intensive treatment.
4. The course and outcome of common psychiatric conditions is that of the "three thirds": one third suffer a single episode, one-third have recurrent episodes, and one-third are chronic and unresponsive to "cure."

Furthermore, Fry divided the topics most amenable to single practice research into the categories of studies of the way in which the practice is run, including such topics as volume, types, and problems of patients, referrals, home visits, use of diagnostic facilities, and prescribing information; long-term studies of patients with specific diseases; studies of the course and prognosis of common disorders; and studies of the impact of social, personal, and family factors. Hodgkin and Fry did their practice-based research without benefit of computers. Imagine what could be done today with benefit of automated information systems.

Care must be taken, however, in generalizing the results from studies conducted in one or just a few facilities using a population that may not be representative of the general public. The ability to generalize findings is compromised when the study population is not representative of the population or, at least, of an identifiable population subgroup. Generalizability is a challenge in any kind of research, but it is particularly problematic in primary care because the characteristics of the particular setting are so influential that they become a constellation of factors that themselves must be considered. Therefore, a promising alternative approach to research in primary care involves collaborative, multicenter research in office-based practice.

Collaborative, multicenter research

Collaborative efforts offer much greater potential to conduct health services research and clinical research because different clinical settings will almost certainly have different types of structural (e.g., personnel, organization, financing) and process characteristics. Good prototypes of such collaborative efforts (Niebauer and Nutting, 1994) include the Ambulatory Sentinel Practice Network (ASPN) in the United States and Canada, Pediatric Research in Office Settings (PROS) in the United States, (Wasserman, 1998) and the European General Practice Research Network.

The ASPN, initiated in the late 1970s by the North American Primary Care Research Group, consists largely of family physicians (Culpepper and Froom, 1988). In the mid-1980s, the American Academy of Pediatrics organized a similar network, PROS. Both networks involve practices across the country in conducting research on topics derived from experience in practice and address topics important to primary care practitioners. In both networks academically based physicians are of value in research management and in providing the research skills necessary for the conduct of scientific research. Their steering committees also include active practitioners who participate in the choice of topics for study.

A few regional networks complement these national networks. The Cooperative Information Project (COOP), is a network of practitioners in New England who have carried out collaborative research in conjunction with Dartmouth Medical School for over a decade. Another regional network is the Pediatric Practice Research Group (PPRG) in Chicago, a joint effort of the Children's Memorial Hospital and its Institute for Education and Research, Northwestern University, together with physicians in office practice. This network has undertaken and published the results of studies on infant growth, the exposure of children to environmental hazards, the office management of foreign body ingestion, cholesterol screening, and the acceptance of new infant formulas (Christoffel et al., 1988).

PROS and its precursor based in practices in California have conducted studies of vision screening practices, iron-deficiency anemia, and fever in infants. ASPN studies have provided new information on various characteristics of a number of important problems in primary care, including chest pain, pelvic inflammatory disease, spontaneous abortion, and headache (Rosser et al., 1990; Freeman et al., 1988; Green et al., 1988; Becker et al., 1988). COOP projects have addressed measurement of functional status in physicians' offices (Nelson et al., 1990), a prospective study of fatigue (Kirk et al., 1990), cancer control in primary care practice (Dietrich et al., 1990), the use of antibiotics in primary care, and many other topics (Dartmouth COOP Project Bibliography, 1991).

Notable European collaborative practice-based networks are EUROSENTINEL (Leurquin et al., 1995) and the European General Practice Research Network (Jones, 1991). These initiatives are encouraged and supported by the European Union in the form of grants (COMAC-HSR and BIOMED).

Over the years, many local collaborations between academics and office-based practitioners have contributed important information for primary care. Most of these collaborative efforts have been outgrowths of the interests of particular researchers based in medical centers and have therefore focused on topics that were generated within the centers; few efforts survived after the particular researcher moved on or found other interests. Nevertheless, the potential for broader and more stable linkages between the academic primary care physician and the office-based practitioner, with enhanced roles for the practitioners in generating important research topics, is evident from the existing national and regional networks.

System-wide research to inform policies for primary care

This type of research is directed specifically at answering questions to inform decision-making about organization and delivery of services as well as the adequacy of preparation and deployment of health services personnel. Because these policies are generally made at national or regional levels, the research that informs them must produce information that is generalizable and applicable throughout the jurisdiction. Thus, it cannot be conducted in only one health center or even in a group of health centers unless they are known to be a representative sample. Depending on the nature of the specific question asked, the research requires an information system that contains data collected in a uniform manner from clinical facilities or systematic surveys from community samples or health services facilities. For example, assessment of the adequacy of primary care received by a population requires information collected in a standard way from the population or a representative sample of it; characterization of the adequacy of primary care provided by health facilities or centers requires information collected in a standard way from the universe of facilities or a representative sample of them. Clinical databases are not uncommon in health care facilities in many countries, but no country has yet achieved the ability to aggregate data from all facilities because the databases from different facilities are not uniform. In the United States, efforts are underway to specify a minimum core dataset both for individuals and for their encounters with the health services system, and to do so in a way that it is possible to transmit comparable data for planning and evaluation (National Center for Health Statistics, 1996).

Challenges of Primary Care Research

Credible research on primary care, be it basic research, clinical research, health services research, or evaluations of education programs, whatever the level of the research, requires that researchers be trained in the techniques of research. Their expertise must be specific to the task; it must include disciplines such as epidemiology, social sciences techniques, economics, and decision analysis. In addition, training for research should include techniques for collecting nonquantitative data using the skills of the anthropologist and related disciplines. Much is to be gained from analyses that have become increasingly refined and are in good usage in conjunction with the more traditional quantitative techniques and biostatistical applications (Norton et al., 1990). For example, qualitative analyses have revealed reasons for referral that may be missed by more traditional quantitative classifications. Referral behavior may appear to be irrational and therefore difficult to categorize (Wilkin and Dornan, 1990). Training in formal techniques for qualitative analysis are available for teaching as well as for use in ongoing research (Patton, 1980; Miles and Huberman, 1984).

It is accepted practice in the clinical subspecialties for trainees to undertake postdoctoral study under mentoring from senior researchers. Fellowships for postdoctoral training in health services research, including those related specifically to primary care, are available from the Agency for Health Care Policy and Research in the U.S. Department of Health and Human Services. National Research Services Awards for research on primary care issues may also be available from other agencies in the same department.

The challenge of primary care research is exciting. It may well be that its rewards are greater than those of other research. Primary care has the heuristic value of contributing to knowledge common to all research but has the added reward of contributing to research on the cutting edge of developments in health services. Biomedical research has been responsible for the enormous advances that have led to an understanding of the mechanisms of disease and for developments of technology to manage it and to prolong life. Today the cutting edge lies in the organization and delivery of services to make these advances available where they are needed, in the development of ways to determine where these needs are greatest, and in the focusing of more attention on documenting the impact of technology and other services on aspects of health status other than disease processes alone. Research on primary care and translation of research findings into policy and clinical practice are essential ingredients to the achievement of the two main goals of any health services system: to optimize the health of the population by employing the most advanced state of knowledge of disease causation, illness management, and health maximization and to minimize the systematic disparities in health status associated with differential access to the benefits of this knowledge.

References

Becker L, Iverson D, Reed F, Calonge N, Miller R, Freeman W. Patients with new headache in primary care: A report from ASPN. J Fam Prac 1988; 27(1):41–7.

Boerma W, van der Zee J, Fleming D. Service profiles of general practitioners in Europe. Br J Gen Pract 1997; 47:481–6.

Christoffel K, Binns J, Stockman J, McGuire P, Poncher J, Unti S, Typlin B, Lasin G, Seigel W, Pediatric Practice Research Group. Practice-based research: Opportunities and obstacles. Pediatrics 1988; 82(pt 2):399–406.

Culpepper L, Froom J. The international primary care network: Purpose, methods, and policies. Fam Med 1988; 20(3):197–201.

Dartmouth COOP Project Bibliography. COOP Annual Meeting. Hanover, NH: Department of Community and Family Medicine, Dartmouth Medical School, February 1991.

Dietrich A, O'Connor G, Keller A, Carney-Gersten P, Levy D, Nelson E, Simmons J, Barrett Jr J, Landgraf J. Will community physicians participate in rigorous studies of cancer control? The methodology and recruitment of a randomized trial of physician practices. Prog Clin Biol Res 1990; 339:337–81.

Freeman W, Green L, Becker L. Pelvic inflammatory disease in primary care. Fam Med 1988; 20(3):192–6.

Fry J. Profiles of Disease: A Study in the Natural History of Common Diseases. London: E & S Livingstone Ltd., 1966.

Fry J. Single practice research—Longterm research. Scand J Prim Health Care 1993; 11(suppl 2):28–30.

Gold M. Common sense on extending DRG concepts to pay for ambulatory care. Inquiry 1988; 25:281–9.

Green L, Becker L, Freeman W, Elliott E, Iverson D, Reed F. Spontaneous abortion in primary care. J Am Board Fam Pract 1988; 1:15–23.

Groves T. Primary care: Opportunities and threats. What the changes mean. BMJ 1997; 314: 436–8.

Hartog M. Medical outpatients. J R Coll Phys Lond 1988; 22:517.

Hodgkin K. Towards Earlier Diagnosis: A Family Doctor's Approach. London: E & S Livingstone, Ltd., 1963.

Iezzoni L (ed). Risk Adjustment for Measuring Health Care Outcomes. 2nd ed. Chicago: Health Administration Press, 1997.

Jones R. European General Practice Research Workshop. Fam Pract 1991; 8:111.

Kirk J, Douglass R, Nelson E, Jaffe J, Lopez A, Ohler J, Blanchard C, Chapman R, McHugo G, Stone K. Chief complaint of fatigue: A prospective study. J Fam Pract 1990; 30(1): 33–41.

Lanier D, Clancy C. The changing interface of primary and specialty care. J Fam Pract 1996; 42:303–5.

Leurquin P, van Casteren V, de Maeseneer J. Eurosentinel Study Group. Use of blood tests in general practice: A collaborative study in eight European countries. Br J Gen Pract 1995; 45:21–5.

McDowell I, Newell C. Measuring Health. A Guide to Rating Scales and Questionnaires. New York: Oxford University Press, 1996.

Miles M, Huberman A. Qualitative Data Analysis: A Source book of New Methods. Beverly Hills, CA: Sage, 1984.

National Center for Health Statistics. Core Data Elements. Washington, DC: U.S. Government Printing Office, 1996.

Nelson E, Landgraf J, Hays R, Wasson J, Kirk J. The functional status of patients: How can it be measured in physician's offices? Med Care 1990; 28(12):1111–26.

Niebauer L, Nutting PA. Primary care practice-based research networks active in North America. J Fam Pract 1994; 38(4):425–6.

Norton P, Stewart M, Tudiver F, Bass M, Dunn E. Primary Care Research: Traditional and Innovative Approaches. Newbury Park, CA: Sage Publications, 1990.

Patton M. Qualitative Evaluation Methods. Beverly Hills, CA: Sage, 1980.

Rosser W, Henderson R, Wood M, Green L. An exploratory report of chest pain in primary care. J Am Board Fam Pract 1990; 3(3):143–50.

Salem-Schatz S, Moore G, Rucker M, Pearson S. The case for case-mix adjustment in practice profiling: When good apples look bad. JAMA 1994; 272(11):871–4.

Starfield B. Child health status and outcomes of care: A commentary on measuring the impact of medical care on children. J Chron Dis 1987; 40(suppl):109s-15s.

Starfield B. Primary care research, a view from pediatrics [invited lecture]. Conference on Primary Care Research: Agenda for the 1990s, March 18, 1990. Colorado Springs: Agency for Health Care Policy and Research, 1990.

Starfield B. A framework for primary care research. J Fam Pract 1996; 42:181–5.

Starfield B, Powe N, Weiner J, Stuart M, Steinwachs D, Scholle S, Gerstenberger A. Costs versus quality in different types of primary care settings. JAMA 1994; 272(24):1903–8.

Starfield B, Weiner J, Mumford L, Steinwachs D. Ambulatory care groupings: A categorization of diagnoses for research and management. Health Serv Res 1991; 26(1):53–74.

Tucker A, Weiner J, Honigfeld S, Parton R. Profiling primary care physician resource use: Examining the application of case-mix adjustment. J Ambulatory Care Manage 1996; 19:60–80.

Tyrer P. Psychiatric clinics in general practice: An extension of community care. Br J Psychiatry 1984; 145:9–19.

Wasserman RC, Slora EJ, Bocian AB, Fleming GV, Baker AE, Pedlow SE, Kessel W. Pediatric research in office settings (PROS): I. A national practice-based research network to improve children's health care. Pediatrics 1998; in press.

Weiner J, Dobson A, Maxwell S, Coleman K, Starfield B, Anderson G. Risk-adjusted Medicare capitation rates using ambulatory and inpatient diagnoses. Health Care Financing Rev 1996; 17(3):77–99.

Wilkin D, Dornan C. GP Referrals to Hospital: A Review of Research and Its Implications for Policy and Practice. University of Manchester, Center for Primary Care Research, July 1990.

World Organization of National Colleges, Academies, and Academic Associations of General Practitioners/Family Physicians. ICPC-2 (International Classification of Primary Care. 2nd Ed.) Oxford: Oxford University Press, 1998.

Yanos E, Fink A, Hirsch S, Robbins A, Rubenstein L. Helping practices reach primary care goals: Lessons from the literature. Arch Intern Med 1995; 155: 1146–56.

— 18 —

Health Policies to Achieve Effectiveness and Equity

The Alma-Ata Declaration (see Chapter 1) recognized that primary care "reflects and evolves from the economic conditions and socio-cultural and political characteristics of a country and its communities" (World Health Organization, 1978). The characteristics of each primary care system are therefore unique. No two countries will ever configure their systems in identical ways, and the primary care system may even differ within countries if there are regions with different historical, political, cultural, and economic characteristics.

Because countries differ in these characteristics, they differ in their policy agendas. There are, however, some generic issues that must be faced by all countries, whatever the type of primary care system. In many countries, especially in western Europe, the principle of "solidarity" permeates health policy. That is, there is a recognition that the common good is best served when the well being of all population groups is maximized. It is most recently reflected in the Ljubljana Charter of 1996 which, reaffirmed some basic assumptions about health systems. In the same year, the Declaration of Buenos Aires, which addressed Family Medicine and Health Care Reform, proposed a set of principles, many of which are virtually identical to the principles enunciated in the Ljubljana Charter (Ceitlin and Gomez Gascon, 1997) (Table 18.1).

In 1996, The World Health Organization undertook an initiative to focus on reducing disparities in health status and in health services between social groups characterized by different levels of social or economic privilege. The initiative addresses disparities both among countries as well as within them. The initiative is based on evidence of the existence and widening of gaps in almost all countries, the adverse impact of economic structural adjustments mandated by donor agencies in developing countries leading to cuts in social spending and privatization of formerly public functions, and the long-term adverse effects on society of social and health inequalities.

> The pursuit of growth and financial adjustment without a reasonable concern for equity is ultimately socially destabilizing.
>
> Robert McNamara (when head of the World Bank)

Table 18.1. Recent Health Care Reform Policies

Ljubljana Charter (early 1996)
1. Driven by values of human dignity, equity, solidarity, professional ethics
2. Targeted to protecting and promoting health
3. Centered on people, allowing citizens to influence health services and take responsibility for their own health
4. Focused on quality, cost effectiveness
5. Based on sustainable finances to allow universal coverage and equitable access
6. Oriented toward primary care

Declaration of Buenos Aires 9/96: Family Medicine and Health Care Reform
1. Political decisions must parallel executive action
2. Health care reform must accomplish
   Universality
   Equity
   Accessibility
   Efficiency
   Quality
   Solidarity
   Social participation
   Decentralization
   Intersectorial collaboration
   (An additional 14 principles address family medicine specifically)

Source: Ceitlin and Gomez Gascon (1997).

Health systems in almost all nations are undergoing reform. In many places, these reforms are oriented toward enhancing the role of the market in the organization and financing of health services. The consequences of this change are not clear. In most countries of western Europe, they are superimposed on systems with long histories of universal access to services and with explicit attention to improving equity or "solidarity" in the provision of services. In the main, market-oriented western European reforms are not being permitted to compromise these principles. In fact, by 1997, some aspects of reform were abandoned in countries such as the United Kingdom and New Zealand because their effects were incompatible with the principles. In some countries, such as Australia, health care reform efforts consisted of strengthening primary care (Webster, 1996). In many countries where there is no historical precedent toward equality or equity of access to health services or to primary care, reforms may even further undermine their attainment.

Equity—or justice—is one of the principles of ethics. Any health system—or any health policy—that purports to be ethical must consider equity. Although eastern and western nations differ somewhat in their approach to achieving the other aspects of ethics (autonomy and beneficence), western nations tend to be similar to each other in their approach to these two ethical principles. The same cannot be said of the principle of justice. Justice means fairness: equals should be treated similarly. There are two opposing views of *fairness*: the egalitarian and the libertarian. From the egalitarian viewpoint, equity is achieved when resources are distributed according to needs. That is, more resources are made available to populations that need more services because of their greater social or health disadvantage. The egalitarian views "similarly" as meaning the state of humankind, such that everyone has the right to strive to equal health status. The libertarian views things under the assumption that "equal" applies to merits; resources are distributed according to merits, that is, to those who deserve them by some specified criteria. In the libertarian's view, health care should be distributed according to minimum standards and financed according to willingness to pay. Under the libertarian approach, health policy sets a basic minimum of services, and those who have the means to do so help finance services for those who do not, up to that basic minimum. According to this latter view, equality in health status for all human beings need not be a central priority (Wagstaff and Van Doorslaer, 1993a).

Within the western industrialized world, there is no common understanding of the relative importance of egalitarian and libertarian viewpoints. As noted earlier, egalitarian views tend to prevail in western Europe and are embodied in documents such as the European Goals for Health; equity is the first of the 38 targets. But even in western Europe, there are large differences in the extent to which equity is achieved.* The differences are due partly to differences in financing of services and partly to differences in provision of services.

Many countries make some attempt to finance health services according to egalitarian principles. That is, individuals with higher incomes pay a greater share of their income for health insurance. Because income tax systems in most industrialized countries are usually somewhat progressive, countries with income tax–based health insurance systems are more egalitarian in the financing of their health services. Health systems financed by social insurance, that is, by employer–employee payments, tend to be less egalitarian because these taxes are generally less progressive than general income taxes. Private health insurance, such as is common in the United States, is retrogressive, because it is not related to income and is often more expensive for those with the least ability to afford it (Wagstaff and Van Doorslaer, 1993b; Bodenheimer and Sullivan, 1998). Co-insurance for services, such as deductibles and co-payments, are a regressive means of financing because it is usually unrelated to ability to pay.

Just as countries vary in the extent to which financing of health systems is egalitarian, so they vary in the extent to which they are egalitarian in the delivery of services as reflected in their attempt to distribute resources according to needs. As noted in Chapter 1, this variability has a large impact on the achievement of important outcomes of health systems: more efficient services in terms of lower costs for value achieved and better outcomes in terms of health status indicators.

Protection from increasing inequity and from unfilled expectations about savings in costs of care with sacrifices in quality of care depends on concerted efforts

---

*The terms *equality* and *equity* are not synonymous. Achieving "equality" in health requires that systematic inequities in the determinants of health (including but not limited to access to and provision of appropriate health services) be reduced. The means of doing so might require different approaches in different social groups according to their different needs. Equity in provision of resources takes underlying needs into consideration in deciding on the appropriate levels of resources to be made available for each population subgroup to reduce systematic inequalities in health status across population groups distinguished by differences in social advantage.

to systematically evaluate health system reforms according to predetermined criteria agreed on by the population of each country and according to the principles arrived at by international covenants.

Learning From International Comparisons Concerning Health System Financing and Delivery

Many nations and many international organizations of nations have developed health goals; some of these are described in Chapters 13 and 14. Most of these goals are not, however, framed as equity goals. Of the 638 unduplicated health objectives for the United States as set out in the revised objectives in 1996 (National Center for Health Statistics), over 200 relate specifically to minority races and ethnic groups. Although a greater proportion of individuals in minority groups are low income, the majority of low-income individuals and families are not from these groups. Despite this, only 30 objectives specifically address improving the health status of low-income individuals. These goals are stated in terms of percentage improvement in current states of health, with the intended improvement for those in disadvantaged groups greater than for the population as a whole. As a result, at least a few of the U.S. goals are aimed at reducing the relative differences in health between more deprived and less deprived population groups. No goals are set for income disparities. Thus, the health system is expected to reduce inequalities in health without reducing social inequalities. Whether this is possible is a moot question; if it is possible, it will occur through improving primary care as a policy strategy.

The examples of a few other nations may be instructive. Some relatively poor countries have succeeded in greatly improving the health of their populations despite their relatively low average income. Cuba, with its population of 11 million people and being a still developing country, has reached health levels almost equivalent to many industrialized nations; as noted earlier, it made a major commitment to developing a strong primary care infrastructure with family physician–nurse teams living and working in the communities of 200–400 people. In rural areas especially, their responsibilities include public health activities in these communities as well as clinical activities. Each family physician is required to see every patient in his or her catchment area at least twice a year. The physician's record is reviewed at least monthly with a clinical supervisor who is an academically based family physician. Computerized surveillance has been implemented at all provincial levels and is being extended to cities and local rural areas (Waitzkin et al., 1997). It would be instructive to determine how much of the improvements in health in countries that have made great strides over the past few decades is a result of reducing inequalities in health, rather than merely increasing health levels among the more privileged.

This book makes repeated reference to the improvement of health through primary care, which has been considered the means to improve both effectiveness of health services and equity in the provision of health services. Ample evidence of the former exists; the latter is more theoretical and lies in the assumption that greater efficiencies that accrue from a strong primary care infrastructure release resources that can be made available to those with greater needs. However, there is no assurance that this will be the case, especially in countries where savings may be passed on primarily to the wealthy in the form of returns on investments in profit-making health services. A more compelling justification comes from the attributes of primary care, two of which (comprehensiveness and coordination) require attention to population needs. This is especially the case for comprehensiveness, which cannot be achieved unless the needs of the population are explicitly recognized in the planning and delivery of services. Thus, populations with greater needs would have more services provided. A further justification lies in the community orientation of health systems that are especially advanced in their organization of primary care policy and delivery of services. Community orientation derives its impetus from the recognition of needs of communities. If it is done honestly, communities with greater needs should receive more services to compensate for their greater need.

In the cross-national comparison described in Chapter 1, it was shown that countries with a strong primary care base to their health system achieve better outcomes, and at lower costs, than countries in which the primary care base is weaker. This latter group of countries, which have higher costs, do not necessarily have more hospital beds, greater hospitalization rates, or longer lengths of stay in the hospital—traditionally the most expensive components of health system costs. In fact, the United States with its very high costs, has among the lowest figures for all three characteristics (Starfield, 1993). High-cost countries do not have more physicians per capita than other countries, although they do tend to have higher visit rates in ambulatory care settings. Notable, however, is the average physician per capita rate and the relatively low ambulatory care visit rate in the United States, the country with by far the highest costs.

Although intensity of services once people reach them is higher in countries with less equitable distribution of resources (most notably the United States), there is also no assurance that this is associated with greater use among the more needy. Available data indicate that costs for inpatient stays and for ambulatory care services are much higher in high-cost countries. The rate of use of coronary artery bypass surgery in the United States is over eight times that of the next higher country. Renal dialysis rates are higher in the United States and Germany than in other countries (Rublee, 1992). When countries are ranked according to their rates of use of various technologies, the excess in use of technology in the United States is primarily concentrated in that group of technologies that are machine intensive. (see Fig. 10.1). In contrast, its rates of person-intensive technology, such as allogeneic bone marrow transplant, is only average in rank, and comparisons have shown that the deployment of this technology is much more inequitable than is the case in other countries (Silberman et al., 1994).

This inequity in distribution of technology is mirrored by an inequity in health policies related to primary care. The absence of a policy to distribute health personnel and facilities to areas of greatest need leads to a concentration of these resources in areas of least need because they are the areas that are most in a position to pay for their presence. The absence of policies to ensure universality and public accountability for financing of health services leads to a situation wherein those who are able to pay for services get the most services. Furthermore, the absence of a policy to reimburse those who provide primary care services equal to those who provide subspecialty services leads to a situation where there are powerful incentives to choose a specialty other than primary care among medical trainees. Thus, these health policies, which are reflected in health services practices, are not conducive to improving the health of the more deprived. The privileges of power and influence are so compelling that nothing short of firm goals and working toward them will suffice to improve equity. Left to itself, inequity will worsen, as it has over the past few decades in most industrialized countries. Most privileged populations are unable to see the advantages of greater social and health equalities; it requires a very long-term view to see that ultimate best interests, perhaps of their descendants, are in a society with shared aspirations and shared opportunities. Equity, like entropy, naturally falls to lower levels; it requires energy to maintain and improve it.

The data reported in Chapter 1 concerning the relationship between the strength of primary care and health levels using 14 different indicators of health suggest that health system factors also might make their own contribution to explaining the differences in the relationship between socioeconomic factors and health, particularly because countries with the strongest primary care are not necessarily those countries with the most equitable distribution of wealth. Table 18.2 provides the primary care scores for the 11 countries in the comparison, their rank for the 14 health indicators, and the ranks for equity in distribution of income as derived from the work of the Luxembourg Income Studies (Atkinson et al., 1995). As shown,

Table 18.2. Primary Care, Health, and Income Equity*

Country	Primary Care Rank	14 Health Indicators	Equity in Distribution of Income‡
Sweden	6	1	3
Netherlands	2	2	5
Canada	6	3	8
Spain	5	4	9
Australia	8	5	10
United States	11	6 (9§)	11
Denmark	2	7	4
Finland	2	8 (6§)	1
West Germany	9	9 (8§)	6
United Kingdom	1	10	7
Belgium	9	11	2

*Late 1980s, early 1990s.
† Best ranking is 1, worst is 11. See Chapter 1 for description of the international comparison.
‡ Derived from Smeeding (1996).
§ Rank if life expectancy at age 80 is excluded.

there are notable differences in ranks for primary care and ranks for equitable distribution of income particularly for the United Kingdom and Belgium (both of which rank worse for health than they do for income inequalities) and Spain, Canada, the Netherlands, and Australia (which rank higher for health than they do for income inequalities).

The situation in the United Kingdom is anomalous because its ranking for primary care is best but its rankings for health status are not near the top. The country has spent relatively little on its health system, and there were systematic cutbacks from these low levels in the decade of the 1980s. To the extent that health systems in general and primary care in particular require at least a basic minimum of financial support, the United Kingdom has suffered from serious undercapitalization of its health system for many years. Moreover, the country, like the United States, spends a relatively small proportion of its central government funding on social welfare and education. Thus, in the presence of lack of support for housing, education, and other social programs, even primary care is unlikely to compensate for threats resulting from the other determinants of health.

Finland's relatively poor ranking for health indicators results from poor performance at older age groups. Because Finland's orientation to primary care is a relatively recent phenomenon, it may be that poor health status at older ages reflects the effects of the prior health system orientation. It also may be related to high-fat diets.

The United States is unique in having low ranks for all three characteristics, particularly when life expectancy at age 80 is removed from consideration. Lifestyle factors do not play a major role in influencing the low ranking of the United States because its rates of smoking are among the lowest of all the nations, as is the proportion of individuals who consume alcohol. Moreover, its rate of death from motor vehicle accidents per million miles driven is the lowest of all the countries (U.S. Congress, 1993). Furthermore, removing all violent causes of death does not change the country's poor position with regard to years of potential life lost (analyses from the data of Desenclos and Hahn [1992], U.S. Congress [1993], and Centers for Disease Control and Prevention, [1990].)

The role played by health policies in general, and with regard to primary care in particular, in reducing the impact of social disparities in health is poorly explored. Two findings make such a role plausible. The first is the finding that some states have much better health levels than would be expected given the extent of social disparities in income in the state. The most dramatic example of this is Hawaii, the only state in the nation to have had mandated employer contributions to health insurance coverage for over 20 years (since 1974). States such as New York and Minnesota also do better then other states because their social and health policies partly compensate for income inequities. Other states with high income inequality (e.g., Mississippi and Louisiana) show even poorer health than would be expected on the basis of the average relationship between income inequality and health because their health policies do not compensate for the effect of income inequality (Kennedy et al., 1995; Kaplan et al., 1996).

The second line of evidence derives from a reanalysis of the data from the study by Shi (1994) (see Chapter 1), which showed a highly significant relationship between the primary care physician to population ratio and health levels in the population of states. When measures of income inequality are added in the analysis, the importance of primary care remains significant for all measures and the strength of the relationship between income inequality and health is reduced (but not elim- inated). Thus, it appears that a primary care orientation can in part overcome the severe adverse impact of income inequalities on health, even in the United States (Shi et al., manuscript 1998 preparation).

The third line of evidence is the relatively privileged position of the elderly in the United States. In the face of almost uniformly poor relative performance on most health indicators, the United States ranks very high for life expectancy at age 80. This is the only population group in the country as a whole to have had basic income support after retirement (since 1935) and to have had universal coverage for medical expenses (Medicare) since 1965. Of all the age groups, the elderly have the closest reported relationship with a primary care physician and, except for very young children, the highest rate of first-contact visits with their primary care phy- sician (Forrest, 1995).

It is also possible that this is the age group that is most likely to benefit from advanced and expensive technology designed to maintain survival in the presence of life-threatening illness; analyses (unpublished) of data (U.S. Congress, 1993) on rates of death among the elderly (over age 75) from different causes indicate that the relative advantage of the United States is in survival with cardiovascular dis- ease, cancer, and accident rates (among females only). Rates of death from *other* causes in the elderly, including those that reflect acute conditions such as infections, are no lower in the United States than elsewhere.

The relatively better ranking for health indicators in the United States relative to its ranking on social inequality may also be a result of the "safety-net" measures enacted in the mid-1960s in the form of Medicaid, which provides financing for health services primarily for mothers and children in very-low-income families and in the form of a network of primary care–oriented community health centers located in geographic areas lacking other health services. Although neither of these pro- grams ever reached the majority of very-low-income individuals (largely as a result of differences in eligibility policies in the different states), the range of services provided are at least as good as if not better than those associated with most private health insurance plans in the country. Reductions in benefits associated with both Medicare and Medicaid consequent to changes in national policy in the mid-1990s, by removing the protective effect of these "safety-net" programs, may worsen the already poor relative position of the United States and heighten the already adverse impact of social disadvantage on health differentials in the country.

The tremendous variety of approaches to various aspects of primary care throughout the world provides an opportunity for each nation to identify alterna- tives to current modes of operation. Some of these approaches, such as limitations of specialists to hospital practice, are ingrained within systems, and some are in- novative solutions in response to specific priorities, such as encouragement of pre- ventive care. It is not necessary for each country to "reinvent" each approach; wise policy study can take advantage of knowledge deriving from already existing "demonstrations" in other countries.

Policy Issues for Primary Care

As time passes, we can expect the relevance of studies conducted in one country to have increasing relevance to other countries because the nature of their challenges is converging. The challenges include at least the following:

Increasing costs

Rising rates of technology use

New concepts of health and the role of health services, particularly the increasing acceptance of the biopsychosocial rather than the biomedical model

The imperative toward medical practice based on evidence rather than personal experience

Greater sharing of information within and across countries as a result of electronic communications

Increased economic cooperation with its concomitant need for improving standards and quality control

Demographic shifts with concomitant changes in the relative frequency of different types of disease and dysfunction

Changing epidemiological patterns of disease with, on the one hand, greater burdens of chronic illness and, on the other hand, heightened threats of communicable disease as a result of increased travel, commerce, and communication

Increasing expectations and demands of populations

Increasing needs for accountability in the provision of services

Erosion of professional autonomy

The move toward increased competition rather than cooperation

Greater interest in risk and cost-sharing

Because the principles of primary care are the same everywhere, knowledge gleaned in one country is likely to be of relevance in other countries as well. The importance of the four unique features of primary care has been documented by at least moderate if not definitive evidence. This evidence derives from relatively small-scale research in individual facilities and increasingly in groups of facilities as well as from cross-national comparisons that examine the strength of primary care against a variety of important facets of health. The issue for policy is the extent to which standards for their attainment are instituted.

Two structural components of health systems that are undergoing scrutiny in the context of health care reform are cost-sharing and "gatekeeping" as an empowering rather than a punitive strategy. Both are highly related to the achievement of primary care attributes.

Cost-sharing

Unobstructed access to primary care for all who need it is a basic principle in most industrialized nations. In practicality, limitations on resources often lead to the imposition of barriers to services. Many countries have explicit policies regarding the appropriate balance between incentives and impediments to use of services.

Cost considerations may make it desirable to require patients to pay some of the costs of primary care services. However, studies have shown that such policies reduce the number of visits and that the reduction is indiscriminate because it influences both necessary and more discretionary utilization. More constructive are policies that improve utilization of valued services (such as those related to pre-vention of illness) by reducing or eliminating requirements for payment or by paying bonuses to physicians to encourage them to provide services. Any barriers to access will have a greater impact on socioeconomically disadvantaged popula-tions and will therefore risk increasing the disparities in health status between more advantaged and less advantaged population subgroups. The issue for policy debate concerns the extent to which constraints on resources, particularly those related to costs of care, should dictate restrictions on access and degree of tolerance to the consequences of these restrictions for achievement of equity.

Evidence is clear on the perverse impact of cost-sharing at the point of contact with health services. Cost-sharing consisting of deductibles or more than a very small co-payment interferes with access to care and is a decidedly regressive form of taxation because it disproportionally affects those with lesser ability to pay and interferes as much with needed care as with discretionary care. In many countries, those with lesser ability to pay are exempt from cost-sharing, but administrative costs may be high and accompanied by threats to human dignity when dependency on public largesse is highly visible.

Gatekeeping

Gatekeeping, when it is conducted as a method of enhancing the appropriate use of non-primary care health services, is an empowering strategy for primary care because it applies resources at levels of care where they are most justified. When used as a barrier to needed services, however, the strategy becomes a means of interfering with the achievement of equity because those who are financially able to buy extra care will do so.

Several other structural features under consideration in health care reform ef-forts are of unknown impact on the adequacy of achievement of high level primary care. Efforts at reform should be regarded as opportunities for experimentation, with appropriate evaluation according to achievement of the goals of the reform and possible unintended side effects.

1. Methods of reimbursing physicians. Little is known about the impact of different methods of paying primary care physicians and specialists. Health care reform efforts are converging on mixtures of types of payments (usually capitation and/or salary with fee for services) in many countries, but only in one have changes been accompanied by systematic evaluation. Evaluations in Denmark found that a change to part fee-for-services payment led to an increase in diagnostic and therapeutic services and a decrease in referrals. Interestingly, the increase in provision of ser-vices was greatest for those where the evidence for their utility was most lacking, that is, for diagnostic compared with curative services (Krasnik et al., 1990). Thus, where fee for service is to be instituted for other than clearly indicated services, it should be done with consideration of its possible effect on increasing unnecessary services.

2. Indications for referral and impact of differences in referral strategy on costs and outcomes. As noted earlier in this book, methods for determining what is appropriately managed entirely within primary care, the indications for short-term consultation with specialists for advice and guidance, the types of problems that are most amenable to shared management by primary care physicians and other specialists, and the types of problems that are best managed mainly by other specialists themselves are unexplored territory. Informed decisions about the need for referral await studies on the distribution of different types of problems in primary care, types and frequencies of complications of common diagnoses, and descriptions and comparisons across different practitioners and different health facilities and plans. Thus, research conducted by individual practitioners on their own practices could provide useful descriptive information; information obtained from collaborative research could further inform the issue by analyzing correlates and determinants of variability across practices and plans. The subject itself is also of considerable policy relevance because planning for the training and deployment of specialist resources depends on better knowledge about the need for their services, as well as for considerations of how they are best reimbursed for their services. For example, if (as is likely) the vast majority of needs for most care by other specialists are for short-term consultation and primarily for the purpose of providing advice to the primary care physician, the organization of their work, its location, and its payment are likely to be different than if a considerable proportion of the need for their services is for long-term direct care of complex or rare conditions.

3. Free choice of physician. In many countries, particularly the United States, much has been made of the importance of free choice of physician by citizens. In European health systems in which primary care services are provided in individual or small group offices rather than in large health centers, free choice of primary care physician is the rule. In countries in which primary care services are delivered in large health centers, the health center itself (rather than an individual physician or physician team) often serves as the primary care source. Empirical evidence indicates that identification with a specific health center (rather than with no specified regular source of care) is associated with benefits, including better receipt of indicated preventive care and better appointment keeping. As noted earlier, however, identification with a particular physician or physician team provides additional benefits: better concordance between physician and patient, better problem recognition, fewer hospitalizations, and lower overall costs. Because most of these benefits are likely to accrue from long-term associations leading to better knowledge of physicians about their patients and greater confidence of patients that their physician understands their situation and needs, free choice of primary care physician provides an opportunity for patients to identify physicians with whom they are likely to develop a long-term relationship. Ironically, in the United States (with its clear preference for free choice of physician), an increasing proportion of people lack free choice because their employers permit only a limited choice of health plans, a problem that is further compounded by the tendency of employers to change health plans from year to year.

Free choice of specialists is likely to be more limited in most countries because the number of available specialists in any given geographic area is usually determined by planning and governmental regulation. The same is increasingly true in the United States, where health plans that contract to provide services to defined populations generally limit the range of specialists to whom patients can be referred. Collaborative and especially system-wide research that identifies the role of free choice of primary care physicians, and its impact on the achievement of longitudinality and its consequent benefits, would contribute to informed policies for allowing citizens to choose their physician. The frequency with which changes are made, the number of options that are permitted, the reasons why changes are perceived as desirable, and possible interventions to reduce the perceived need for change on the part of patients would also benefit from informed policy deliberations. More information is also needed on the impact of free choice of other specialists on both the processes of care and its outcomes.

4. Teamwork Although primary care is generally considered a "team" activity, with linkages between physicians and nurses and often other health professionals as well, there is little empirical evidence of the specific benefits achieved by these linkages. Although nurses have long been employed as "managers" of treatment for a variety of conditions common in primary care, including the now-popular disease-management arrangements, the nature of the nurses' work in relationship with that of physicians is unknown, and information that would help plan for the rational training and deployment of health professionals is lacking. Collaborative research could provide a strong basis for identifying the main issues to be addressed in subsequent policy decisions.

5. Hospital versus community-based specialists. The work of specialists is poorly understood everywhere. In classic regionalization, specialist services are organized into secondary and tertiary levels, with secondary levels located at community hospitals and tertiary levels located at teaching hospitals in large regions. Planning for the location of these levels is based on the population to be covered under the assumption that the frequency of problems requiring specialty services should determine how many specialists are needed in a given area (White, 1973). Community hospitals would be expected to provide short-term services when primary care physicians encounter a problem for which they needed advice or a patient had a medical or surgical problem requiring short-term specialized intervention, whereas specialists in large medical centers would care for the most unusual, rare, or complex conditions that would be uncommon in the population and require very specialized expertise, often on an ongoing basis.

New forms of organization of services are challenging old assumptions, particularly in countries where markets rather than central planning determine the location and types of services made available to people. While specialists continue to practice primarily in the hospital in most countries, community-based specialists are still common in others. As health systems move more toward consolidation of facilities from single or small practices to larger health centers and even to "integrated health systems," specialists may increasingly move from the hospital into the community in more and more areas. In some places, this may result in types of organizations resembling the polyclinics that characterized eastern European nations under their socialist regimes; in this form of arrangement, specialists of various types are located primarily in the health center, and patients may even consult them directly. This is particularly common in the case of obstetrics/gynecology, dermatology, ophthalmology, and otorhinolaryngology. In other places, specialists may continue to be based primarily in the hospital but attend regularly in the primary care health center, to consult with the primary care physician on diagnostic or therapeutic conundrums, to provide continuing education sessions, to provide services directly to groups of patients who might benefit from periodic visits with a specialist, or under formal arrangements for the sharing of care.

Little is known about the relative benefits to patient care and outcomes, to physicians' knowledge and skills, and to the overall costs of care of the various options for the organization, delivery, and payment for subspecialist services. When subspecialists worked in the hospital they were largely paid by salary; now that primary care facilities may contract for their services, they may be paid a capitation for their clinical work or paid a fee for service as had conventionally been the case when they were community based and working in fee-for-service health systems. Policy decisions will have to be based on more accurate knowledge about how much of their work is devoted to short-term advice rather than long-term ongoing care of patients. Decisions will also have to be made concerning the benefits and deficiencies of care provided in hospital facilities rather than in community practices and about the relative merits of various modes of reimbursing for services provided by subspecialists.

6. Role of primary care physicians in the care of their hospitalized patients. As a matter of policy in most countries such as those described in Chapter 15, primary care physicians do not bear responsibility for the care of their patients when they are in the hospital, although some may do so in rural areas (as in Australia and Canada) or where they care for patients with chronic illness and respite care in small hospitals especially designed for these purposes (as in Finland). Primary care physicians, regardless of whether they are family physicians, general internists, or general pediatricians, often are the "physician of record" for their hospitalized patients. The potential for a primary care physician role as at least a participant in inpatient care would appear to have great merit, not only to enhance coordination of care but also because the primary care physician's greater knowledge of the patient could add a useful dimension to decision-making. Wachter and Goldman (1996) proposed that the United States consider the training of "hospitalists," who would be specialists in internal medicine (and, presumably, pediatrics) responsible for managing the care of hospitalized patients. Although a new idea in the United States, where patients are often cared for by non-primary care specialists who are managing the patient's problems associated with the hospitalization, such physicians have had a role in hospital care in many other countries. Regardless of whether it is the non-primary care physician who bears responsibility for the patient or a "hospitalist" who does so, there appears to be a rationale for an additional role for the primary care physician as a member of the "team" in all countries, thus making this an important area of consideration for policy.

> I performed an autopsy on a 60-year-old man who had died following surgery for a pituitary adenoma. He had a long history of acromegaly, presumably because the tumor had been secreting growth hormone. His post-surgical course was complicated by hypothermia. The hypothermia resolved, but the patient continued to do poorly and died. The neurosurgeon called me just as I was about to start the autopsy to tell me that he didn't have a clue about the cause of death.
>
> At autopsy, I found a "textbook" picture of bronchopneumonia. I had never before and have never since seen such a classic case. The patient died with a normal body temperature only because of the opposing effects of hypothermia (a complication of the surgery) and hyperthermia from infection. Apparently, the neurosurgeons never listened to the patient's lungs and never considered that he might have a problem outside the realm of neurosurgery.   Dr. K.R., a pathologist

7. Impact of primary care on equity. Differences in the health status of populations in different countries could be a result of differences in average health or, alternatively, of differences in distribution of health in which some subpopulations have better or similar health whereas others have much worse health. Literature deriving from studies in many countries documents the direct relationship between social class and health; other studies document the different degrees of social inequities in different countries. Although existing research indicates that countries oriented more strongly toward primary care have better health, it is not known whether this is accomplished by improving average health levels or, rather, by reducing disparities across social class groups. Most countries now have a mechanism to classify social class of residential areas so that individuals living in those areas can be characterized as to their likely social class. Improvements in computerized information systems that can link medical care to area of residence should provide data that answer questions about which subpopulations benefit most from improved primary care. The international comparison of primary care mentioned in Chapter 1 demonstrated that primary care appears to be most beneficial for children and youth; in old age (particulary very old age) the incidence and prevalence of illnesses become so much greater that higher, and perhaps even direct, use of some subspecialty care might be justifiable in defined instances. Research that explores the differential impact of primary care on different population groups, particularly those characterized by differences in age and social advantage, could help policy makers make more informed judgments about the type and nature of services needed in different geographic areas.

8. Quality and outcomes of care. When research demonstrates the superiority of certain practices, the policy debate focuses on the advisability of incentives for employing them or, alternatively, dis-incentives for using the less adequate alternatives. There are several policy options, including educational efforts of various types and intensities, peer or group pressure, denial of payment, or more drastic sanctions such as publicity or penalties for improper actions. Although the type of option will depend on the nature and severity of the contraindicated action, the policy debate will focus on the need for rewards and sanctions and the rapidity with which they are implemented after the scientific evidence of superiority becomes accepted.

Incentives to encourage the involvement of both practitioners and patients in developing both indicators and criteria for quality of care is another consideration for a policy agenda. There is increasing evidence of the relationship between patients' knowledge and attitudes toward their care and its outcomes as measured by improvement in well being. Approaches that enhance the agreement between patients and practitioners concerning the goals of care would be expected to improve the overall outcomes of care. Local councils or other third party payers that pay for care might consider providing incentives to practices that involve patients in setting goals and objectives, with such financial incentives earmarked for improvements in a practice resulting from joint planning of patients and practitioners.

Outcome assessment is an important component of accountability of health services. Effectiveness of services and equity in their provision are critical in primary care as well as for health services in general. Outcomes can be considered at the individual level as well as at the health system level. Conventional outcomes assessments address the extent to which clinical services provided to individuals achieve end results that are commensurate with the expectations of the medical care provided and are often assessed by medical record review or interview of patients. Rutstein et al. (1976, 1980) and Charlton et al. (1983) set the stage for considering the impact of health services on health (primarily on deaths), but a plethora of studies failed to find much of an impact (Mackenbach et al., 1990). None of these studies examined the relationship between the strength of the primary care system in either the countries or the areas where the studies were conducted. A challenging area of research involves the selection of indicators that reflect primarily the impact of primary care services rather than the health system in general, as discussed in Chapter 13. Because many of the indicators of primary care effectiveness are heavily related to and influenced by low social class, any comparisons of their attainment by different health systems should take into account and control for differences in social class (and other social disadvantages) of the populations served by them.

By its very nature, health systems research involves basic research strategies (to develop appropriate measures of outcome), collaborative research strategies (to test the feasibility of the measures and to develop information systems to ascertain the outcomes), and system-wide research (to develop appropriate interventions to progressively improve performance).

Developing a Strategy To Achieve the Derivative Features of Primary Care

Neither family-centeredness nor community orientation is a focus of primary health care systems in most countries. In some countries, a family orientation is implicit as a result of the designation of family physicians as the primary care practitioners.

However, no country insists on accountability for family orientation. Community orientation is an ideal rather than a reality everywhere, except perhaps in a few localized areas. Although there is intuitive appeal and apparent validity of the concepts of family and community orientation, evidence of their universal practicality does not exist. Policy makers will have to decide whether to encourage research to obtain the evidence, to proceed with planning for implementation, or to disregard the concepts as of low priority. The merits of the three alternative approaches deserve debate in the policy arena.

The thrust of the Declaration of Alma-Ata is toward community orientation, and many countries, particularly in the developing world, implement policies designed to achieve it. Descriptions of its characteristics are not generalizable, and there is little known about what kinds of information are useful and how they may be applied to improving care. Various initiatives, such as the World Health Organization's Healthy Cities project and the "goals for the nation" of several countries, suggest some directions for study, although these are directed more at health systems in general than primary care in specific. Policy-oriented research that is designed to test different approaches to reaching defined community goals and to evaluate different approaches to meeting them would be of use to all systems striving to achieve community orientation.

Furthermore, it is evident that policies (including those for medical education) intended to improve community-oriented primary care should involve collaboration with public health professionals because the boundaries between public health and clinical medicine are becoming increasingly blurred as health centers are taking on responsibility for the health of defined populations—traditionally the province of public health agencies and professionals.

If community orientation emerges as a priority for policy, there will have to be incentives for the development of community data systems linked to clinical data systems that can be used for setting priorities, planning, and evaluation. Presently existing vital statistics, reporting systems, and clinical data reporting can be adapted to make the data systems and their linkages more useful at the level of the communities in which the practices exist. New data systems will have to be developed to supplement information on causes of death and disease with documentation of functional status as well. This may require the conduct of periodic surveys in communities, an effort that will require additional resources. Local referenda concerning the importance accorded to such an approach will help provide the justification for the expenditure of additional funds.

Ethical Issues Concerning the Use of Resources

A major policy concern is the use of expensive technology when the procedures are clearly unjustified. Mechanisms are generally available to deny reimbursement if a policy to do so exists. When expensive procedures are scientifically justified, the concern for policy makers is the extent to which they can be justified on grounds of cost effectiveness. Some jurisdictions have already begun developing public commissions to deliberate the costs and benefits of medical care procedures and to deny those that are found to have the lowest justifiability according to cost/benefit considerations. Rationing is a heatedly debated issue in many countries, and the debate focuses as much on primary care level services as on heroic tertiary care services (McKee and Figueras, 1996; Doyal, 1997; Coast, 1997). When applied to entire populations, such an approach can have merit. Serious ethical questions would arise, however, if the process results in a situation where certain equally needy segments of the population are denied access to services available to other segments of the population (Heath, 1997). The policy debate must consider these ethical issues as well as the more general issue of the advisability of using cost effectiveness as a basis for making decisions about what services and procedures are to be provided or paid for by the health system.

Encouragement and Support of Research in Primary Care

Because the vast majority of health-related research is conducted by subspecialists in medical centers, the base of knowledge of primary care practice is underdeveloped. Policy should encourage the conduct of such research, preferably with the direct involvement of primary care physicians who have a better grasp of the nature of the problems in primary care than do other specialists or non-physician researchers. Governmental and private research organizations should set an agenda for research and invite proposals. Professional societies should provide extra continuing education credits or present certificates of merit to physicians who become involved in such research. Collaborative efforts in which primary care physicians develop networks to define and conduct research have particular promise because properly conducted research occurring in a wide variety of settings has greater generalizability than does research in only one or a few settings. Involvement of researchers in medical centers, even if they are subspecialists, might also be encouraged, because exposure to primary care issues by these researchers will enhance their understanding of the challenges of primary care. However, these specialists should not define the research topics or exert sole control over the analysis or interpretation of the findings.

Encouragement and Support of Primary Care Training

Because the natural tendency for any system is to subspecialize, special efforts have to be made to maintain a viable primary care sector. Primary care training programs will require special financial support to remain viable and attract physicians who not only have interest in it but also are of high caliber. In the face of incentives to specialize because of higher prestige and, in most places, the promise of higher incomes, trainees will gravitate toward subspecialization rather than primary care. The challenge to policy makers is to make primary care training and practice at least as attractive as subspecialty training and practice.

Building a Capacity for Accountability

When responsibility for either the financing or the provision of direct services is undertaken by governmental or by private agencies, there must be some explicit specification of the nature and extent of services that will be undertaken. These specifications are usually in the form of guidelines that are to be followed. These guidelines may set a minimum set of benefits to be provided and may even specify how certain services are to be delivered. For example, they may indicate that children should be seen periodically for well-child care and indicate the periodicity. They may require that certain types of services, such as case-management services, be available to patients.

The technical capacity for accountability today extends beyond the mere specification of requirements. It is possible to set operational goals and measure their attainment. The goals may be expressed as the attainment of certain health levels, the attainment of certain levels of satisfaction of the population, or the attainment of set standards for quality of care.

Today, when the technical capacity for accountability of performance exists, the community of managers and practitioners is neither sufficiently aware of the capabilities or committed to the concept of accountability to undertake the necessary activities to ensure it. Therefore, the challenge to policy is the adoption of a system of incentives to encourage experimentation with methods of ensuring accountability. Bonuses could be given to service organizations that set goals and measure the degree of their attainment. To encourage interest, the organizations might be permitted to choose the area in which they wish to experiment or at least to select from a variety of options. Potential areas for increasing accountability include the implementation of advisory councils of patients, evaluation of changes in health status, linkages with public health agencies that make possible the use of community health data, and involvement in research to generate new knowledge about primary care problems and their management.

References

Atkinson A, Rainwater L, Smeeding T. Income Distribution in Advanced Economies: Evidence From the Luxembourg Income Study. Syracuse, NY: Maxwell School of Citizenship and Public Affairs, Syracuse University, October 1995, Working Paper No. 120.

Bodenheimer T and Sullivan K. How large employers are shaping the health care marketplace. N Engl J Med 1998; 338:1084–87.

Ceitlin J, Gomez Gascon T (eds). Medicina Familiar: la clave para un nuevo modelo. Madrid, Spain: CIMF and SEMFYC, 1997.

Charlton JR, Hartley RM, Silver R, Holland WW. Geographical variation in mortality from conditions amenable to medical intervention in England and Wales. Lancet 1983; 1(pt 1):691–6.

Centers for Disease Control and Prevention. Mortality in developed countries. Morbidity and Mortality Weekly Report, April 6, 1990. p. 206.

Coast J. The rationing debate: The case against. BMJ 1997; 314: 1118–22.

Desenclos J-C, Hahn R. Years of potential life lost before age 65, by race, Hispanic origin, and sex, United States 1896–1988. Morbidity and Mortality Weekly Report, November 20, 1992. pp 18–19.

Doyal L. The rationing debate: Rationing within the NHS should be explicit. BMJ 1997; 314:1114–8.

Forrest C. Opening the Gate to Primary Care; How First Contact Care Influences Costs for Ambulatory Episodes of Care. Dissertation. Baltimore, MD: Johns Hopkins University Press, 1995.

Heath I. Threat to social justice. BMJ 1997; 314:598–9.

Kaplan GA, Pamuk ER, Lynch JW, Cohen RD, Balfour JL. Inequality in income and mortality in the United States: Analysis of mortality and potential pathways.BMJ 1996; 312: 999–1003.

Kennedy BP, Kawachi I, Prothrow-Stith D. Income distribution and mortality: Cross sectional ecological study of the Robin Hood index in the United States. BMJ. 1996; 312(7037):1004–7.

Krasnik A, Groenewegen PP, Pedersen PA, von Scholten P, Mooney G, Gottschau A, Flierman HA, Damsgaard MT. Changing remuneration systems: Effects on activity in general practice. BMJ 1990; 300:1698–701.

Ljubljana Charter on reform health care. BMJ 1996; 312:1664–6.

Mackenbach JP, Bouvier-Colle MH, Jougla E. "Avoidable" mortality and health services: A review of aggregate data studies. J Epidemiol Community Health 1990; 44:106–11.

McKee M, Figueras J. For debate: Setting priorities: Can Britain learn from Sweden? BMJ 1996; 312:691–4.

National Center for Health Statistics. Healthy People 2000 Review, 1995–1996. Hyattsville, MD: Public Health Service, 1996.

Rublee D. International Health Care Systems: A Chartbook Perspective. Center for Health Policy Research. Chicago, IL: American Medical Association, 1992.

Rutstein D, Berenberg W, Chalmers T, Child C 3d, Fishman A, Perrin E. Measuring the quality of medical care: A clinical method. N Engl J Med 1976; 294(11):582–8.

Rutstein D, Berenberg W, Chalmers T, Fishman A, Perrin E, Zuidema G. Measuring the quality of medical care: Second revision of tables of indexes. N Engl J Med 1980; 302(20):1146.

Shi L. Primary care, specialty care, and life chances. Int J Health Serv 1994; 24(3):431–58.

Silberman G, Crosse M, Peterson E, Weston R, Horowitz M, Applebaum F, Cheson B. Availability and appropriateness of allogeneic bone marrow transplantation for chronic myeloid leukemia in 10 countries. N Engl J Med 1994; 331:1063–7.

Smeeding T. America's income inequality: Where do we stand? Challenge 1996; (Sept–Oct). 45–52.

Starfield, B. Primary care. J Ambulatory Care Manage 1993; 16(4):27–37.

U.S. Congress. Office of Technology Assessment, International Health Statistics: What the Numbers Mean for the United States. Background Paper, U.S. GPO, OTA-BP-H-116. Washington, DC: U.S. Congress, November 1993.

Wachter R, Goldman L. The emerging role of "hospitalists" in the American health care system. N Engl J Med 1996; 335:514–7.

Waitzkin H, Wald K, Kee R, Danielson R, Robinson L. Primary care in Cuba: Low- and high-technology developments pertinent to family medicine. J Fam Pract 1997; 45:250–8.

Wagstaff A, Van Doorslaer E. Equity in the Finance and Delivery of Health Care: Concepts and Definitions. In Van Doorslaer E, Wagstaff A, Rutten F (eds): Equity in the Finance and Delivery of Health Care: An International Perspective. Oxford: Oxford University Press, 1993a. pp 7–19.

Wagstaff A, Van Doorslaer E. Equity in the Delivery of Health Care: Methods and Findings. In van Doorslaer E, Wagstaff A, Rutten F (eds): Equity in the Finance and Delivery of Health Care: An International Perspective. Oxford: Oxford University Press, 1993b. pp20–48.

Webster I. General practice—a rising phoenix. Med J Aust 1996; 164:709–10.

White KL. Life and death and medicine. Sci Am 1973; 229:23–33.

World Health Organization. Primary Health Care. "Health for All" Series, No. 1. Geneva: World Health Organization, 1978, p 4.

World Health Organization. Equity in Health and Health Care: A WHO Initiative. WHO/ARA/96.1. Geneva: World Health Organization, 1996.

EPILOGUE

Long before the technological era began, the noted cellular pathologist Rudolf Virchow observed that "The improvement of medicine would eventually prolong human life but improvement of social conditions could achieve this result more rapidly and successfully." These sentiments led him to the position that "medicine is a social science, and politics is nothing more than medicine on a larger scale."

The ensuing century brought developments, which continue unabated to this day, in the ability of physicians to intervene in heretofore unimaginable ways to reduce the adverse impact of diseases. Health systems and practitioners will still be faced, however, with the reality that much of ill health is not associated with specific deseases. Pleiotropism, etiological heterogeneity, and variable penetrance will continue to thwart a mechanistic approach to illness and health. Not everyone with a given biological defect will succumb to the disease with which it is associated, and similar diseases will occur even in its absence. The genetic revolution that is widely equated with biological determinism will be accompanied by a realization of the pervasive influence of social and environmental factors on experiences of illness and the ability of people to achieve health and personal satisfaction, just as it was in the days of Virchow.

The role of primary care will become even more critical with increasing recognition of the interplay of biology and the social and physical environment. The challenge of primary care is to understand and interpret this interplay and to help individuals modify their life circumstances to maximize their potential for health and achievement. As the role of medicine moves from the goal of cure to prevention of disease and then to protection and promotion of health, its contribution to health will assume increasing importance. As the only branch of medicine to focus primarily on people rather than on their illnesses, primary care is pivotal in the advancement of the science and art of health services in modern society. If this book has stimulated thinking about the challenges posed by Virchow and the role of primary care in undertaking them, it will have achieved its goals.

APPENDIX
The Child Health Systems Primary Care Assessment Survey Tool

The Child Health Systems Primary Care Assessment survey instruments are designed to assess the extent of primary care provided consistent with each of the domains and subdomains of primary care as described in this book. The domains include the four unique attributes of primary care—first contact, continuity, comprehensiveness, and coordination—and the three derivative attributes—family-centeredness, community orientation, and cultural appropriateness. The survey is designed to provide scores for each subdomain and domain. The instruments are not designed to measure health status per se.

This appendix provides the questions that are included in the survey instrument. The survey forms themselves are formatted and include categories for recording and coding the responses.

The Consumer/Client Survey is designed to collect information from individuals regarding their experiences using health care resources. The survey can be administered through either telephone or face-to-face interviews.

The Facility/Provider Survey is designed to collect information about specific operational characteristics and practices related to primary care employed by direct care providers (office-based solo or graoup practices, private or public clinics, health maintenance organizations or hospital outpatient facilities, and so forth). The survey can be implemented by mail or by face-to-face or telephone interviews.

Data collected through pilot testing provided estimates of reliability and validity of the scales in each domain, including inter-scale correlations, item means, inter-item correlations, and internal consistency. These tests are critical to the process of producing a valid and reliable tool.

If you wish to consider using either of the questionnaires, please communicate with one of the undersigned.

Sincerely,

Holly Allen Grason, MA
Director
Women's and Children's
Health Policy Center

Barbara Starfield, MD, MPH
University Distinguished Service Professor
Department of Health Policy & Management
410-955-3737
bstarfie@jhsph.edu

Appendix

Child Health Systems Primary Care Assessment Tool

Developed by

Barbara Starfield, MD, MPH

Charlyn E. Cassady, RN, PhD

Women's and Children's Health Policy Center

Johns Hopkins School of Public Health

Department of Maternal and Child Health

For the

Maternal and Child Health Bureau

Health Resources and Services Administration

Public Health Service

U.S. Department of Health and Human Services

and

The Henry J. Kaiser Family Foundation

Development of this document was supported by two Cooperative Agreements (MCU 243A19 and MCU 249386) from the Maternal and Child Health Bureau (Title V, Social Security Act), Health Resources and Services Administration, Department of Health and Human Services. Additional funding for this Provider Survey was provided by the Kaiser Family Foundation (grant 94-1499).

Provider Survey

Please respond to the survey reflecting the care you provide as an *individual practitioner.*

1. Type of practice

2. Your specialty

3. Of children and adolescents served by your practice, what is the approximate percent in the following types of plans?

4. About what percent of your child and adolescent patients are in insurance plans where your income is affected by the number of referrals or costs you generate?

5. About what percent of your child and adolescent patients have health coverage that limits referrals, limits to whom you can refer, or requires approval for referrals?

6. About what percent of your child and adolescent patients have health coverage that requires pre-approval for non-emergency hospitalizations?

7. Is your practice open on Saturday or Sunday?

8. Is your practice open on weekday evenings until 8 p.m.?

9. When your practice is open and a child gets sick, would someone from your practice see the child that day?

10. When your practice is closed on Saturday or Sunday and a child gets very sick, would someone from your practice be able to see the child that day?

11. When your practice is closed during the night and a child gets very sick, would someone from your practice be able to see the child that night?

12. Can a family easily get an appointment for routine well-child check-ups at your practice?

13. When your practice is closed, do you have a phone number families can call when a child gets sick?

14. On average, do patients have to wait more than 30 minutes after arriving before they are examined by the doctor or nurse?

15. At your practice, do children see the same clinician each time they make a visit?

16. Do you think the children (if old enough) or families in your practice understand what you ask them or say to them?

17. Do you believe you give families enough time to talk about their worries or problems?

18. Do you believe families feel comfortable telling you about their worries or problems?

19. If a family has a question, can they call and talk to the doctor or nurse who knows the child best?

20. Do you believe you know the families in your practice "very well"?

21. Do you believe you understand what problems are most important to the families you see?

22. Does your practice ask to meet with family members to discuss a health or family problem?

23. What percent of your practice's child and adolescent patients are "enrolled" or are assigned to receive all their non-referred care at your practice?

24. What percent of your child and adolescent patients do you think use your practice for *all* their well and sick health care needs (with the exception of true emergencies and referred care)?

25. About what percent of your child and adolescent patients must pay a fee or co-payment at each visit?

26. What percent of your patients have long-term medical or behavioral problems or disabilities?

27. On average, about how long does a child stay with your practice?

28. Does your practice have a geographically defined population that it is intended to serve?

29. During visits to your practice are the following subjects discussed with the child and parent/guardian?

    a. Ways to keep children healthy, such as nutritional foods or getting enough sleep?

    b. Ways to keep children safe, like . . .

        1. (Under 6)—teaching them to cross the street safely; using child safety seats in cars?

2. (Ages 6–12)—staying away from guns; using seatbelts and bicycle helmets?

3. (Over 12)—safe sex; saying no to drugs; not drinking and driving?

c. Home safety, like using smoke detectors and storing medicines safely?

d. Ways to handle problems with child's behavior?

e. Changes in growth and behavior that parents can expect at certain ages?

30. If a child needs any of the following services, would they be able to get them on-site at your practice?

a. Nutrition counseling by a nutrition specialist or professional

b. Immunizations

c. Eligibility screening for social service programs or benefits

d. WIC services (supplemental milk and food program)

e. Dental check-ups

f. Dental treatment

g. Family planning or birth control services

h. Substance or drug abuse counseling or treatment

i. Counseling for behavior or mental health problems

j. Tests for lead poisoning

k. Suturing for a minor laceration

l. Counseling and testing for HIV/AIDS

m. Tympanocentesis

31. Do you use the following methods to ensure that indicated services are provided?

a. Flow sheets in patients charts for lab results

b. Printed practice guidelines in patients' records

c. Periodic medical record audits

d. Problem lists in patients' records

e. Medication lists in patients' records

f. Other (please specify) _____

32. Are parents/guardians expected to bring their child's medical records, such as immunizations or medical care they received in the past?

33. Would you allow a family to look at the child's medical record if they wanted to?

34. When a patient needs a referral, do you discuss different places the family might go to get help with their problem?

35. Does someone at your practice help the family make the appointment for the referral visit?

36. Do you think you know about all the visits that your patients make to specialists or special services?

37. Do you receive useful information about your referred patients back from the specialists or special services?

38. After the visit, do you talk with the parent/guardian/child about the results of the visit(s) they had with the specialist or special service?

39. How often are each of the following included as a routine part of your health assessment?

    Use of:

    a. Familiograms, family APGAR

    Discussion of:

    b. Family health risk factors, e.g., genetics

    c. Family economic resources

    d. Social risk factors, e.g., loss of employment

    e. Living conditions, e.g., working refrigerator, heat

    f. Health status of other family members

    g. Parenting

    Assessment of:

    h. Signs of child abuse

    i. Indications of family in crisis

    j. Impact of child's health on family functioning

    k. Developmental level

40. Do the doctors and nurses at your practice ask the parents/guardians about *their* ideas and opinions when planning treatment and care for a child?

41. Does your practice make home visits?

42. Do you think your practice has adequate knowledge about the health problems of the communities it serves?

43. Does your practice use the following types of data to determine what programs/ services are needed by the communities you serve?

    a. Mortality data (data on deaths)

    b. Public health communicable disease data (e.g., STDs, TB)

    c. Community immunization rates

    d. Public health data on health or occupational hazards

    e. Clinical data from your practice

    f. Other (please specify) _____

44. Are you able to change the health care services or programs you offer in response to specific health problems in the communities?

45. Does your practice use the following methods to monitor and/or evaluate the effectiveness of your services/programs?

    a. Surveys of your patients

    b. Community surveys

    c. Feedback from community organizations or community advisory boards

    d. Feedback from practice staff

    e. Analysis of local data or vital statistics

    f. Systematic evaluations of your programs and services provided

    g. Community health workers

    h. Have a family member on the board of directors or advisory committee

    i. Other (please specify) _____

46. Does your practice use any of the following methods to address the cultural diversity in your patient population?

    a. Training of staff by outside instructors

    b. In-service programs presented by staff

    c. Use of culturally sensitive (language, visual images, religious customs) materials/pamphlets

    d. Staff reflecting the cultural diversity of the population served

    e. Translators/interpreters

    f. Planning of services that reflect cultural diversity

    g. Other (please specify) _____

47. Does your practice use any of the following activities to reach out to populations in the communities you serve?

    a. Networks with state and local agencies involved with culturally diverse groups

    b. Linkages with religious organizations/services

    c. Involvement with neighborhood groups/community leaders

    d. Outreach workers

    e. Other (please specify) _____

48. Do you consider your practice to be accessible to people who do not speak English well?

49. Are you able to incorporate a family's special beliefs about health care, or use of folk medicine, such as herbs/homemade medicines, into the treatment plan?

50. Are you able to incorporate a family's request to use alternative treatment, such as homeopathy or acupuncture, into the treatment plan?

51. Does your practice offer "sliding scale" or long-term payment plans for patients with financial difficulties?

52. Are your professional earnings mainly:
    Salary only
    Capitation only
    Fee-for-service only
    Capitation and fee-for-service
    Salary and fee-for-service
    Salary, capitation, and fee-for-service
    Share of practice earnings
    Other (please specify) _____

53. Are you eligible for bonuses or subject to withholds depending on your utilization experience?

54. Are you eligible for bonuses if you achieve certain guidelines or outcomes?

55. In your practice, what are the current number of visits

    a. Per day?

    b. Per week?

56. What is the approximate percentage of visits by age?

57. Is your practice currently accepting new patients?

58. Is your practice able to determine how many patients (not visits) you have seen in a year?

Consumer/Client Telephone Survey

P1. To what doctor or place does (Name of child) usually go if (s)he is sick or advice is needed about (his/her) health?

P2. What is the *name* of the doctor or place?

P3. What is the *name* of the doctor or place that *knows* (Name of child) *best* as a person, aside from any special health problem that (s)he has?

P4. What is the *name* of the doctor or place where you would take (Name of child) if (s)he got a completely new health problem that wasn't an emergency?

P5. Can you tell me the address of (Doctor/Place P) or where it is?

P6. What kind of place is it?

P7. Do(es) the doctor(s) at (Place P) take care of children only or both children and adults?

P8. Do(es) the doctor(s) at (Place P) mainly take care of children with certain kinds of problems or most kinds of problems?

O5. About *how many times total* has (Name of child) been to (Doctor/Place P)?

O16. How long has (Doctor/Place P) been your source of care?

O17. Did you choose (Doctor/Place P) or were you assigned to it?

O18. Could you change from (Doctor/Place P) anytime you wanted to?

O19. Would you change from (Doctor/Place P) to somewhere else if it was easy to do?

F1. Is (Doctor/Place P) open on Saturday or Sunday?

F2. Is (Doctor/Place P) open on weekday evenings until 8 p.m.?

F4. When (Doctor/Place P) is *open* and (Name of child) gets sick, would the doctor/place see (him/her) the same day?

F5. When (Doctor/Place P) is *closed* on *Saturday or Sunday* and (Name of child) gets sick, would the doctor/place see (him/her) or talk with you the same day?

F6. When (Doctor/Place P) is *closed* and (Name of child) gets sick *during the night,* would someone from there see (him/her) or talk with you that night?

F7. Do you have to wait a long time or talk to too many people to make an appointment at (Doctor/Place P)?

F19. Is it easy to get an appointment for routine well-child check-ups at (Doctor/Place P)?

F20. When (Doctor/Place P) is closed, do they have a phone number you can call when (Name of child) gets sick?

F23. When (Name of child) has to go to (Doctor/Place P), does someone have to take off from work or school to take (him/her)?

F16. Once you get to (Doctor/Place P), do you have to wait more than 30 minutes before (Name of child) is checked by the doctor or nurse?

F21. Is it difficult for you to get medical care for (Name of child) when you think it is needed from (Doctor/Place P)?

O1a. Has (Name of child) ever had a regular check-up?

O1b. Where did (Name of child) go the *last* time for a *regular check-up* when (s)he was not sick?

O1c. When was the *last* visit there for a *check-up?* (month and year)

O2a. Has (Name of child) ever had immunizations (''shots'')?

O2b. Where did (Name of child) go the *last* time for *immunizations (''shots'')?*

O2c. When was the *last* visit there for *immunizations (''shots'')?* (month and year)

O3a. Has (Name of child) ever been seen by a doctor or nurse because (s)he was sick?

O3b. Where did (Name of child) go the *last* time (s)he was sick?

O3c. When was the *last* visit there for sickness? (month and year)

06. When you take (Name of child) to (Place P), is (s)he taken *care* of by the same doctor or nurse each time?

07. Do you think that doctor or nurse *understands what you say or ask?*

08. Are your questions to the doctor or nurse *answered in ways that you understand?*

O14. If you have a question, can you call and talk to the doctor or nurse at (Doctor/Place P) who knows (Name of child) best?

O21. Does (Doctor/Place P) seem interested in (Name of child) as a *person,* rather than as someone with a medical problem?

O23. Does (Doctor/Place P) give you enough time to talk about your worries or problems?

O24. Do you feel comfortable telling (Doctor/Place P) about your worries or problems?

O26. Do you think (Doctor/Place P) knows your family ''very well''?

O27. Does (Doctor/Place P) understand what problems are most important to you and your family?

K6. Would (Doctor/the doctors and nurses at Place P) meet with members of your family if you thought it would be helpful?

O20. Does (Doctor/Place P) have to get approval from someone else to refer to a specialist?

M15. When you go to (Doctor/Place P), do you bring any of (Name of child)'s medical records, such as records of shots or reports of medical care (s)he has received?

M16. Would (Doctor/Place P) let you look at (Name of child)'s medical record if you wanted to?

M1. Has (Name of child) ever had a visit to any kind of specialist or special service?

M3. When was the *last* time (Name of child) had a visit to a specialist or special service? (month and year)

M2. What was this specialist or special service?

M3a. Was this visit for a physical, mental, or behavioral problem, such as a condition that doesn't go away or lasts longer than a year?

M3b. Had (Name of child) ever visited that specialist or special service before this last visit?

M17. Did the (Doctor/the doctor or nurse at Place P) know about visits you made to the specialist or special services?

M4. Did the (Doctor/the doctor or nurse at Place P) discuss with you different places you could have gone to get help with that problem?

M7. Did someone at (Doctor/Place P) help you make the appointment for that visit?

M10. After going to the specialist or special service, did (Name of doctor/someone from Place P) talk with you and (Name of child) about what happened at the visit?

M11. Does (Doctor/the doctor at Place P) know what the results of that visit were?

M13. Does (Doctor/the doctor at Place P) seem interested in the quality of care (Name of child) gets from that specialist or special service?

M14. Is (Name of child) taking any medicines that the doctor at (Place P) does *not* know about?

C3. I'm going to read a list of services that your child or family might need at some time. For each one, tell me if you can get them at (Doctor/Place P).

   a. Answers to questions about nutrition or diet

   b. Immunizations or "shots"

   c. Checking to see if your family is eligible for any social service programs or benefits

   d. WIC services (supplemental milk and food program)

   e. Dental check-up

   f. Treatment by a dentists

   g. Family planning or birth control

   h. Substance or drug abuse counseling or treatment

   i. Counseling for behavior or mental health problems

   j. Tests for lead poisoning

   k. Sewing up a cut that needs stitches

   l. Counseling and testing for HIV/AIDS (optional)

C1. In visits to (Doctor/Place P) with (Name of child), are any of the following subjects discussed with you and (Name of child)?

    a. Ways to keep your children healthy, such as nutritional foods; or getting enough sleep?

    b. Ways to keep your children safe, like . . .

        1. (Under 6)—teaching them to cross the street safely and using child safety seats in cars?

        or

        2. (Ages 6–12)—staying away from guns and using seatbelts and bicycle helmets?

        or

        3. (Over 12)—safe sex, saying no to drugs, and not drinking and driving?

    c. Home safety, like using smoke detectors and storing medicines safely?

    d. Ways to handle problems with your child's behavior?

    e. Changes in growth and behavior that you can expect at certain ages?

K1. Do the (Doctor/the doctors and nurses at Place P) ask you about *your* ideas and opinions when they are planning treatment and care for (Name of child)?

R1. Does anyone at (Doctor/Place P) ever make home visits?

R3. Does (Doctor/the doctor or nurse at Place P) know about all of the important health problems of your neighborhood?

K5. How does (Doctor/Place P) get opinions and ideas from people that will help them provide better health care? Do they . . .

    a. Do surveys of their patients to see if their services are meeting people's needs?

    b. Do surveys in the community to find out about health problems that (Doctor/Place P) should know about?

    c. Ask family members to be on the board of directors or advisory committee?

H2. Would you recommend (Doctor/Place P) to a friend or relative?

H1. Would you recommend (Doctor/Place P) to someone who does not speak English well?

H3. Would you recommend (Doctor/Place P) to someone who uses folk medicine, such as herbs or homemade medicines, or has special beliefs about health care?

B7. How much of the past 12 months was (Name of child) covered by *any* type of health insurance, including Medicaid?

B1. During the last 12 months, was any of (Name of child)'s health care paid through:

    a. HMO (health maintenance organization)

    b. Some other private health insurance company

    c. Medicaid or Medical Assistance

d. Some governmental health department clinic

e. Any other way? (Specify)_____

B10a. In the last year, did you have trouble paying for health care for (Name of child)?

B8. When you make a visit to (Doctor/Place P), do you have to pay something at the visit?

B9. Do you get most or all of this money back from any health insurance program?

D1. Is (Name of child):
African-American
White
Hispanic or Latino
Native African
Native American/American Indian/Alaskan Native
Asian, Asian-American, or Pacific Islander
Other (Specify) _____

D2. What is (Name of child)'s country of origin?

D4. What languages are usually spoken in your home?

D5. How much does your family pay a month in rent or mortgage?

D6. Finally, I would like to ask you about your household income. Which of the following most closely describes the level of income for your household?

INDEX